The Natural Immune

The Neutrol

The Natural Immune System

The Neutrophil

Edited by
JON S. ABRAMSON
Bowman Gray School of Medicine,
Winston-Salem, North Carolina

and

J. GARY WHEELER
Arkansas Children's Hospital,
Little Rock, Arkansas

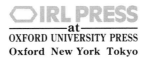

OXFORD UNIVERSITY PRESS
Oxford New York Tokyo

Oxford University Press, Walton Street, Oxford OX2 6DP
Oxford   New York   Toronto
Delhi   Bombay   Calcutta   Madras   Karachi
Kuala Lumpur   Singapore   Hong Kong   Tokyo
Nairobi   Dar es Salaam   Cape Town
Melbourne   Auckland   Madrid
and associated companies in
Berlin   Ibadan

Oxford is a trade mark of Oxford University Press

Published in the United States
by Oxford University Press Inc., New York

A catalogue record for this book is available from the British Library

Library of Congress Cataloging in Publication Data
The Neutrophil / edited by Jon S. Abramson and J. Gary Wheeler.
(The natural immune system)
Includes bibliographical references and index.
1. Neutrophils.   I. Abramson, Jon S.   II. Wheeler, J. Gary.
III. Series
[DNLM: 1. Neutrophils–pathology.   2. Neutrophils–physiology.
WH 200 N4958]
QR185.8.N47N457   1993   616.07′9–dc20   92–48202
ISBN 0–19–963374–6 (hbk.)
ISBN 0–19–963373–8 (pbk.)

Typeset by
Footnote Graphics, Warminster, Wiltshire
Printed in Great Britain by
Information Press Ltd., Eynsham, Oxford

To our wives, Cynthia and Rebecca,
and children, Seth, Rebecca, Melissa, Emily, and Abigail.

Preface

The creation of a new volume on the neutrophil was driven by two forces. The first was the need to provide a cogent update on basic neutrophil research and its new clinical applications. Because of a rapidly expanding data base, an interval summation for scientists and clinicians seemed necessary.

The second force was the need to provide accessible information to a wider, more connected audience, a community of lay and professional individuals with all manner of backgrounds. In the past the layman, the bioscientist, and the clinician lived in different worlds. In the 1990s computer literature access, improving scientific literacy, and cable TV have 'defeudalized' science, enabling better exchange of information among all interested parties. *The neutrophil* has therefore been written to speak to a wide spectrum of people including the graduate student, the practising physician, the laboratory scientist, and the interested layman.

Walker Percy in *Message in the bottle* (1) describes a liberal arts student who finds a dogfish on the beach and marvels at the magnificence of its biological organization. He also relates the boredom of the biology student forced to dissect the dogfish in the laboratory. The point is made that a novel perspective on a subject, particularly when caught off guard, can yield great insight and pleasure and can feed the imagination. By using case presentations to highlight basic and clinical points, we hope that the bench scientist will better appreciate the human impact of neutrophil-related disease and that the clinician will discover the intricacies of the pathophysiology. At the very least we hope to make palpable the remarkable relevance of current medical bench research.

The neutrophil is organized so that basic cell biology is presented first (Chapters 1–4), followed by neutrophil pathology (Chapters 5–7), and finally therapeutic solutions (Chapter 8). Chapter 1 covers the neutrophil in the human newborn, both its development and maturation from marrow precursors and its role in disease as a functional (albeit immature) cell. Chapter 2 paints a role for the neutrophil as a co-participant in the immune response. Chapter 3 describes the role of signal transduction and cell activation in allowing for the movement of neutrophils to the site of infection and the killing of microbial invaders. Chapter 4 describes the normal phagocytic process.

The following chapters define the neutrophil gone awry. Chapter 5 describes acquired immune deficiencies induced by either infectious agents or pharmacologicals, and Chapter 6 details the primary immune deficiencies of neutrophils. Chapter 7 provides a review of the consequences of overly activated neutrophils.

In Chapter 8 therapeutic solutions to several neutrophil disorders are presented including both upregulation and downregulation of neutrophil responses.

We are extremely grateful to the individual contributors in this volume who were kind enough to pause in the midst of their active research to share with us the current developments in their respective fields. We would especially like to thank our families and colleagues for accommodating our schedules to produce this work and for the guidance and inspiration of our mentors: Paul Quie, Cash McCall, David Bass, and the late Lawrence DeChatelet. We would also like to express our gratitude to Joe and Marianna Wheeler for their assistance in this project and Oxford University Press for the encouragement to pursue its conception and completion.

Reference

1 Percy, W. (1975). *Message in the bottle*. Farrar, Strauss, and Giroux, New York.

Winston-Salem   J.S.A.
Little Rock   J.G.W.
May 1992

Contents

2   Neutrophil receptors and modulation of the immune response

C. ROSALES AND E. J. BROWN

3   Signal transduction in neutrophil oxidative metabolism and chemotaxis

L. C. McPHAIL and L. HARVATH

4   Neutrophil phagocytosis and killing: normal function and microbial evasion

J. VERHOEF AND M. R. VISSER

5   Microbial and pharmacological induction of neutrophil dysfunction

J. G. WHEELER AND J. S. ABRAMSON

Contributors

J. S. Abramson Bowman Gray School of Medicine, Wake Forest University, Medical Center Blvd, Winston-Salem, NC 27157, USA

L. A. Boxer Pediatric Hematology/Oncology, C. S. Mott Children's Hospital, University of Michigan, Rm F6515, Box 0238, Ann Arbor, MI, USA

E. J. Brown Department of Internal Medicine, Division of Infectious Diseases, Washington University School of Medicine, Campus Box 8051, 660 S. Euclid Ave, St Louis, MO 63110, USA

M. S. Cairo Pediatric Hematology/Oncology, Children's Hospital of Orange County, PO Box 5700, Orange, CA 92613–5700, USA

L. Harvath Center for Biologics Evaluation and Research, FDA, Division of Hematology, Bldg 29, Room 331, 880 Rockville Pike, Bethesda, MD 20892, USA

V. S. Kanwar Hematology/Oncology Research, Children's Hospital of Orange County, PO Box 5700, Orange, CA 92613–5700, USA

J. A. Leff Webb-Waring Institute, Department of Medicine, University of Colorado Health Sciences Center, Denver, CO 80262, USA

L. C. McPhail Bowman Gray School of Medicine, Wake Forest University, Medical Center Blvd, Winston-Salem, NC 27157, USA

E. Mills Pediatrics and Microbiology/Immunology, McGill University, and Montreal Children's Hospital, Division of Infectious Diseases, 2300 Tupper St, Montreal, PQ Canada H3H 1P3

F. Noya Pediatrics and Microbiology/Immunology, McGill University, and Montreal Children's Hospital, Division of Infectious Diseases, 2300 Tupper St, Montreal, PQ Canada H3H 1P3

J. E. Repine Webb-Waring Institute, Department of Medicine, University of Colorado Health Sciences Center, Denver, CO 80262, USA

C. Rosales Department of Internal Medicine, Division of Infectious Diseases, Washington University School of Medicine, Campus Box 8051, 660 S. Euclid Ave, St Louis, MO 63110, USA

R. F. Todd III Taubman Center, Rm 3118, Box 0374, Ann Arbor, MI 48109, USA

J. Verhoef Afdeling Klinische Microbiologie and Lab, Infectieziekten, Academisch Ziekenhais Utrecht, Postbus 85500, 3508 GA Utrecht, The Netherlands

M. R. Visser Afdeling Klinische Microbiologie and Lab, Infectieziekten, Academisch Ziekenhais Utrecht, Postbus 85500, 3508 GA Utrecht, The Netherlands

J. G. Wheeler Arkansas Children's Hospital, 800 Marshall St, Little Rock, AR 72202, USA

Abbreviations

A1PI	α_1-proteinase inhibitor (formerly α_1-anti-trypsin)
AA	arachidonic acid
ADCC	antibody-dependent cell-mediated cytotoxicity
ANC	absolute neutrophil count
ARDS	acute respiratory distress syndrome
BM	bone marrow
B/PI	bactericidal/permeability-increasing protein
cAMP	cyclic adenosine monophosphate
CBC	complete blood count
CD	cluster of differentiation
CF	cystic fibrosis
CFU	colony-forming unit
CFU-G	CFU-granulocyte
CFU-GEMM	CFU-granulocyte, erythroid, monocyte, megakaryocyte
CFU-GM	CFU-granulocyte macrophage
CFU-S	CFU-spleen
CGD	chronic granulomatous disease
CLCP	chymotrypsin-like cationic protein
CMV	cytomegalovirus
CNP	circulating neutrophil pool
CR_1	complement receptor 1 (binds C3b)
CR_3	complement receptor 3 (binds iC3b)
CT	cholera toxin
CVF	cobra venom factor
DAG	diacylglycerol
DMTU	dimethylthiourea
EBV	Epstein–Barr virus
ECM	extracellular matrix
ELAM-1	endothelial leukocyte adhesion molecule
ERK	extracellular signal-regulated kinase
F-actin	filamentous actin
FcR	receptor for the crystallizable (non-variable) portion of immunoglobulins
FMLP	N-formylmethionyl-leucylphenylalanine
G_i	G protein, inhibitory pathways
G_q	G protein, not inhibitable by pertussis toxin
G_s	G protein, stimulatory pathways
G-actin	globular actin

GAP	GTPase-activating protein
G-CSF	granulocyte colony-stimulating factor
GDI	guanine nucleotide dissociation inhibitor
GDP	guanosine diphosphate
GM-CSF	granulocyte-macrophage colony-stimulating factor
GNRP	guanine nucleotide release proteins
gp	glycoprotein
G proteins	guanosine-binding proteins (e.g. GTP, GDP)
GTP	guanosine triphosphate
GTPase	guanosine triphosphate phosphatase
HA	haemagglutinin
HETE	hydroxyeicosatetraenic acid
HLA	human lymphocyte antigen
HR	high responder
IAP	integrin-associated protein
ICAM-1(-2)	intracellular adhesion molecule-1(-2)
IL	interleukin
INF	interferon
IP_3	inositol triphosphate
I/R	ischaemia/reperfusion
i.v.	intravenous
K	killer cell
KDO	2-keto-3-deoxy-D-mannooctulonic acid
LAD	leukocyte adhesion deficiency
LAM-1	leukocyte adhesion molecule
LBP	LPS-binding protein
LeCAM	lectin adhesion molecule
LeuCAM	leukocyte cell adhesion molecule
LFA	lymphocyte function-associated antigens
LHR	long homologous repeat
LPS	lipopolysaccharide
LR	low responder
LRG	ligand–receptor–G protein complex
LRI	leukocyte-response integrin
LRX	inactive ligand–receptor complex
LTB_4	leukotriene B_4
mAb	monoclonal antibody
MAC-1	CD11b–CD18 complex on PMN
MARCKS	myristoylated, alanine-rich, C-kinase substrate
M-CSF	macrophage colony-stimulating factor
MEP	mucoid exopolysaccharide
MNP	marginated neutrophil pool
MPO	myeloperoxidase
MR	mannose-resistant

MS	mannose-sensitive
MW	molecular weight
NADPH	reduced form of nicotinamide-adenine dinucleotide
NK	natural killer cell
NPP	neutrophil proliferative pool
NSAID	non-steroidal anti-inflammatory drugs
NSP	neutrophil storage pool
OAG	1-oleoyl-2-acetylglycerol
p22	22 kDa protein
PA	phosphatidic acid
PAF	platelet-activating factor
PC	phosphatidylcholine
PE	phosphatidylethanolamine
PhOX	gene product which is a phosphorylated oxidase component
PIP_2	PI-4,5-biphosphate
PIP_3	phosphatidyl-inositol-3,4,5-triphosphate
PKC	protein kinase C
PLA_2, C, D	phospolipases A_2, C, D
PMA	phorbol myristate acetate
PMN	polymorphonuclear leukocytes
PRP	polyribosyl-ribitol phosphate
PT	pertussis toxin
Rh	recombinant human
Rm	recombinant murine
ROS	reactive oxygen species
RSV	respiratory syncytial virus
SCF	stem cell factor
SCN	severe congenital neutropenia
SCR	short consensus repeat
SDS	sodium dodecyl sulphate
SLPI	secretory leukoproteinase inhibitor
TGF	transforming growth factor
TIMP	tissue inhibitors of metalloproteinases
TNF	tumour necrosis factor
VCAM	vascular cell adhesion molecule
VLA	very late activation antigen
WGA	wheat germ agglutinin

Introduction

In George Bernard Shaw's 1909 comedy *The doctor's dilemma* (1), three schools of scientific thought are played against each other. The 'humoral' school proposes that all disease is cured with induced or passive anti-toxins:

Find the germ of the disease; prepare from it a suitable anti-toxin; inject it three times a day quarter of an hour before meals. (Act 1)

The 'surgical' school believes that disease must be removed:

Walpole: (swiftly) I know what's the matter with you. I can see it in your complexion. I can feel it in the grip of your hand.
Ridgeon: What is it?
Walpole: Blood poisoning.
Ridgeon: Blood poisoning! Impossible.
Walpole: I tell you, blood poisoning. Ninety-five percent of the human race suffer from chronic blood poisoning, and die of it. It's as simple as A. B. C. Your nuciform sac is full of decaying matter—undigested food and waste products—rank ptomaines. Now you take my advice, Ridgeon. Let me cut it out for you. You'll be another man afterwards. (Act 1)

And finally, the 'immune potentiation' school:

There is at bottom only one genuinely scientific treatment for all diseases, and that is to stimulate the phagocytes. Stimulate the phagocytes. Drugs are a delusion. (Act 1)

In the centuries which preceded the publication of *The doctor's dilemma*, debates over infection had a theological bent reflecting the philosophical perspectives of the day. During this period disease was attributed to moral flaws or violation of taboo. With the introduction of the scientific method and the development of the germ theory, theories of infection and inflammation became radically modified to accommodate the facts of the day, but still generated diverse opinions as reflected in Shaw's play. Fervent arguments on the role of neutrophilic inflammation in disease persist today as investigators grapple with how multiple immune components interact and are mutually regulated.

In a delightful essay written in 1937 (2), E. B. Krumbhaar chronicled the medical history of inflammation pathology up to his time. He outlined several periods in which a particular scientific observation or theory was dominant. In the earliest period, Hippocrates (400 BC) and Celsus (AD 25) argued their seminal theories that pus is derived from blood. According to

Galen (AD 170), stagnation of evil humours accounted for this process. For the next millennium and a half, inflammation theory lay dormant while moral issues were debated and the Dark Ages ensued. Finally, in the early 19th century, a better picture of the inflammatory process emerged. Purulence was argued as either a good (laudable pus) or bad (disease-producing) force. As outlined in *The neutrophil* we now recognize that the neutrophil has both capabilities. An interesting theory then emerged that pus was a result of abnormalities in the blood vessels, such as passive congestion, friction, and the like. This concept developed in the absence of a theory of cellular pathology which was later proposed by Virchow in the 1800s. On the basis of his theories, he argued that cellular degeneration accounted for inflammation and was independent of vascular tissues. The pre-Virchow pathologists were interpreting with the instruments available to them at the time what they could observe; that is, focal oedema and engorgement surrounding arterioles and venules. Cruveilhier argued that abnormal secretions from blood vessels promoted inflammation and therefore induced the plethoric state. It is of interest to the student of human thought that while misdirected in the precise details of vascular inflammation, Cruveilhier's ideas bear some similarities to the new descriptions of endothelial membrane changes in the upregulation of selectins, ICAMs, and other proteins described in Chapter 2. While just a few years ago it was assumed that vascular tissues were simple bystanders in the movement of neutrophils into tissues, current information attributes inflammation to upregulation of both phagocytic and endothelial adhesion molecules. In addition, endothelial cells may be a prominent source of modulating factors for these same receptors. These new discoveries have provided us with important keys to understanding chemotaxis and to explain the early and fundamental observations of Addison of extravascular pus corpuscles.

Not surprisingly, certain technologies have precipitated changes in scientific thought regarding inflammation. The microscope, the cellular staining techniques of Paul Ehrlich, analytical biochemical methods of the mid 20th century, and the birth of practical molecular biology techniques in the 1980s have led to newer perceptions of the inflammatory response. Similarly, the development of specific *in vitro* systems such as the cell-free oxidase system (described in Chapter 3) and the isolated perfused lung model (described in Chapter 7) have provided a means to elucidate new mechanisms of neutrophil activation and neutrophil-mediated injury.

Modern ideas of neutrophil activation are increasingly focused on gene regulation with that regulation being a complicated product of autocrine, paracrine, and endocrine factors as well as the products of pathogenic microbes. However, it is of great interest that many of our ideas on the role of phagocytic cells are not conceptually different from our scientific predecessors, even though the details of our concepts are better defined. We continue to redress old notions (e.g. the host versus the environment) in new clothes suitable to the facts of our day (theories of immunologic recognition). Admittedly, we appear to be moving more efficiently towards solutions to clinical problems, and even now we are beginning to control neutrophil genesis (with recombinant colony-stimulating factors) and neutrophil activation/deactivation (with interferon gamma/anti-adhesion molecules). If the sheer weight of our knowledge does not overwhelm us and create in itself an intellectual ceiling, it would appear that a colourful tapestry of basic science knowledge and rational therapy is about to be woven. The chapters that follow should provide appropriate companions for the student of the neutrophil as we embark into this exciting time.

References

1 Shaw, G. B. (1988). *The doctor's dilemma.* Penguin USA, New York.
2 Krumbhaar, E. B. (1962). *Pathology.* Hafner Publishing Co., New York.

1 Neonatal neutrophil maturation, kinetics, and function

V. S. KANWAR and M. S. CAIRO

1 Clinical case: neonatal sepsis and neutropenia

A 3450 g male infant was born to a 19-year primigravida female following an uneventful pregnancy. At 2 hours of age, he was noted to be tachypnoeic. A chest X-ray revealed bilateral diffuse infiltrates. A CBC demonstrated a haemoglobin count of 13.2 g/dl, white cell count 4.0×10^9/l (differential of 12 per cent neutrophils, 8 per cent bands, 56 per cent lymphocytes, 10 per cent monocytes), absolute neutrophil count 0.8×10^9/l, an immature to total neutrophil ratio (I:T) of 0.4, platelets 83×10^9/l. Blood, urine, and CSF cultures were obtained and ampicillin and gentamicin were started.

The infant deteriorated within a few hours, requiring intubation and mechanical ventilation. A tibial bone marrow aspirate demonstrated a neutrophil storage pool (bands + metamyelocytes + neutrophils/total nucleated cells) of 5.6 per cent. He subsequently received a total of five adult donor granulocyte transfusions administered twice daily over the next 3 days.

He continued to receive full supportive care for the next 48 h. His initial blood cultures were positive for group B streptococcus. On the third day his respiratory status began to improve, and he subsequently recovered.

When seen 1 year later in follow-up, he appeared developmentally normal, without evidence of any neurological or pulmonary sequelae.

2 Introduction

The adequate production and distribution of normally functioning neutrophils is vital to neonatal host defence (1). Production and distribution involve a series of dynamically interlinked pools of cells (2) (Fig. 1.1). The progenitor pool is the most primitive pool and contains stem cells and other progenitors not totally committed to neutrophil production. The neutrophil proliferative pool (NPP) is more mature and contains committed

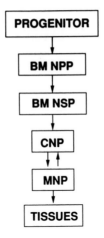

Fig. 1.1 The maturational process of myeloid progenitor and mature effector neutrophil pools. BM NPP, bone marrow neutrophil proliferative pool; BM NSP, bone marrow neutrophil storage pool; CNP, circulating neutrophil pool; MNP, marginated neutrophil pool.

neutrophil precursors capable of cell division, i.e. myeloblasts, promyelocytes, and myelocytes. The neutrophil storage pool (NSP) consists of neutrophils and non-dividing precursors, i.e. metamyelocytes and band cells. The NPP and NSP may be determined from a differential count of 500–1000 cells of a bone marrow aspirate. In the infant described above, the NSP was documented at 5.6 per cent. NSP deletion by <7 per cent has been associated with a poor outcome during neonatal sepsis (3).

The circulating neutrophil pool (CNP) is the product of the total blood volume and the absolute neutrophil count (ANC) and is commonly depleted during neonatal sepsis. Manroe *et al.* previously defined the normal range of ANC for a healthy newborn (4). The lower limit of ANC during the newborn period fluctuates between $1.8 \times 10^6/l$ and $7.2 \times 10^6/l$ (Fig. 1.2). Neutropenia is a hallmark finding in neonatal sepsis and reflects increased consumption and decreased production of neutrophils. During sepsis, there is an increased tendency to release immature precursors into the circulating pool. The ratio of immature neutrophils (bands + metamyelocytes + myelocytes) to total neutrophils in the peripheral blood may exceed 0.16 as above. This increase in the I:T ratio has also been used for the early diagnosis of neonatal septicaemia (4).

Neonatal neutrophils may also demonstrate biochemical, structural, and functional abnormalities (5, 6). Activation, chemotactic factor–receptor interaction, and signal transduction are all impaired. Poor deformability and decreased mobilization of surface receptors as well as unsatisfactory adhesion, aggregation, phagocytosis, and bactericidal activity have all been demonstrated (7). Neonatal neutrophils have also been shown to

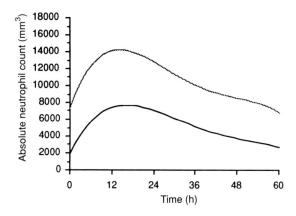

Fig. 1.2 The normal range of the absolute neutrophil count (ANC) of term newborn infants in the first 60 h after birth.

have decreased expression of the complement receptor for iC3b (CR_3) (8). All of these factors predispose infants like the one described above to rapidly overwhelming bacterial infection.

The immaturity of granulopoiesis and neonatal phagocytic immunity will be the subject of the following chapter and is summarized in Table 1.1. Altered neutrophil kinetics, a propensity to develop peripheral neutropenia, and the functional abnormalities of mature neutrophils during the neonatal period will be reviewed. Therapeutic modulation including polymorphonuclear leukocyte (PMN) transfusions, intravenous immunoglobulin (i.v. Ig), and cytokine treatment of the above-mentioned abnormalities will also be addressed.

3 Neutrophil production

3.1 Progenitor pools

The myeloid progenitor pool contains cells in a continuum of developmental stages starting with stem cells and developing into progressively more

Table 1.1 Neonatal phagocytic abnormalities

Quantitative	Qualitative
Decreased myeloid progenitor pools (CFU-GM)	Deformability—chemotaxis
Increased myeloid progenitor rates	Adherence—C3bi expression
Decreased myeloid storage pools	Phagocytosis
Decreased myeloid response to sepsis	Bacterial killing
Predisposition to neutropenia	Oxidative metabolism

committed cells such as CFU-GEMM (colony-forming unit-granulocyte, erythroid, monocyte, megakaryocyte), CFU-GM (colony forming unit-granulocyte macrophage), through to CFU-G (colony forming unit-granulocyte). Haematopoietic stem cells are pluripotential cells with the capacity for self replication as well as differentiation. They are thought to originate in the embryonic yolk sac, subsequently migrating to the liver and spleen and eventually residing in the bone marrow (1). Isolation of these cells has proved difficult in humans and until recently our knowledge of stem cells was based mainly on experiments with murine spleen colony and repopulation assays. Stem cells are thought to be small cells with a large nucleus, prominent nucleoli, and basophilic cytoplasm, somewhat resembling lymphocytes in appearance.

Till and McCullogh (9) were the first to infuse bone marrow into irradiated mice and demonstrate colonies of donor cells forming in the recipients' spleens. These colonies, containing a mixture of neutrophils, monocytes, erythrocytes, megakaryocytes, eosinophils, and basophils were shown as arising from single haematopoietic progenitors—denoted as colony forming units-spleen or CFU-S. These progenitors were subsequently isolated from *in vitro* cultures and designated CFU-GEMM (10). CFU-GEMM are pluripotential but no longer retain the capacity for self-renewal, although they are almost identical to stem cells in their morphology. In addition to the cluster of differentiation (CD) phenotypic cell marker, CD34, they also express CD33 and HLA-DR.

CFU-GM is a more mature progenitor cell capable of differentiating only into granulocytes or monocytes. These cells are morphologically distinct from stem cells, being larger with a more open nucleus as well as more cytoplasm. CFU-GM expresses CD13 in addition to CD34, CD33, and HLA-DR. The later stage CFU-G loses cell-surface markers for CD34, but begins to express CD15 and CD11b (Fig. 1.3).

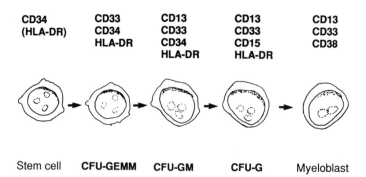

CD34	CD33	CD13	CD13	CD13
(HLA-DR)	CD34	CD33	CD33	CD33
	HLA-DR	CD34	CD15	CD38
		HLA-DR	HLA-DR	

| Stem cell | **CFU-GEMM** | **CFU-GM** | **CFU-G** | Myeloblast |

Fig. 1.3   Schematic diagram of myeloid antigen expression during normal myelopoiesis.

Studies in neonatal rats have demonstrated that the amount of CFU-GEMM/g body weight is decreased compared to adult rats. However, CFU-GEMM and CFU-GM in neonatal rats show extremely high rates of division as assayed by thymidine suicide rates when compared with adult rats (11). High rates of thymidine suicide correspond to rapid cell division. One study demonstrated neonatal rats to have a thymidine suicide rate around 80 per cent compared with 10 per cent or less in adult rats.

In adults, the progenitor pool is located almost entirely within the bone marrow. Only a small number of progenitor cells egress into the peripheral blood. Ganser *et al*. found 22 ± 7 CFU-GEMM/ml blood in samples from eight healthy adults (12). In contrast, newborn umbilical cord samples have been demonstrated to contain a very high concentration of both CFU-GM and CFU-GEMM (>2000/ml) (13, 14). Studies by Christensen *et al*. in fetal rats during the third trimester have shown a similarly high concentration of multipotent progenitor cells in peripheral blood. The pool of progenitor cells per unit body weight in fetal rats was, however, only 20 per cent that of adult animals (11). Similarly, the CFU-GM proliferative rate is already at 75–80 per cent of maximum compared to a 25 per cent rate in adult animals (11).

3.2   Neutrophil proliferative pools (NPP)

The first three committed cell stages in myelopoiesis are the myeloblast, promyelocyte, and myelocyte. They are all capable of division and together with the progenitor pool, constitute the neutrophil proliferative pool. Myeloblasts and promyelocytes undergo one or two divisions. However, myelocytes undergo three to four divisions, and there is speculation that they may undergo up to six divisions in the fetus. The additional cell divisions observed in fetal neutrophils are associated with a decrease in primary granules (see Section 4.1) and may account for the sharply decreased myeloperoxidase activity seen in fetal neutrophils.

There is evidence from neontal rat studies that the neonatal proliferative pool is not only smaller compared to adult values, but is also operating at near maximum capacity. At birth the neutrophil proliferative pool in the neonatal rat is only 25 per cent of adult animals and requires 4 weeks to reach adult values.

3.3   Neutrophil storage pool (NSP)

The non-dividing stages of myelopoiesis constitute the neutrophil storage pool. This pool consists of metamyelocytes, bands, and neutrophils, and is located within the bone marrow and the liver/spleen in neonates. Precise estimates of pool size are not available, but it is thought to constitute $4-7 \times 10^9$ cells/kg in adult rats (15).

During experimental infection in adult rats, the storage pool turnover increases from 1.6×10^9 to 6.0×10^9 neutrophils/kg/day. However, their myeloid proliferative rate has the capacity to increase by 300 per cent and NSP depletion is not usually seen. The neonatal rat only has a storage pool approximately 25 per cent of the adult rat ($1-2 \times 10^9$ cells/kg). There is little reserve proliferative capacity. During experimental sepsis, neonatal rats fail to increase their NSP or progenitor pool. Under these circumstances, a septic newborn rat usually becomes neutropenic with increased neutrophil consumption (16, 17).

Recent human neonatal sepsis studies, however, have demonstrated the neutrophil storage pool to be reasonably well maintained, and severe NSP depletion occurs in less than 15 per cent of septic neonates (18). This finding was confirmed by Engle *et al.* (3) who found similar NSP depletion in only 6 per cent of their sick neonates. In prior series the incidence of severe NSP depletion in neonatal sepsis had previously been estimated to be 15–62 per cent (19–21).

3.4   Neutrophil egress

As neutrophils mature they become more deformable, alter their surface charge, acquire new cell membrane receptors and demonstrate motility (22). It has been proposed that the acquisition of these properties helps the mature neutrophils actively migrate or 'egress" through *trans*-endothelial pores in the marrow sinusoids to reach the bloodstream. Interleukin-1 (IL-1) and complement factors such as C3e and C3d.g appear to act as positive modulators for this process (23). C3d.g fragments have recently been shown to enhance the egress of neutrophils from neonatal rat marrow. During group B streptococcal sepsis, the degradation of C3b to C3d.g may be responsible for neutrophil egress (23).

We have recently demonstrated that RhG-CSF administered to neonatal rats is associated with a profound neutrophilia, presumably by inducing neutrophil egress (24). RhG-CSF, administered intraperitoneally to newborn rats for a total of 7 days, induced a sustained increase in the circulating ANC, starting first with a sharp increase in the ANC on the first day secondary to neutrophil egress and subsequently increasing secondary to an expansion of the marrow NSP.

Other agents have been associated with an acceleration in neutrophil egress. Administration of IVIG has recently been shown to enhance neutrophil egress in the neonatal rat (25). The administration of glucocorticoids also leads to increased neutrophil egress with reduced neutrophil emigration into tissues and a relatively prolonged half-life of PMNs in the circulating pool.

3.5   Circulating neutrophil pool (CNP) and marginated neutrophil pool (MNP)

Athens *et al.* demonstrated that neutrophils in the peripheral blood consist of a freely circulating pool and a marginated pool (26). Both pools are of approximately equal size. The circulating pool (CNP) contains approximately 0.3×10^9 cells/kg. Estimates of CNP size can be determined by multiplying the neutrophil count per mm^3 of blood by the known circulating blood volume. When attempts were made to confirm this value by autologous reinfusion of neutrophils labelled with difluorphosphate[32] or ^{51}Cr, a value was obtained twice that of the estimated CNP. The difference between these two figures was due to the marginated neutrophil pool.

The marginated neutrophil pool (MNP) is thought to total 0.4×10^9 cells/kg (27). It consists of cells still within the vascular space, but adherent to the walls of small vessels. Adhesion is thought to be modulated by interaction between LFA-1 (CD11a–18 complex) on the surface of the neutrophil with ICAM-1, ELAM-1, and other similar receptors on the vessel endothelium (28–32). Rather than adhering in a static manner to the vessel endothelium, these cells gradually roll along until reaching an area of tissue damage or inflammation. Upon doing so, diapedesis occurs and they enter the tissues.

In the last decade, the availability of Tc 99- and In 111-labelled neutrophils has allowed anatomic imaging to be performed. Using animal and human subjects, it appears that injected neutrophils selectively marginate in the lung, liver, and spleen (33).

Neutrophils from the MNP can be released into the general circulation by a suitable stimulus such as epinephrine (and epinephrine-releasing stimuli, e.g. exercise), other beta-agonists, and interleukin-6. Demargination is thought partly to account for the neutrophilia seen within the first 48 h of birth. The exact mechanism by which neutrophils leave the MNP to enter the CNP remains unclear. Demargination involves disruption of the bond between the endothelium and leukocyte adhesion receptors, presumably modulated by cytokines.

The circulating pool in the newborn shows more heterogeneity with regard to a wide variety of characteristics than has previously been recognized. Between 20 and 70 per cent of neonatal neutrophils sampled from peripheral blood are non-motile. Krause *et al.* (34), using a 31D8 monoclonal antibody, identified a population of cells that were less mature and poorly motile. Neonates appear to have a larger population of such cells ($31D8^+$) compared to adults.

3.6   Cytokine regulation

Cytokines modulating granulopoiesis may be divided into two classes. Class I factors affect proliferation and differentiation of progenitors and other early precursors (e.g. CFU-GEMM) whereas Class II factors influence more lineage-specific precursors (e.g. CFU-G). These cytokines are also referred to as 'colony-stimulating factors' because of their *in vitro* effect on hematopoietic progenitor colonies (see Table 1.2). Class I factors include interleukin-3 (multi-CSF), granulocyte-macrophage colony-stimulating factor (GM-CSF), interleukin-6, and stem cell factor (SCF). Examples of Class II factors are granulocyte colony-stimulating factor (G-CSF), monocyte colony-stimulating factor (M-CSF), and erythropoietin (35).

Human G-CSF is a glycoprotein which was first purified from the bladder carcinoma cell line 5637. It is composed of 174 amino acids and has a MW of 18 000 daltons. G-CSF stimulates CFU-G proliferation and induces peripheral neutrophilia. It also acts on mature cells enhancing n-formyl-methionyl leucyl-phenylalanine (FMLP) binding, chemotaxis, and antibody-dependent cellular cytotoxicity (ADCC) (36).

Human GM-CSF was first identified from the Mo-T lymphoblastoid cell line as a glycoprotein with MW 22 000 daltons with 127 amino acids. It stimulates proliferation of CFU-GM and CFU-GEMM. GM-CSF additionally enhances (i.e. primes) neutrophil oxidative metabolism, chemotaxis, degranulation, and ADCC (37).

Human interleukin-3, first isolated from the Gibbon T cell line MLA-

Table 1.2   Cytokines influencing myelopoiesis

Cytokine	MW (daltons)	Source	Target progenitor pool
Granulocyte colony-stimulating factor (G-CSF)	18 000 glycoprotein	Human bladder carcinoma cell line 5637 medium	CFU-G CFU-GM
Granulocyte-macrophage colony-stimulating factor (GM-CSF)	22 000 glycoprotein	Mo-T lymphoblastoid cell line	CFU-GM CFU-GEMM
Interleukin-3 (IL-3)	14 600 glycoprotein	Gibbon cell line MLA-144	CFU-GEMM CFU-GM
Interleukin-6 (IL-6)	26 000 glycoprotein	Fibroblastoid cells	CFU-GEMM
Stem cell factor (SCF)	26 000 glycoprotein	Buffalo rat liver cells BRL-3A	CFU-Blast

144, stimulates very early progenitor cells. It is documented as enhancing proliferation of myeloid progenitors as well as erythroid and megakaryocytic cell lines. It has a MW of 14 600 daltons and is composed of 152 amino acids (38).

4 Maturation of neutrophils

4.1 Granule maturation

Bainton *et al.* (39) meticulously described the origin and content of azurophil and specific granules during myelopoiesis. There are now known to be at least three and possibly four types of granules in the neutrophil (40).

Primary or azurophilic granules are first seen in the promyelocyte (Fig. 1.4). They are thought to be a special type of primary lysosome and are budded off from the concave surface of the Golgi complex. They contain myeloperoxidase and lysozyme, as well as cationic proteins, proteases, and acid hydrolases. Myeloperoxidase is often used as a specific marker for these granules.

Secondary or specific granules appear in both myelocytes and meta-

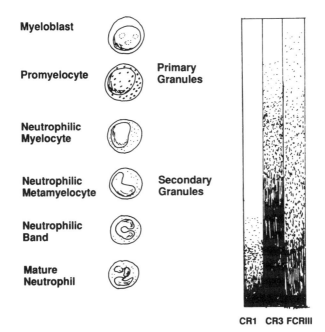

Fig. 1.4 The expression of intracellular granules and surface adhesion receptors during myelopoiesis. The figure on the right demonstrates the increase in receptor density as the cell matures from the myeloblast form to the differentiated PMN.

myelocytes. They are smaller, less dense, and stain heavily for glycoprotein. They arise from the convex surface of the Golgi complex. They are known to contain lysozyme, collagenase, lactoferrin, B12-binding protein, plasminogen activator, and cytochrome *b*.

The myelocyte exhibits a mixture of large reddish-purple azurophilic granules as well as smaller pinkish specific granules. Throughout this stage, specific granules are produced. No further primary granules are produced, and as the myelocytes divide the number of primary granules per cell progressively declines. In adults, myelocytes divide up to four or five times. Preterm infants appear to employ additional divisions, and the resulting reduction in the number of primary granules per mature neutrophil may contribute to a functional myeloperoxidase deficiency (41); however, the degree of decrease in myeloperoxidase present needs to be compared to assays of bacterial killing to determine its 'functional' significance.

In the mature neutrophil, only one-third of its granules are primary granules. Maturation of these granules alters their staining characteristics and they no longer retain the red-purple colour that makes them so prominent in the promyelocyte, but instead appear light pink and virtually invisible to the light microscope.

Tertiary granules have not been visualized as a separate entity except under electron microscopy. They are thought to be similar to specific granules, although slightly less dense, and are rich in gelatinase. They are thought to appear during the myelocyte stage.

4.2   Appearance of membrane receptors

The mature neutrophil has receptors for complement: CR_1 and CR_3, as well as Fc receptors for IgG namely, Fc gamma I, II and III. CR_3 receptors are a family of at least three different glycoproteins each consisting of an identical beta subunit (CD18) non-covalently linked to different alpha subunits (CD11a, CD11b, CD11c, corresponding to LFA-1, MAC-1 and p150,95) (42; see Chapter 2 for further discussion of the function of these various receptors).

Glasser and Fiederlein have studied the appearance of receptors during myelopoiesis (43). CR_1 initially appears in a small proportion of band cells and is more widely represented in mature neutrophils. CR_3, however, is first detected at the promyelocyte stage and is present in over half of metamyelocytes, and almost all bands and mature neutrophils. Bainton *et al.* (44) has suggested that CD11a/CD18 may be the earliest receptor to appear. Intracellular pools (peroxidase-negative granules) containing MAC-1 and p150,95 are first detected at the myelocyte stage (45).

FcR gamma III is present on one-third of all promyelocytes, one-half of all metamyelocytes and four-fifths of bands and mature neutrophils.

The expression of membrane receptors in neonatal neutrophils has recently been of major interest. There is evidence that following FMLP stimulation, expression of CR_1, CR_3 and FcR III are all impaired in neutrophils from preterm infants (46). In term infants following FMLP stimulation, CR_1 appeared to have normal expression although CR_3 and FcR III were moderately impaired (7).

5 Neonatal neutrophil function

The following discussion addresses specific aspects of neonatal PMN function. The reader is directed to Chapters 2–4 for complete descriptions of signal transduction and PMN functions in normal PMN.

5.1 Activation and signal transduction

Hill (6) demonstrated that exposure of neonatal neutrophils to low levels of chemotactic factors failed to result in enhanced motility or respiratory burst activity. This was originally attributed to a decreased ability to produce leukotriene B_4 (LTB_4). Subsequently, Kikawa *et al.* (47) demonstrated that neonatal neutrophils produce normal levels of LTB_4.

Anderson *et al.* (48) have demonstrated that neonatal neutrophils have a normal number of receptors for FMLP. Using a calcium-sensitive probe, they were also able to demonstrate lower levels of intracellular calcium in neonatal versus adult neutrophils following FMLP binding. In addition they reported that neonatal neutrophils have a poor hyperpolarization response. Further work is needed to determine the molecular basis for these observations.

5.2 Adherence, aggregation, and motility

Neonatal neutrophils adhere poorly, which has been attributed to a failure to upregulate the surface expression of adhesive glycoproteins (49). Olson *et al.* (50) also demonstrated that neonatal neutrophils not only have a poor aggregation response but also fail to undergo disaggregation, leading to increased morbidity.

Neonatal neutrophils fail to deform normally following chemotactic stimulation (51). Neonatal neutrophils do not mobilize surface receptors for Con A following microtubule disruption by colchicine. Anderson *et al.* (48) reported impaired movement of membrane receptors from the head to the tail of migrating neutrophils, as well as failure to orient or assemble microtubules normally in a chemotactic gradient. It has been postulated that neonatal neutrophils contain rigid cytoskeletal elements that prevent normal deformation and hinder mobility. Neonatal neutrophils also appear to have a normal, or slightly elevated content of filamentous (F)-actin. The defect may lie in decreased cellular ATP affecting actin–myosin dissociation.

5.3   Phagocytosis and bactericidal activity

Bruce *et al.* (8) reported diminished upregulation of C3bi receptors following exposure of neonatal neutrophils to FMLP. Neutrophils from 'well' neonates were shown to have normal phagocytic and bactericidal capabilities. However, several studies have suggested that neutrophils from 'stressed' neonates consistently show decreased phagocytic and bactericidal activities (52). The mechanism for this remains uncertain but it may be related to decreased lactoferrin in specific granules, with subsequent decreased production of bactericidal hydroxyl radicals (6).

6   Therapy of neonatal neutrophil disorders

This section contains information about the treatment of PMN dysfunction in neonates. Chapter 8 reviews therapies for older infants and children.

6.1   White cell transfusions

Santos *et al.* (53) first demonstrated the efficacy of PMN transfusions during experimental sepsis in neonatal rats. Neonatal rats inoculated with group B streptococcus and randomized to receive 2×10^6 adult human neutrophils, had a 25 per cent mortality rate compared with 100 per cent without transfusions. Christensen *et al.* (54) reported that newborn puppies inoculated with *Staphylococcus aureus* demonstrated a mortality rate of 16 per cent in the group receiving neutrophil transfusions compared with 100 per cent in the untreated group.

Several other groups have examined the efficacy of neonatal transfusions during neonatal sepsis, and the results are summarized in Table 1.3 (19–21, 55, 56). It is difficult to compare most of these studies because of the differences in patient populations, the small numbers of patients, the different methods of acquiring the neutrophils used, and marked intergroup differences in the NSP. Nevertheless, the combined data suggests significantly improved survival for the septic neonates receiving neutrophil transfusions.

Our institution has recently completed a prospective randomized trial comparing adult granulocyte transfusions versus i.v. Ig administration in the treatment of neonatal sepsis (55). Thirty-five septic newborns were randomized to receive either neutrophil transfusions or i.v. Ig. Criteria for

Table 1.3 Summary of PMN transfusions for septic newborns

Study (year)	Method	Dose of PMN	Neutrophil storage pool (NSP) depletion	Survival control versus PMN (percentages)
Christensen[19] (1982)	Continuous flow centrifugation	0.7×10^9	16/16	Increased** 1/9 versus 7/7 (11 versus 100)
Baley[20] (1987)	Fresh buffy coat	0.35×10^9	9/25	No change 9/13 versus 7/12 (69 versus 58)
Wheeler[21] (1987)	Fresh buffy coat	0.4×10^9	9/28	No change** 2/5 versus 2/4 (40 versus 50)
Cairo[55] (1992)	Continuous flow centrifugation	0.75×10^9	5/75	Increased 18/33 versus 41/42 (54 versus 98)
Laurenti[56] (1981)	Continuous flow centrifugation	$0.5–1.0 \times 10^9$	–/38*	Increased 5/18 versus 18/20 (28 versus 90)
Totals	Buffy and Leuko	$0.35–1.0 \times 10^9$	39/144	Increased 35/78 versus 75/85 (45 versus 88)

* NSP not examined.
** Only patients with NSP depletion were randomized to PMN transfusions versus supportive therapy alone.

entrance included weight >800 g, age <28 days, and signs of overwhelming bacterial sepsis. Neutrophils were obtained from normal adult donors by continuous flow centrifugation leukapheresis. To avoid graft versus host disease, neutrophils were irradiated with 1500 rad. Transfusions were administered within 4 h of diagnosis and a total of five transfusions, each 15 cm^3/kg (i.e. ~1 × 10^9 neutrophils/transfusion) was administered over 3 days. Neonates randomized to i.v. Ig received 1000 mg/kg over 4–6 h daily for a total of 3 days.

There was a significant difference in survival between the two groups. One-hundred per cent of those infants receiving neutrophil transfusions survived as opposed to 64 per cent in the i.v. Ig group (P <0.03). In the group receiving transfusions, there was no evidence of graft versus host disease, fluid overload, pulmonary insufficiency, or transfusion-associated infections (55).

6.2   Immunoglobulin therapy

Neonates are deficient in circulating levels of immunoglobulin and specific antibody production compared to infants and children. This immaturity also predisposes to a significant delay between exposure of bacterial organisms and release of neutrophils from bone marrow NSP. In addition, antibody-deficient neonates have a significantly increased interval between release of neutrophils from NSP and their localization at the site of bacterial infection.

Recent studies have suggested that antibody therapy in the neonate with presumed sepsis will aid in the release of PMN from storage pools. Harper *et al.* (57) demonstrated that i.v. Ig administered to neonatal rats experimentally infected with either group B streptococcus or *Escherichia coli* reduced the mortality rate by modulating neutrophil kinetics. Christensen *et al.* (25) documented that administration of 750 mg/kg of i.v. Ig to septic neonates resulted in an increase in neutrophil egress from the marrow and an elevation of the circulating I:T ratio within 1 h of administration and complete resolution of neutropenia by 24 h. The mechanism by which i.v. Ig induces neutrophil egress from the marrow is currently under study.

The dose of i.v. Ig administered is important and excessive levels of serum IgG may cause binding of non-specific antibody to neutrophil receptors, thus preventing specific opsonophagocytic antibody from initiating phagocytosis. However, Marodi *et al.* (58) reported that administration of appropriate doses of i.v. Ig (300 mg/kg/day) enhanced *in vitro* neonatal neutrophil opsonophagocytosis of *S. aureus*.

6.3   Cytokine modulation

IL-3, IL-6, SCF, GM-CSF, and G-CSF are all capable of modulating neutrophil production. The latter two factors also have significant effects on neutrophil function. Recent experience has suggested that each of these cytokines may also modulate neonatal myelopoiesis and/or neonatal neutrophil function.

IL-3 appears to stimulate early progenitors, including multipotent progenitor cells. Administration of recombinant murine IL-3 for 7 days to neonatal rats increased the neonatal bone marrow myeloid progenitor pool (59). IL-6 given prior to G-CSF therapy induced an increase in peripheral neutrophilia compared with G-CSF treatment alone (60).

Administration of rmGM-CSF for 7 days to neonatal rats increased the marrow NSP and resulted in an increase in peripheral neutrophilia with enhanced neutrophil egress (59). GM-CSF also primes and modulates neonatal neutrophils, resulting in enhanced motility, C3bi expression, adherence, and aggregation (61). GM-CSF has also been demonstrated to enhance neonatal neutrophil oxidative metabolism and bacterial killing (62).

Administration for 7 days of recombinant human (RL) G-CSF to newborn rats has been demonstrated to increase significantly the bone marrow (BM) NSP as well as peripheral ANC. Pulse Rh G-CSF or a more prolonged 7 day administration of Rh G-CSF in newborn rats resulted in a synergistic increase in survival during experimental group B streptococcal sepsis (24, 63).

SCF has been demonstrated to act synergistically with G-CSF, GM-CSF, and IL-3 during *in vitro* myeloid progenitor studies (64). Simultaneous as well as sequential administration of Rh G-CSF and Rh SCF for 14 days to newborn rats caused a significant increase in BM neutrophil storage pool and the peripheral ANC (65).

The number and equilibrium binding of G-CSF and GM-CSF receptors on mature neutrophils do not differ significantly between adult and neonatal cells (66). However, stimulation of cord blood mononuclear cells results in markedly decreased production of G-CSF, GM-CSF, and IL-3 compared with adult mononuclear cells (66, 67). Exogenous administration of G-CSF or other cytokines might thus be beneficial in the prevention or treatment of sepsis in the neonate. A Phase I trial is currently underway to determine whether G-CSF is a safe and effective therapy for neonatal sepsis (68).

7   Conclusions

Neutrophil production and distribution involves sequential proliferation and differentiation of a series of interlinked pools. Neonatal progenitor and proliferative pools divide at near maximal capacity but contain comparatively small storage pools. During neonatal sepsis, decreased production and increased consumption of neutrophils rapidly leads to neutropenia. Tibial BM aspiration in the neonate may help in determining the size of the NSP and in differentiating NSP depletion from increased consumption. Depletion of the NSP is an adverse prognostic factor during neonatal sepsis. Neonatal neutrophils also demonstrate various functional abnormalities. These includes poor motility, adherence, a tendency towards irreversible aggregation, and diminished upregulation of C3bi receptors following FMLP exposure. Phagocytic and bactericidal activity in neutrophils from 'stressed' neonates is also diminished.

These deficits in neonatal neutrophil function and distribution may be ameliorated by using adult neutrophil transfusions, i.v. Ig therapy, or cytokine therapy. Studies to date suggest that the first two modalities may be of clinical benefit. Cytokines now available include IL-3, SCF, G-CSF, and GM-CSF. Clinical trials with G-CSF in neonatal sepsis are currently underway. Studies in neonatal animals suggest that optimal responses may be obtained by combination cytokine therapy.

The case presented at the beginning of this chapter illustrates the pathophysiology of sepsis-induced neutropenia in the newborn. In this particular case, overwhelming bacterial sepsis resulted in a depletion of BM NSP reserves, an early release of early myeloid cells, an increase in the I:T ratio, and the development of neutropenia. Although this patient appeared to benefit from PMN transfusions, future therapy with i.v. Ig or colony-stimulating factors may also potentiate the newborn immune response and reduce sepsis-induced morbidity and mortality.

References

1 Christensen, R. (1989). Hematopoiesis in the fetus and neonate. *Pediatr. Res.*, **26**, 531–5.

2 Cronkite, E. and Fliedner, T. (1964). Granulocytopoiesis. *N. Engl. J. Med.*, **270**, 1347–52.

3 Engle, W., McGuire, W., Schreiner, R., and Yu, P. (1988). Neutrophil storage pool depletion in neonates with sepsis and neutropenia. *J. Pediatr.*, **113**, 747–9.

4 Manroe, B., Weinberg, A., Rosenfeld, C., and Browne, R. (1979). The neonatal blood count in health and disease. *J. Pediatr.*, **95**, 89–98.

5 Cairo, M. S. (1989). Neonatal neutrophil host defense. *Am. J. Dis. Child.*, **143**, 40–6.

6 Hill, H. (1987). Biochemical, structural and functional abnormalities of polymorphonuclear leukocytes in the neonate. *Pediatr. Res.*, **22**, 375–82.

7 Christensen, R. (1989). Neutrophil kinetics in the fetus and neonate. *Am. J. Pediatr. Hematol. Oncol.*, **11**, 215–23.

8 Bruce, M., Baley, J., and Medvik, K. (1987). Impaired surface membrane expression of C3bi but not C3b receptors on neonatal neutrophils. *Pediatr. Res.*, **21**, 306–11.

9 Till, J. and McCulloch, E. (1961). A direct measurement of the radiation sensitivity of normal mouse bone marrow cells. *Radiat. Res.,* **14,** 213–22.

10 Suda, T., Suda, J., and Ogawa, M. (1983). Single cell origin of mouse hemopoietic colonies expressing multiple lineages in variable combinations. *Proc. Natl Acad. Sci. USA,* **80,** 6689–93.

11 Christensen, R. and Rothstein, G. (1984). Pre- and post-natal development of granulocyte stem cells (CFUc) in the rat. *Pediatr. Res.,* **18,** 599–602.

12 Ganser, A., Eistner, E., and Hoelzer, D. (1985). Megakaryocytic cells in mixed haemopoietic colonies (CFU-GEMM) from the peripheral blood of normal individuals. *Br. J. Haematol.,* **59,** 627–33.

13 Christensen, R., Harper, T., and Rothstein, G. (1986). Granulocyte-macrophage progenitor cells in term and preterm neonates. *J. Pediatr.,* **109,** 1047–51.

14 Christensen, R. (1987). Circulating pluripotent hematopoietic progenitor cells in neonates. *J. Pediatr.,* **110,** 622–5.

15 Marsh, J., Boggs, D., Cartwright, G., and Wintrobe, M. (1967). Neutrophil kinetics in acute infection. *J. Clin. Invest.,* **46,** 1943–53.

16 Christensen, R., Shigeoka, A., HIll, H., and Rothstein, G. (1980). Circulating and storage neutrophil changes in experimental type II group B streptococcal sepsis. *Pediatr. Res.,* **14,** 806–8.

17 Christensen, R., Hill, H., and Rothstein, G. (1983). Granulocytic stem cell (CFU-C) proliferation in experimental group B streptococcal sepsis. *Pediatr. Res.,* **17,** 278–80.

18 Cairo, M. (1989). Neutrophil transfusions in treatment of neonatal sepsis. *Am. J. Pediatr. Hematol. Oncol.,* **II,** 227–34.

19 Christensen, R., Rothstein, G., Anstall, H., and Bybee, B. (1982). Granulocyte transfusions in neonates with bacterial infection, neutropenia, and depletion of mature neutrophils. *Pediatrics,* **70,** 1–6.

20 Baley, J., Stork, E., Warkentin, P., and Shurin, S. (1987). Buffy coat transfusions in neutropenic neonates with presumed sepsis: a prospective randomized trial. *Pediatrics,* **80,** 712–20.

21 Wheeler, J., Chauvenet, A., Johnson, C., Block, S., Dillard, R., and Abramson, J. (1987). Buffy coat transfusions in neonates with sepsis and neutrophil storage pool depletion. *Pediatrics,* **79,** 422–5.

22 Wallace, P., Packman, C., and Lichtman, M. (1987). Maturation-associated changes in the peripheral cytoplasm of human neutrophils: a review. *Exp. Hematol.,* **15,** 34–45.

23 Shigeoka, A., Gobel, R., Janatova, J., and Hill, H. (1988). Neutrophil mobilization induced by complement fragments during experimental group B streptococcal (GBS) infection. *Am. J. Pathol.,* **133,** 623–9.

24 Cairo, M., Plunkett, J., Mauss, D., and van de Ven, C. (1990). Seven-day administration of recombinant human granulocyte colony-stimulating

factor to newborn rats: Modulation of neonatal neutrophilia, myelo-poiesis, and group B streptococcus sepsis. *Blood,* **76,** 1788–94.

25 Christensen, R., Brown, M., Hall, D., Lassiter, H., and Hill, H. (1991). Effect on neutrophil kinetics and serum opsonic capacity of intravenous administration of immune globulin to neonates with clinical signs of early-onset sepsis. *J. Pediatr.,* **118,** 606–14.

26 Athens, J. (1981). Leukocytes. In *Clinical Hematology* (ed. M. Wintrobe), pp. 208–13. Lea and Febiger, Philadelphia.

27 Dancey, J., Deubelbeiss, K., Harker, L., and Finca, C. (1976). Neutrophil kinetics in man. *J. Clin. Invest.,* **58,** 705–15.

28 Leeuwenberg, J., Jeunhomme, G., and Buurman, W. (1990). Adhesion of polymorphonuclear cells to human endothelial cells. Adhesion-molecule-dependent, and Fc receptor-mediated adhesion-molecule-independent mechanisms. *Clin. Exp. Immunol.,* **81,** 496–500.

29 Smith, C., Marlin, S., Rothlein, R., Toman, C., and Anderson, D. (1989). Cooperative interactions of LFA-1 and Mac-1 with intercellular adhesion molecule-1 in facilitating adherence and transendothelial migration of human neutrophils in vitro. *J. Clin. Invest.,* **83,** 2008–17.

30 Cybulsky, M., McComb, D., and Movat, H. (1989). Protein synthesis dependent and independent mechanisms of neutrophil emigration. Different mechanisms of inflammation in rabbits induced by interleukin-1, tumor necrosis factor alpha or endotoxin versus leukocyte chemo-attractants. *Am. J. Pathol.,* **135,** 227–37.

31 Smith, C., Rothlein, R., Hughes, B., Mariscalco, M., Rudloff, H., Schmalstieg, F., and Anderson, D. (1988). Recognition of an endothelial determinant for CD18-dependent human neutrophil adherence and transendothelial migration. *J. Clin. Invest.,* **82,** 1746–56.

32 Spertini, O., Kansas, G., Munro, J., Griffin, J., and Tedder, T. (1991). Regulation of leukocyte migration by activation of the leukocyte adhesion molecule-1 (LAM-1) selectin. *Nature,* **349,** 691–4.

33 Saverymuttu, S., Peters, A., Danpore, H., Reavy, H., Osman, S., and Lavender, J. (1983). Lung transit of [111]indium-labelled granulocytes: Relationship to labelling techniques. *Scand. J. Haematol.,* **30,** 151–60.

34 Krause, P., Kreutzer, D., Eisenfeld, L., Herson, V., Weisman, S., Bannon, P., and Greca, N. (1989). Characterization of nonmotile neutrophil subpopulations in neonates and adults. *Pediatr. Res.,* **25,** 519–24.

35 Cairo, M. (1991). Hematopoietic growth factors: A new frontier in immunotherapy. *J. Pediatr.,* **118,** S1–S3.

36 Welte, K., Platzer, E., Lu, L., Gabrilove, J., Levi, E., Mertelsmann, R., and Moore, M. (1987). Purification and biochemical characterization of human pluripotent hematopoietic colony-stimulating factor. *Proc. Natl Acad. Sci. USA,* **82,** 1526–30.

37 Wong, G., Witek, J., Temple, P., Wilkkens, K., Leary, A., Luxem-

burg, D., *et al.* (1985). Human GM-CSF: Molecular cloning of the complementary DNA and purification of the natural and recombinant proteins. *Science,* **228,** 810–15.

38 Yang, Y., Ciarletta, A., Temple, P., Chung, M., Kovacic, S., Witek-Giannotti, J., *et al.* (1986). Human interleukin-3 (multi-CSF): Identification by expression cloning of a novel hematopoietic growth factor related to murine IL-3. *Cell,* **47,** 3–10.

39 Bainton, D., Ullyot, J., and Faarquhar, M. (1971). The development of neutrophilic polymorphonuclear leukocytes in human bone marrow. *J. Exp. Med.,* **134,** 907–34.

40 Boxer, L. and Smolen, J. (1988). Neutrophil granule constituents and their release in health and disease. *Hematol./Oncol. Clinics of N. Am.,* **2,** 101–34.

41 Christensen, R. and Rothstein, G. (1985). Neutrophil myeloperoxidase concentration: Changes with development and during bacterial infection. *Pediatr. Res.,* **19,** 1278–82.

42 Springer, T., Thompson, W., Miller, L., and Anderson, D. (1984). Inherited deficiency of the Mac-1, LFA-1, p150,95 glycoprotein family and its molecular basis. *J. Exp. Med.,* **160,** 1901.

43 Glasser, L. and Fiederlein, R. (1987). Functional differentiation of normal human neutrophils. *Blood,* **69,** 937–44.

44 Bainton, D., Miller, L., Kishimoto, T., and Springer, T. (1987). Leukocyte adhesion receptors are stored in peroxidase-negative granules of human neutrophils. *J. Exp. Med.,* **166,** 1641–53.

45 Foy, M. and Simchowitz, L. (1988). Recent developments in leukocyte research. In *The Year in Immunology* (ed. J. Cruse and R. J. Lewis), Vol. 4, pp. 208–17. Karger, Basel.

46 Smith, J., Campbell, D., Ludomirsky, A., Polin, R., Douglas, S., Garty, B., and Harris, M. (1990). Expression of the complement receptors CR1 and CR3 and the type III Fcg receptor on neutrophils from newborn infants and from fetuses with Rh disease. *Pediatr. Res.,* **28,** 120.

47 Kikawa, Y., Shigematsu, Y., and Sudo, M. (1986). Leukotriene B_4 biosynthesis in polymorphonuclear leukocytes from blood of umbilical cord, infants, children, and adults. *Pediatr. Res.,* **20,** 402–6.

48 Anderson, D., Hughes, B., and Smith, C. (1981). Abnormal mobility of neonatal polymorphonuclear leukocytes: Relationship to impaired redistribution of surface adhesion sites by chemotactic factor or colchicine. *J. Clin. Invest.,* **68,** 863–74.

49 Anderson, D., Freeman, K., Hughes, B., and Buffone, G. (1985). Secretory determinants of impaired adherence and motility of neonatal PMNs. *Pediatr. Res.,* **19,** 257A.

50 Olson, T., Ruymann, F., Cook, B., Burgess, D., Henson, S., and Thomas, P. (1983). Newborn polymorphonuclear leukocyte aggregation:

A study of physical properties and ultrastructure using chemotactic peptides. *Pediatr. Res.,* **17,** 993–7.

51 Miller, M. (1975). Developmental maturation of human neutrophil motility and its relationship to membrane deformability. In *The Phagocytic Cell in Host Resistance* (ed. J. Bellanti and D. Dayton), pp. 295–307. Raven Press, New York.

52 Miller, M. (1969). Phagocytosis in the newborn infant: Humoral and cellular factors. *J. Pediatr.,* **74,** 255–9.

53 Santos, J., Shigeoka, A., and Hill, H. (1980). Functional leukocyte administration in protection against experimental neonatal infection. *Pediatr. Res.,* **114,** 1408–13.

54 Christensen, R., Bradley, P., Priebat, D., Anstall, H., and Rothstein, G. (1982). Granulocyte transfusion in septic canine neonates. *Pediatr. Res.,* **16,** 571–5.

55 Cairo, M., Worcester, C., Rucker, R., Hanten, S., Amlie, R., Sender, L., and Hicks, D. (1992). Randomized trial of granulocyte transfusions versus intravenous immune globulin therapy for neonatal neutropenia and sepsis. *J. Pediatr.,* **120,** 281–5.

56 Laurenti, F., Ferro, R., Isacchi, G., Panero, A., Savignoni, P., Malagnino, F. *et al.* (1981). Polymorphonuclear leukocyte transfusion for the treatment of sepsis in the newborn infant. *J. Pediatr.,* **98,** 118–22.

57 Harper, T., Christensen, R., and Rothstein, G. (1986). Effect of intravenous immunoglobulin G on neutrophil kinetics during experimental group B streptococcal infection in neonatal rats. *Rev. Infect. Dis.,* **8(suppl),** S401–8.

58 Marodi, L., Kalmar, A., and Szabo, I. (1989). Opsonic activity in serum from septic infants treated with intravenous immunoglobulin. *Arch. Dis. Child.,* **64,** 530–4.

59 Cairo, M., Mauss, D., Plunkett, J., Gillis, S., and van de Ven, C. (1991). Modulation of neonatal myelopoiesis in newborn rats following 7-day administration of either GM-CSF or IL-3 (granulocyte-monocyte colony stimulating factor or interleukin-3). *Pediatr. Res.,* **29,** 504–9.

60 Cairo, M., Plunkett, J., Nguyen, A., Clark, S., and van de Ven, C. (1991). Sequential administration of interleukin-6 and granulocyte-colony-stimulating factor in newborn rats: Modulation of newborn granulopoiesis and thrombopoiesis. *Pediatr. Res.,* **30,** 554–9.

61 Cairo, M., van de Ven, C., Toy, C., Suen, Y., Mauss, D., and Sender, L. (1991). GM-CSF primes and modulates neonatal PMN motility: Upregulation of C3bi (Mo1) expression with alteration in PMN adherence and aggregation. *Am. J. Pediatr. Hematol. Oncol.,* **13,** 249–57.

62 Cairo, M., van de Ven, C., Toy, C., Mauss, D., and Sender, L. (1989). Recombinant human granulocyte-macrophage colony stimulating factor primes neonatal granulocytes for enhanced oxidative metabolism and chemotaxis. *Pediatr. Res.,* **26,** 395–9.

63 Cairo, M., Mauss, D., Kommareddy, S., Norris, K., van de Ven, C., and Modanlou, H. (1990). Prophylactic or simultaneous administration of recombinant human granulocyte colony stimulating factor in the treatment of group B streptococcal sepsis in neonatal rats. *Pediatr. Res.,* **27,** 612–16.

64 Bernstein, I., Andrews, R., and Zsebo, K. (1991). Recombinant human stem cell factor enhances the formation of colonies by CD34$^+$ and CD34$^+$lin$^-$ cells, and the generation of colony-forming cell progeny from CD34$^+$lin$^-$ cells cultured with interleukin-3, granulocyte colony-stimulating factor, or granulocyte-macrophage colony-stimulating factor. *Blood,* **77,** 2316–21.

65 Cairo, M., Plunkett, J., Zsebo, K., Hammoch, V., Nguyen, A., and van de Ven, C. (1991). In vivo modulation of neonatal rat hematopoiesis by rat stem cell factor (R-SCF) ± human G-CSF (RhG-CSF): Significant enhancement of neonatal myelopoiesis. *Blood,* **78,** 76A.

66 Cairo, M., Plunkett, J. M., Nguyen, A., and Cairo, M. S. (1992). The effect of stem cell factor with and without G-CSF on neonatal hematopoiesis: *In vivo* induction of newborn myelopoiesis and reduction of mortality during experimental group B streptococcal sepsis. *Blood,* **80(1),** 96–101.

67 Cairo, M., Suen, Y., Knoppel, E., Dana, R., Park, L., Clark, S., *et al.* (1992). Decreased G-CSF and IL-3 production and gene expression from mononuclear cells of newborn infants. *Pediatr. Res.,* **31(6),** 574–8.

68 Gillan, E., Christensen, R., Kuenn, K., Hunter, D., van de Ven, C., and Cairo, M. (1992). A phase I (biological dose response) study of rh G-CSF in newborns with presumed sepsis: Significant induction of peripheral neutrophilia. *Clin. Res.,* **40,** 5A.

2 Neutrophil receptors and modulation of the immune response

C. ROSALES and E. J. BROWN

1 Clinical case: leukocytoclastic vasculitis

A 30-year-old white male with no previous medical illness began to experience pain in his abdomen which was associated with anorexia and was unrelieved by antacids. One week later he developed myalgias involving his upper and lower extremities, and 3 days thereafter he developed low grade fever. Laboratory examination showed a white blood cell count of 15 000 with 87 per cent neutrophils and normal amylase, lipase, CPK, urine analysis, and liver functions. Abdominal CT revealed markedly thickened walls of small bowel, with possible haemorrhage into the bowel wall, and an oedematous mesentery. One week later, a petechial symmetrical rash was noted around his ankles and soles. The erythrocyte sedimentation rate was 30 mm/min and the CPK had risen to 350 U/l. Approximately 3 weeks into his illness, the patient developed gastrointestinal (GI) bleeding. At that time physical examination also revealed prepatellar, olecranon, and Achilles' tendon warmth, swelling, and tenderness. Palpable purpura was present on feet, legs, groins, and buttocks. Skin biopsy showed inflammation of the blood vessel walls with intense accumulation of polymorphonuclear leukocytes (PMN), oedema, and fibrinoid necrosis (leukocytoclastic vasculitis). Immunofluorescence showed perivascular immunoglobulin deposition. Repeat urine analysis remained normal. The patient was treated with high doses of glucocorticoids, with improvement.

This illustrates the close link of PMN with the process of inflammation, in this case as an autoimmune phenomenon. PMN can become activated by a variety of inflammatory stimuli and can also release a number of substances which augment the inflammatory response. In this chapter we focus on recent advances in understanding the PMN receptors involved in activation at sites of inflammation and the effects of activation on chemotactic, phagocytic, and metabolic activities of PMN. Readers are directed to Chapter 3 for a more complete description of the signal transduction processes involved in PMN activation.

2   Introduction

The immune response is a host-protection mechanism which is engaged when the body encounters an antigen recognized as foreign. The subsequent events involve a highly regulated and co-ordinated response of several cell types. Traditionally, the most important cells in immune reactions have been thought to be the lymphocytes, since these cells are responsible for the specificity of the immune response. However, it is clear that lymphocyte function is modulated by the products of many cells, including other lymphocytes and macrophages. The details of the interactions among lymphocytes and macrophages have been the subject of several recent reviews (1–4). Importantly, lymphocytes are inefficient at removing the infectious or inflammatory agents which elicit the immune response, and other cells are needed to eradicate micro-organisms. Neutrophils (PMN) play a prominent role in these effector functions. They are important in phagocytosis and destruction of the invading pathogens and in elicitation and maintenance of the inflammatory state. Interestingly, many of the mediators of inflammation in neutrophils exist presynthesized and stored in secretory granules which are released only upon PMN activation at sites of inflammation. In recent years it has become increasingly clear that PMN are also more capable of protein synthesis than previously thought and can contribute significantly to immune reactions by *de novo* protein synthesis as well.

It is our purpose in this review to survey new developments in the understanding of neutrophils as effectors of the immune response. We will concentrate on two areas in which the advance of knowledge has been particularly rapid: the molecular mechanisms of regulation of neutrophil adhesion at sites of inflammation and the structure and function of IgG Fc receptors.

3   Interaction with endothelial cells

Near sites of inflammation PMN undergo a series of morphologic changes associated with adhesion to the endothelium. These include assuming a spherical shape and rolling along the blood vessel walls, cessation of movement and flattening, membrane ruffling, and modulation of membrane receptors. The PMN then migrate through endothelial cell junctions apparently without disrupting the electrical resistance of the endothelial monolayer and travel to the actual inflammatory site by amoeboid movements still under the influence of chemoattractants. Many recent studies have concentrated on the molecules that mediate the selective adhesion of leukocytes at the sites of inflammation, describing several receptors and their ligands. This has led to a clearer picture of the ways PMN and other blood cells are directed to the inflamed areas.

The three types of leukocytes—neutrophils, monocytes, and lymphocytes—migrate to inflamed areas in an orderly fashion. PMN, the most abundant white blood cells, are recruited within minutes of an inflammatory stimulus. Monocytes and lymphocytes arrive within hours, and depending on the severity of the infection or damage, new mononuclear cells may be recruited for days. Later, if the offending stimulus cannot be cleared, granulomas or chronic inflammatory reactions are formed with the presence of many macrophages, lymphocytes and plasma cells. One of the major advances in understanding this orderly local appearance of inflammatory cells has been the unravelling of the active role of the local endothelium in interactions with the circulating leukocytes both for their initial adhesion and for their exit from the circulation to sites of inflammation or infection.

Resting post-capillary venule endothelium generally has little capacity to recognize circulating leukocytes. However, stimulation of the endothelium with a variety of inflammatory agents such as lipopolysaccharide (LPS), tumour necrosis factor-α (TNFα), IL-1, or with proteases of the clotting cascade such as thrombin, can induce expression of endothelial surface molecules which specifically enhance interaction with circulating leukocytes. Current data suggest that the orderly, regulated appearance of these molecules on the endothelial plasma membrane accounts for much of the kinetics of the extravascular inflammatory events. Adhesion molecules which mediate binding of PMN appear on the endothelium after an inflammatory stimulus before molecules specific for monocyte or lymphocyte adhesion, perhaps acounting for the earlier ingress of neutrophils than mononuclear cells.

Molecules currently known to be involved in leukocyte–endothelium interactions belong to three structural groups: the immunoglobulin (Ig) gene superfamily, the integrin family, and the selectins family (5).

3.1   The Ig family

The Ig family contains many molecules involved in adhesion and transmembrane signalling in leukocytes. They all contain at least one Ig domain, consisting of 70–110 amino acids with a disulphide bridge spanning 50–70 residues that folds the domain in the typical tertiary structure present in antibodies (6). Intercellular adhesion molecule-1 (ICAM-1), ICAM-2, and vascular cell adhesion molecule-1 (VCAM-1) belong to this family and are expressed on endothelial cells. ICAM-1 and VCAM-1 are expressed minimally on resting endothelium; in contrast ICAM-2 seems to be constitutively present. All these Ig family members bind to ligands on leukocytes to mediate adhesion and migration, as discussed later in this chapter.

3.2   Integrins

Counter-receptors for ICAMs and VCAM-1 belong to the growing integrin family (7, 8). Members of this family mediate cell to cell and cell to extracellular matrix interactions. Integrins are plasma membrane receptors composed of two gene products, termed α and β chains, which are linked in a noncovalent but very stable structure (heterodimers). Both chains are required for normal receptor expression and for ligand binding. Currently, more than 10 α chains are known and at least eight β chains have been characterized (9) (Fig. 2.1). Most β chains have the ability to combine with more than one α chain, to make a variety of heterodimers with varying function. This is also true for some α chains. These various combinations of

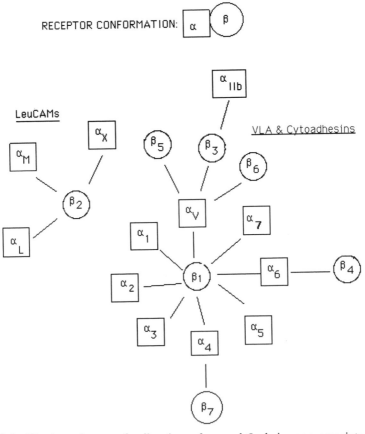

Fig. 2.1 The integrin superfamily. Any of several β chains can associate with a specific α chain to generate a great diversity of heterodimer integrin receptors with different specificities. β_4 to β_7 chains are not known to be expressed on neutrophils.

α and β increase the diversity of integrin receptors, which in turn increases the number of ligands which can be recognized and the number of functions performed by receptors in this superfamily. Classification of the integrins is in some flux, but a common way to subgroup this diverse family is by β chain. Thus, integrins which use the gene product β_1 are known as the VLA (very late activation antigen) family; integrins which use β_2 are known as LeuCAMs (leukocyte cell adhesion molecule); and integrins which use β_3 are known as cytoadhesins. Indeed, it is clear that the limits of the size of the integrin receptor family have not been defined, since there are integrin receptors including one on PMN whose sequence has not been defined (10). Cytoadhesins (the β_3 family) are expressed only at low levels on leukocytes (7, 9, 11) so most studies on leukocytes have concentrated on β_1 and β_2 integrin families.

3.2.1   The VLA family on PMN

Whether or not PMN express VLA integrins has been controversial. Initial reports suggested that they did not (8). However, more recent reports have demonstrated the presence of VLA-6 on PMN and its importance in neutrophil adhesion to laminin (12, 13). Our own data (unpublished) suggest that PMN may also express very low levels of α_3 and α_4. No systematic survey of β_1 expression on PMN has been published. In any case, receptors of this family are expressed at very low levels on PMN. This does not preclude the possibility of their importance in PMN activation in response to inflammation.

3.2.2   LeuCAMs

The most predominant integrins in all leukocytes, including PMN, are in the β_2 (LeuCAM) family. Interestingly, the expression of this family is limited to white blood cells. There are three β_2 integrins: lymphocyte function-associated antigen-1 (LFA-1/designated as CD11a–CD18), MAC-1 (CD11b–CD18) and glycoprotein (gp) 150,95 (CD11c–CD18) (Table 2.1). Each has a unique α chain in combination with β_2 (CD18). Many excellent reviews of LeuCAM structure and function have been published (5, 14, 15). LFA-1 binds specifically to the intercellular adhesion molecules ICAM-1 and ICAM-2 expressed on many different cell types. MAC-1, which also binds ICAM-1 (16) is sometimes referred to as the complement receptor 3 (CR_3) because it binds to the iC3b product of activated complement. The gp150,95 is sometimes called the complement receptor 4 because it may also bind iC3b (17). In contrast to LFA-1 and MAC-1, cellular ligand(s) for gp150,95 are as yet unknown. The importance of the β_2 integrins in PMN function is demonstrated by the congenital leukocyte adhesion deficiency (LAD) syndrome (see Chapter 6). In LAD, white blood cells do not express normal amounts of β_2 integrins due to mutations in the common β_2 chain. Patients have recurring infections and

Table 2.1 The β_2 integrin family

	LFA-1			MAC-1			gp150,95		
Glycoprotein designation	LFA-1			MAC-1			gp150,95		
Heterodimer structure	α_L	β		α_M	β		α_X	β	
Molecular weight (kDa)	180	95		170	95		150	95	
CD designation	CD11a	CD18		CD11b	CD18		CD11c	CD18	
Cell distribution	Granulocytes			Granulocytes			Granulocytes		
	Monocytes			Monocytes			Monocytes		
	Activated macrophages			Macrophages			Macrophages		
	Lymphocytes			NK cells			Activated lymphocytes		
	NK cells						Hairy cell leukaemia		
							Natural killer cells		
Function	Adhesion			Adhesion			Adhesion		
				iC3b receptor (CR3)			iC3b binding		

can be identified in infancy because of elevated levels of circulating PMN and failure to involute the umbilical stump. Neutrophils from these patients fail to respond normally to chemoattractants and are unable to bind and cross the endothelium at sites of infection (15, 18).

3.3   Selectins and ligands

The selectin family includes molecules with an interesting array of structural motifs found in other adhesive molecules (5, 19) (Fig. 2.2). They present in their amino-terminal segments a domain that resembles the carbohydrate-binding domain of calcium-dependent animal lectins. Very recently, sugar determinants on leukocytes have been identified as the ligands for some of these receptors (20, 21). This lectin-like domain is followed by a domain with homology to epidermal growth factor (EGF) and then by several cysteine-rich globular domains homologous to the short consensus repeats characteristic of complement regulatory proteins. Three members of this family have been characterized. Several names have been given to the same molecule by independent groups studying them (Table 2.2). A new nomenclature has recently been proposed for these adhesion molecules (22). We will describe them using their new names to

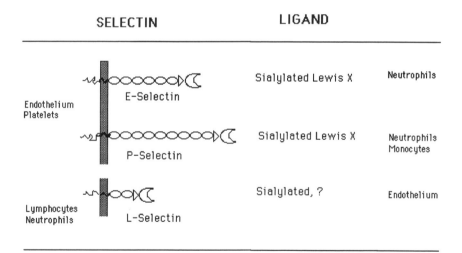

Fig. 2.2   Structure and ligand specificities of the selectins.

Table 2.2 The selectin family

Receptor nomenclature		Cell distribution
Selectin	Other names	
L-selectin	Lymphocyte homing receptor, gp90Mel, Mel-14, LAM-1, LECCAM-1	Lymphocytes Neutrophils
P-selectin	CD62, GMP-140, PADGEM	Endothelial cells
E-selectin	ELAM-1	Endothelial cells Platelets

avoid redundancy and confusion. L-selectin (previously the lymphocyte homing receptor, gp90Mel, Mel-14, LAM-1, LECCAM-1) is found on leukocytes and it is required for lymphocyte binding to endothelium in the peripheral lymph nodes, during lymphocyte recirculation, and also for neutrophil emigration at inflammatory sites. P-selectin (CD62) (previously GMP-140 or PADGEM) is a glycoprotein associated with α granules of platelets and Weibel–Palade bodies of endothelial cells. Its expression is upregulated at the cell surface by thrombin, histamine, and peroxides (23–25). The P-selectin then binds its ligand on circulating leukocytes to enable an early step in leukocyte adhesion to endothelium at sites of inflammation. E-selectin (ELAM-1) is a glycoprotein synthesized by endothelial cells in response to cytokines such as IL-1 and TNF. E-selectin also recognizes a carbohydrate ligand on PMN and possibly other leukocytes and is thought to be important in PMN–endothelial interactions during tissue immune responses. Recent data have implicated this molecule in the homing of T lymphocytes to skin (26). Thus all selectins described so far are thought to mediate adhesion of leukocytes to endothelium during inflammation (5) (Fig. 2.3).

Identification of the cellular ligands for selectins is an area of great interest and active research. The presence of the lectin-like domain in these adhesion receptors has pointed to carbohydrates as the logical candidates for their ligands. Early reports indicated that polysaccharides rich in fucose sulphate or mannose phosphate interfered with binding of lymphocytes to endothelial cells, during their homing to lymph nodes (27). Since the ligand for P-selectin is known to be present on PMN and monocytes, it was first identified by screening anti-leukocyte antibodies for their ability to prevent binding to P-selectin. Only anti CD15 antibodies (which recognize the Lewis × (Le^x) blood group) were inhibitory (28). The same antibodies also inhibited binding of P-selectin to monocytes, the monocytic cell line U937, and COS cells (monkey cells transformed with SV40 viral DNA that produces viral T antigens but lacks an origin of replication)

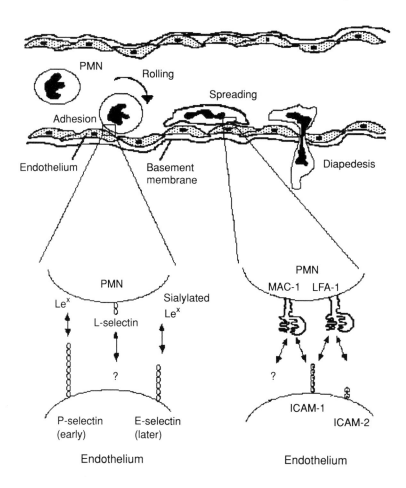

Fig. 2.3 Molecular interactions during neutrophil adhesion to endothelium at sites of inflammation. The bottom half of the figure is an exploded view of the PMN–endothelial cell interface within the rectangle.

transfected with P-selectin cDNA (29). This suggests that Le^x may be an important cell ligand for P-selectin; but these data have not been clearly confirmed (30). Other experiments have indicated that PMN binding to P-selectin is neuraminidase sensitive, suggesting that sialic acid is a component of the carbohydrate ligand. A very recent report suggest that sulphatides, heterogeneous 3-sulphated galactosyl ceramides are also ligands for P-selectin (31). A series of reports have identified sialylated Le^x as part of the ligand for E-selectin (32–34). This has raised the possibility that sialylated Le^x may also be a ligand for both P-selectin and E-selectin. Especially convincing evidence for assigning sialylated Le^x as a ligand for E-selectin came from transfection of α fucosyltransferase (which is responsible for the generation of the Le$^{\times}$ antigen) that resulted in expression of an E-selectin ligand (35, 36). Although the homing receptor, L-selectin was the first selectin reported to recognize carbohydrates (27) its actual ligand remains unknown (Fig. 2.2).

3.4   Molecular interactions between neutrophils and endothelium

PMN are the first phagocytes to arrive at inflamed tissues. How do PMN 'know' that homeostasis is disturbed and that they need to leave the circulation at a particular site? The answer involves recognition of specific endothelial surface molecules expressed near the inflammatory stimulus. Two basic mechanisms activated during inflammation seem to be involved in directing PMN into tissues at sites of inflammation (37). One is immediate and does not require protein synthesis. It involves transient increased adhesiveness of both PMN and endothelium. The other is activated later (1–2 h after inflammation begins) and requires synthesis and expression of new endothelial proteins that promote binding of both activated and resting PMN.

When PMN are exposed to chemoattractants and other active substances including PMA, LPS, and TNF, they very rapidly become much more adhesive for endothelium whether or not the endothelium is stimulated. This interaction seems to be mediated by activation of the β_2 integrins LFA-1 and MAC-1, since it can be blocked by mAb against these LeuCAMs (38, 39). Unstimulated endothelium expresses ICAM-2 but little or no ICAM-1 (CD54). Since LFA-1 can bind both these ligands, ICAM-2 is clearly an important component of PMN–endothelium interaction in this situation. However, MAC-1 does not bind ICAM-2, but apparently is involved in PMN adhesion to unstimulated endothelium (16). In this case, its ligand is unknown. Interestingly this β_2-dependent adhesion results from a qualitative change in integrin avidity during PMN activation and does not require the increase in cell-surface integrin expression which also accompanies activation (40). The molecular nature of the change which leads to increased β_2 integrin avidity is unknown. β_2 phosphorylation has been proposed (41), but at least for LFA-1 definitively disproven (42). Recent experiments have implicated a short peptide sequence in the β_2 cytoplasmic domain, KSATTTV, as essential for avidity regulation (42).

A second model for rapid upregulation of adhesion of PMN to endothelium has been explored by Zimmerman and McEver (24, 43). In this model, thrombin or histamine stimulation of endothelium causes rapid PMN adhesion which is independent of new protein synthesis. Rapid PMN binding to endothelium is mediated by P-selectin, since mAb (43) and soluble P-selectin (44) prevent this adhesion. Unlike integrin-dependent adhesion to ICAMs, PMN binding to P-selectin does not require PMN activation, but is dependent on extracellular Ca^{2+} (43). Even formaldehyde-fixed PMN will adhere in this model. Presumably rapid mobilization of P-selectin to endothelial cell plasma membrane allows it to recognize its carbohydrate ligand on PMN. Recent intriguing data in this model have suggested that thrombin or histamine activation of the endothelium causes release of the lipid mediator platelet-activating factor in addition to secretion of P-selectin. Platelet-activating factor in turn activates the β_2 integrins of the adherent PMN. This activation of β_2 integrins leads to a second phase of enhanced adhesion between PMN and endothelium (45). Thus the adhesive event may be seen as a temporal series of molecular interactions requiring the active participation of both cell types. This model is currently in great favour.

After exposure of endothelium to immune modulators such as INFγ, TNF, or LPS for 4 to 24 h, PMN adhesion is promoted by molecules such as ICAM-1 and E-selectin whose synthesis is induced on endothelial cells. ICAM is induced by INFγ, IL-1, and TNF, and binds to the integrins LFA-1 and MAC-1. Recent work from several laboratories has suggested that LFA-1 binds to sites in the two most amino-terminal Ig domains of ICAM-1 (16, 46, 47). This is consistent with the observation that these two domains are more homologous to ICAM-2, another LFA-1 ligand, than are the other Ig domains of ICAM-1. Interestingly, MAC-1 binds to the third Ig domain of ICAM-1 at a site quite distant from the LFA-1-binding site. Since this domain is not very homologous to ICAM-2, this difference from LFA-1 would explain why MAC-1 does not bind ICAM-2. Furthermore, the existence of distinct binding sites for LFA-1 and MAC-1 on ICAM-1 suggests the interesting possibility that these two integrins on the PMN may recognize the same ICAM-1 molecule.

E-selectin expression goes up more than 100-fold after the endothelium is exposed to TNF and IL-1 but not IFNγ. E-selectin expression peaks earlier (~4 h after IL-1) than ICAM-1 (24 h). Both E-selectin and ICAM-1 seem to be required for migration of PMN across the endothelium (48). It has been hypothesized that these adhesion molecules act sequentially on PMN, since interaction of PMN with E-selectin-bearing endothelial cells activates MAC-1-dependent adhesion by PMN to endothelium (49).

These studies demonstrate the involvement of several adhesion molecules in the binding between PMN and endothelial cells. However, they do not reflect the kinetics of the interactions, since they have been performed under static conditions. Recently, some studies have tried to address kinetics and the effects of shear forces by examining adhesion of PMN to endothelium under flow conditions. Lawrence *et al.* measured CD18-dependent and CD18-independent adhesion of PMN to IL-1-treated endothelium at different shear stresses to mimic venous flow conditions (50). They reported that CD18-independent adhesion resists greater shear forces than CD18-dependent adhesion does, suggesting that a selectin first traps the circulating PMN and then delivers it to ICAM-1 and ICAM-2, resulting in CD18-dependent migration across the endothelium (50). More recently, they showed that PMN roll on a lipid surface containing P-selectin at physiological flow rates. When the surface included ICAM-1, resting or activated PMN did not bind at physiological shear stresses. However, on lipid bilayers containing both P-selectin and ICAM-1, the addition of chemoattractants to activate the CD18 integrins resulted in the arrest of PMN rolling (51). This result mimics *in vitro* the events observed for leukocyte accumulation at inflammation sites *in vivo*, supporting the following model for binding: in the absence of an inflammatory signal, PMN are carried along in the blood at a velocity determined by fluid dynamic considerations. Upon recognition of endothelium at an inflamed site, selectin–carbohydrate interactions lead to PMN adhesion to endothelium. This adhesion results not in spreading and flattening at a single site, but 'rolling' at a much reduced velocity compared with the rate of blood flow. Finally, activation of PMN integrins causes interaction with endothelium ICAMs, resulting in stronger adhesion that stops PMN movement along the endothelium. Smith *et al.* found that under flow conditions CD18-dependent adhesion of PMN to IL-1-stimulated umbilical vein endothelial cell monolayers was minimal, but anti-L-selectin antibodies inhibited adhesion by more than 50 per cent. In contrast migration across the cell monolayer was completely inhibited by anti-CD18 antibodies (52, 53). Since L-selectin is lost from the PMN surface at the same time that β_2 integrins are activated after chemoattractant stimulation (54), these results reinforce the model that PMN interact with endothelial cells first through selectins and then through engagement of CD18-dependent mechanisms that lead to trans-endothelial migration (Fig. 2.3).

As indicated above ICAM-1 promotes strong adhesion of PMN *in vitro*, but P-selectin is the relevant molecule for attachment under conditions of flow. Lawrence and Springer suggest an interesting hypothesis to explain the differences in adherence properties of P-selectin and ICAM-1. They suggest that rapid reaction rates rather than affinity constants determine which molecules are responsible for the initial interactions between neutrophils and endothelium. The authors hypothesize that the selectin works because the rate of reaction with its sugar ligand is faster than the rates involving proteins (51, 55). Supporting these ideas is a report in a completely different system by Foote and Milstein suggesting that antibodies can be selected in a secondary antibody response because they show rapid binding kinetics (56). Leukosialin (CD43), an interesting molecule present at high levels on neutrophils, may be relevant in these interactions. This rod-like molecule protrudes about 45 nm from the plasma membrane and presents about 70 O-linked carbohydrate structures. It is possible that P-selectin may react with leukosialin or another similar (sialyl) Le^x-bearing structure on PMN, and that the high concentration of sugar residues on this molecule is responsible for the rapid reaction rates that are proposed as relevant in the initial steps of cell–cell adhesion (55).

Another important molecule that plays a role in cell adhesion events is CD44 (also known as Pgp-1, Ly-24, Hermes). This is an acidic sulphated membrane glycoprotein that varies in molecular weight from 80 to 200 kDa depending on the degree of glycosylation and contents of chondroitin sulphate (57). CD44 is present in a wide number of cells including T cells, B cells, macrophages, neural cells, epithelial cells, and fibroblasts. cDNAs of CD44 have been cloned (58, 59). The amino-terminal portion of CD44 has homology to the cartilage link proteins which mediate adhesion to collagen and other extracellular matrix proteins. CD44 can bind to hyaluronate, collagen, and fibronectin (60). In some cells it has been shown to associate with the cytoskeleton, which suggests that it may play a role in interactions with the extracellular matrix proteins similar to the ones from integrins. CD44 has a role in lymphocyte homing to lymph nodes. Lymphocyte binding to high endothelial venule epithelium is blocked by anti-CD44 antibodies. It has also been shown to have activation effects on B and T cells (61–63). In humans, memory T cells seem to express higher levels of CD44 than naive cells. Since the presence of CD44 has not clearly been shown on PMN, its role in neutrophil adhesive events remains speculative.

4   Antibody receptors

Antibodies produced as an immune response against invading microorganisms are another important defence mechanism of inflammation. They form immune complexes when they bind to specific microbial antigens and play a major role as opsonins and activators of other effector functions. Immunoglobulins (Ig) are formed by two heavy and two light chains. The amino-terminal portions of one heavy and one light chain generate the antigen-binding sites (two per molecule of IgG) of the antibody. The carboxy-terminal domains of the heavy chains constitute the Fc portion of the molecule that is responsible for initiating several cellular responses through the interaction with specific receptors called Fc receptors (FcR). Fc receptors for all the Ig classes and subclasses of IgG have been found. Thus the great variety of responses mediated by different antibody classes depends, in part, on their interactions with particular FcR on different cell types. Among the best studied FcR are those that bind IgG. FcR for IgG are found on all types of leukocytes and mediate important functions such as clearance of immune complexes (64, 65), generation of the respiratory burst (66), secretion of inflammatory mediators (67), antibody-dependent cell-mediated cytotoxicity (68, 69), and phagocytosis (66, 70). Human phagocytic cells bear at least three distinct types of FcR. They are all members of the Ig gene superfamily, but can be distinguished by size, affinity for ligand, mAb reactivity, and primary sequence (71). In recent years tremendous progress has been made in determining the structure and gene organization of the genes encoding these receptors, which all map to the long arm of chromosome 1 [for review see (72, 73)]. The main characteristics (Table 2.3) of these receptors are described next, using a recently proposed nomenclature (72).

4.1   Structure of Fcγ receptors

FcγRI (CD64) is a 72 kDa glycoprotein with a high avidity for monomeric IgG. It is found mainly on monocytes and macrophages. This receptor contains three Ig domains in its extracytoplasmic portion (Fig. 2.4), and a short charged cytoplasmic tail (73). Treatment with INFγ upregulates its expression on neutrophils and HL-60 cells (74).

FcγRII (CD32), is not a single receptor, but a family of closely related 40 kDa transmembrane glycoproteins with low avidity for monomeric IgG. However, all FcγRII avidly bind IgG aggregates and are apparently important in immune complex clearance *in vivo*. One or other of these receptors are found on monocytes, macrophages, PMN, B cells, and platelets. At least six isoforms (hFcγRIIa1, -a2, hFcγRIIb1, -b2, -b3, and hFcγRIIc) which are encoded by three different genes (hFcγRIIA, -B, and -C) have been identified (75, 76). Note that the genes for FcR have uppercase letters and their protein products are designated with lower-case letters. Comparison of the isolated cDNAs that code for the hFcγRII gene products shows that the distinct forms of this receptor have very similar extracytoplasmic regions with two domains which are structurally homologous to immunoglobulin. Comparison between the members of this family shows more than 90 per cent amino acid homology. The only functionally significant differences in the extracytoplasmic domains of this family result from two alleles of human (h)FcγRII which differ in their ability to support T cell proliferation induced by murine IgG1 antibodies. Monocytes from 70 per cent of the donors supported T cell proliferation, while the rest did not (77). The cause of this HR (high responder)/LR (low responder) polymorphism was identified as being due to a difference of one or two amino acids in hFcγRII (78, 79). In general, mAb which recognize the extracytoplasmic domains of FcγRIIs do not distinguish among members of the family. Interestingly, the cytoplasmic tails predicted by the various FcγRII cDNAs differ considerably from one another. The functional significances of these differences are not well understood at present. The best data have been obtained by comparing murine (m) FcγRIIb1 and -b2 which differ because mFcγRIIb1 has a 47 amino acid insert in the cytoplasmic domain, which is generated by alternative splicing during processing

Table 2.3 IgG Fc receptors

Receptor	CD designation	Binding[a]	Cells	Genes[b]	Protein kDa
FcγRI	CD64	IgG1, G3	Macrophage, monocytes	1	72
FcγRII	CD32	IgG1, G3 > G2, G4	Monocytes, PMN, macrophages, platelets, B cells	3	40
FcγRIII	CD16	IgG1, G3 > G2, G4	Macrophages, PMN, NK cells, T cells	2	50–80

[a] Indicates the preferential binding of FcR to the IgG subclasses.
[b] Represents the number of genes encoding the receptor. These are called FcγRIIA, B, and C, and FcγRIIIA and FcγRIIIB (see Section 4.1 for explanation).

Human

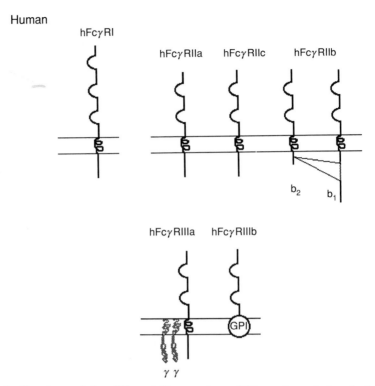

Fig.2.4 Structure of the different Fc receptors. GPI = glycosyl-phosphatidyl-inositol.

of the FcγRIIB gene transcript. mFcγRIIb1 is expressed in lymphocytes and mFcγRIIb2 in macrophages. The inserted domain of mFcγRIIb1 mediates receptor attachment to the cytoskeleton and inhibits localization to clathrin-coated pits (80). Quite recently, portions of the hFcγRIIa and mFcγRIIb2 cytoplasmic tails required for phagocytosis, endocytosis, and release of intracellular Ca^{+2} were defined (81, 82). Now that the extent of the FcγRII family is known, work in the next few years should determine which receptors are responsible for each of the pleotropic effects of IgG binding to the FcγRII family on leukocytes.

FcγRIII (CD16) is found on macrophages, NK cells, and PMN. It is a glycoprotein that runs as a broad band between 50–80 kDa on SDS–PAGE gels. It is a receptor with low affinity for monomeric IgG that preferentially binds immune complexes. FcγRIII has also been implicated in clearance of circulating immune complexes. Two very homologous genes (hFcγRIIIA and -B) have been found for this receptor and cDNAs cloned. FcγRIIIA and -B are closely linked and are expressed specifically in different cell lineages. FcγRIIIB codes for the receptor found on PMN, while FcγRIIIA encodes the receptor found on NK cells and macrophages.

Both products have two Ig domains in their extracytoplasmic portion. The main difference between these two forms of FcγRIII is that the receptor on PMN is attached to the plasma membrane via a glycosyl-phosphatidylinositol (GPI) linkage, while the one on macrophages and NK cells has a typical hydrophobic transmembrane domain and a cytoplasmic tail (83, 84). The two genes are very homologous, but show a critical difference in amino acid 203. FcγRIIIB codes for a serine in this position leading to attachment of a GPI anchor, whereas FcγRIIIA codes for a phenylalanine that determines the retention of the transmembrane and cytoplasmic domains (85, 86). Furthermore, the PMN FcγRIII shows allogenic polymorphism, known as the NA system. The allotypes NA1 and NA2 were defined serologically and the responsible amino acid differences identified (87, 88); it is clear now that only FcγRIIIB encodes these allotypes. The transmembrane form of FcγRIII is expressed in macrophages in association with the γ chain of the high-affinity IgE FcR (89). In NK cells the ζ chain, which is part of the CD3 T cell receptor complex in lymphocytes, is also associated with FcγRIII (90, 91). The possibility that these subunits of the FcR complex might be very important in the signalling mechanisms from distinct receptors is suggested by the finding that the γ chain of Fc receptors is also associated in heterodimers with the ζ chain of the T cell receptor complex in T cells that do not express FcR (92). Besides the FcγRIII present on the surface of cells, a soluble form of the receptor has been detected in serum and appears to be derived from PMN (93). This complex system of IgG FcR is largely reproduced in the murine immune system which is the only other species studied in detail at this point (72, 94, 95).

4.2   FcγR functions

A plethora of biological functions are mediated by interaction of IgG with these FcγR, including removal of immune complexes, activation of the respiratory burst, ADCC, phagocytosis, and release of inflammatory mediators. A great deal about the structure and gene organization of this family of receptors is known, but the functions mediated by each particular type of FcγR are largely unknown. With the use of specific mAb and FcR cDNA transfection studies, elucidation of the roles of individual FcγR is beginning.

4.2.1   Respiratory burst

The three types of FcγR with transmembrane anchors have been shown in different settings to be able to trigger the respiratory burst (96–100). In the case of hFcγRIIIb published reports have been conflicting (98, 99). Differences in the experimental systems, especially the use of different mAb may explain these contradictory results. Details of the activation pathway of the respiratory burst are found in Chapter 3.

4.2.2   Antibody-dependent cell-mediated cytotoxicity (ADCC)

ADCC is another function that has been shown to be mediated by the three main types of transmembrane hFcγR by studies using heteroconjugated antibodies and erythrocytes as targets and by studies with anti-hFcγR mAb-producing hybridomas as targets (10). The hFcγRIIIb on PMN is unable to mediate ADCC (83, 101); however, the transmembrane FcγRIII on NK cells efficiently triggers ADCC (102). Also, it seems that FcγRII is not capable of activating the cytolytic apparatus of the neutrophil (71), but interestingly, treatment of monocytes with INFγ causes increased killing of hybridoma cells via both FcγRI and FcγRII (101). Whether this difference in FcγRII function on various cells reflects different cytoplasmic domains is not known.

4.2.3   Inflammatory mediators

Ligation of FcγR also causes the release of several inflammatory mediators such as leukotrienes, prostaglandins, proteolytic and glycolytic enzymes, IL-1, INFγ, and TNFα from different cell types. The particular type(s) of FcγR mediating each of these responses is unknown, but several studies have been initiated to try and answer this problem. On PMN, both hFcγRII and hFcγRIIIb (GPI-linked) could induce the release of lysosomal enzymes (98). In monocytes hFcγRI ligation is reported to cause release of both TNFα (103) and IL-6 (104), while hFcγRII ligation may be able to induce release of TNFα (103).

4.2.4   Phagocytosis

Phagocytosis is one of the most important functions mediated by FcγR. Studies have been performed to elucidate which type of receptor initiates the ingestion process in various cell types. Anderson *et al.*, using bifunctional antibodies formed by $F(ab')_2$ fragments of anti-erythrocyte IgG linked to $F(ab');_2$ fragments of anti-FcγR mAb, reported that both binding to either hFcγRI or hFcγRII leads to phagocytosis of erythrocytes (105). This study also found that hFcγRIIIa in NK cells could mediate phagocytosis, but that the GPI-linked hFcγRIIIb on PMN was not functional. In contrast to this report, experiments by Salmon *et al.* indicated that phagocytosis of E-ConA and E-IgG occurred via hFcγRIIIb (106, 107). The experimental systems are very different, and some of the phagocytosis seen in PMN in the latter studies may be due to residual FcγRII since the anti-FcγRII mAb IV.3 used to block this receptor on PMN can be dissociated from its ligand by larger immune complexes (76, 108). Our own results indicate that PMN that have been treated with phosphatidylinositol-specific phospholipase C to remove more than 80 per cent of the GPI-linked hFcγRIIIb are able to phagocytose IgG-coated erythrocytes as efficiently as normal PMN expressing both FcγRII and FcγRIII (109). COS-1 cells transfected with

either FcγRI and FcγRII can bind and phagocytose IgG-coated erythrocytes in the absence of any other FcγR (110, 111). The possibility of
receptor co-operativity in phagocytosis has been supported by the observation that ligation of hFcγRIIIb induces actin polymerization in PMN and in
this way 'primes' phagocytosis by hFcγRII (112). Probably the most clear
example of different functions mediated by independent FcγR comes from
the finding that differences in the cytoplasmic tails of murine mFcγRII
isoforms lead to markedly different phagocytic responses. FcγRIIb1 mediates phagocytosis of immune complexes (80) and B cell activation (113),
while FcγRIIb2 mediates endocytosis of immune complexes via clathrin-
coated pits to deliver them into lysosomes (80). In the human system there
are no equivalent data; the existence of even more isoforms than in the
mouse suggests that differences in the responses mediated by each type of
FcγR may be that much more complicated.

Interestingly, two groups have recently reported individuals who lacked
expression of hFcγRIIIb. One described a patient with systemic lupus
erythematosus (114) and the other two healthy individuals (115). In both
cases the defect seems to be due to a defective or completely absent
hFcγRIIIB gene. The fact that the individuals in the second study were
healthy with no signs of abnormal circulating immune complexes or increased susceptibility to infections suggests that *in vivo* FcγRIIIb may not
be essential. This is most probably because at least some functions of the
various IgG FcR overlap or are actually redundant. Further pathophysiologic
correlations regarding phagocytosis are found in Chapter 4.

4.3   Signal transduction

Much has been learned about the signal transduction mechanism from
'chemoattractant' receptors in stimulated phagocytes, described in greater
detail in Chapter 3. Understanding the molecular events which occur after
ligation of IgG Fc receptors has lagged behind, at least in part because of
the complexity of the receptor system and the wide variety of effector
mechanisms engaged upon FcR ligation. With the advent of cloned cDNAs
for various FcR, a lot of information about signal transduction will be
forthcoming in the next few years.

4.3.1   Calcium

Ligation of FcγRI (116), FcγRII (116, 117), FcγRIIIa (118), and FcγRIIIb
(109, 119) mediates a cytosolic calcium increase that primarily comes from
release of calcium from intracellular stores. The rise in cytosolic calcium
concentration ($[Ca^{2+}]_i$) is greatest in the cytoplasm surrounding the new
phagosome (120). This has suggested that the increase in $[Ca^{2+}]_i$ generated
by ligation of the FcR is an important 'second messenger' for phagocytosis.

However, conflicting results have been reported in direct tests of this hypothesis. Mouse peritoneal macrophages (121), and the J774 macrophage-like cell line (122), were able to ingest IgG-opsonized erythrocytes even when an increase in $[Ca^{2+}]_i$ was prevented. In contrast, mouse macrophages (123) and human neutrophils (124) were not able to phagocytose when loaded with the calcium chelator quin-2 to prevent an increase in $[Ca^{2+}]_i$ after FcR ligation. Thus, the role of Ca^{2+} in phagocytosis is not yet clear. One possible reason is that both Ca^{2+}-dependent and -independent mechanisms of ingestion exist in PMN (109).

The mechanisms by which FcR engagement leads to an increase in $[Ca^{2+}]_i$ is unclear. While inositol-(1,4,5)-triphosphate (IP_3) is an intracellular ionophore commonly associated with $[Ca^{2+}]_i$ increases, Walker et al. found that in PMN stimulated by immune complexes the respiratory burst was associated with little formation of IP_3 (125). We have performed experiments directly measuring phosphoinositide turnover after stimulation of $Fc\gamma R$ on PMN with various agonists and found that in contrast to chemoattractant receptor, the $[Ca^{2+}]_i$ rise induced by $Fc\gamma R$ ligation is pertussis toxin-insensitive and completely independent of IP_3 accumulation (126). These data suggest that (i) FcR ligation on PMN does not lead to much phosphoinositide turnover (IP_3 arises from the enzymatic cleavage of phosphoinositide bisphosphate to IP_3 and diacylglycerol) and (ii) the release of Ca^{2+} from intracellular stores by FcR ligation in PMN occurs due to a novel and undescribed mechanism.

4.3.2   Guanine nucleotide-binding proteins

By analogy with the β-adrenergic and FMLP receptors it has been suggested that FcR responses may be coupled via G proteins. Pertussis toxin (PT) inactivates FMLP-induced responses in PMN, but in the same cells, it does not inhibit FcR-stimulated F-actin assembly (127), which is required for phagocytosis to take place (128). PT and cholera toxin (CT) do not affect FcR-mediated phagocytosis in PMN, but PT was found to reduce $Fc\gamma R$-mediated phagocytosis by 68 per cent in monocytes (129). In another report, the enhanced phagocytosis of IgG-coated erythrocytes by PMN stimulated with a cytokine and amphotericin B was inhibited by both PT and CT (130). Moreover, ligation of FcRII on PMN with mAb KuFc79 followed by cross-linking with a secondary $F(ab')_2$ anti-IgG caused superoxide production and degranulation. The former response was completely eliminated with PT, but the latter only by about 50 per cent (131). These reports suggest that at least under some circumstances FcR communicate with the cytoplasm via PT-sensitive G proteins.

4.3.3   Phosphorylation

Thus far, there is no evidence of direct phosphorylation of $Fc\gamma R$ on phagocytic cells. However in B cells the $mFc\gamma RIIb1$ was found to be phosphorylated itself during cell activation (113), and in mast cells the high affinity FcεR is phosphorylated when it binds IgE and dephosphorylated when it dissociates (132). Phosphorylation, probably by activated PKC, of several other proteins after FcγR ligation has been reported. In relation to phagocytosis, a comparative study of IgG- versus complement-mediated phagocytosis by macrophages detected a single protein of 48 000 kDa which was specifically phosphorylated during ingestion of IgG-coated erythrocytes (133). PKC has recently been implicated more directly in Fc-mediated phagocytosis by showing that this enzyme is translocated to phagosome membranes during ingestion of IgG-coated latex beads (134).

5   Complement receptors

The structures of complement receptors and their ligands have recently been reviewed in detail (135). Activation of complement plays an important role in initiating and amplifying inflammation. Products of activated complement cause opsonization, stimulate chemotaxis, and activate leukocytes. C3, the most abundant complement protein in serum (1.3 mg/ml) is converted to C3b, the principal opsonin by either the classic (antibody dependent) or the alternative (antibody independent) pathway. During activation C3 is cleaved into C3a and C3b fragments. A reactive thioester bond in C3b reacts with a hydroxyl group on the target to form a covalent ester bond. C3b can then be converted to iC3b by the action of the enzyme factor I (C3b inactivator). This last reaction requires a co-factor, which can be factor H in serum or the complement receptor type 1 (CR_1) on the surface of many cells. If particles coated with C3b and iC3b are not removed by phagocytosis, these opsonins are converted to C3dg by further action of factor I. C3b and also C4b, the product of C4 activation, are recognized primarily by CR_1 (Table 2.4). iC3b is recognized by three different receptors: CR_2 (CD21), present on B lymphocytes, CR_3 (CD11b–CD18) found on almost all phagocytes and some lymphocytes, and CR_4 (CD11c–CD18) or (gp150,95) on some lymphocytes and phagocytes.

Table 2.4   Complement receptors

Receptor	CD designation	Ligands	Other names
CR_1	CD35	C3b > C4b >iC3b	C3b receptor
CR_2	CD21	C3dg, iC3b > C3b	C3d receptor
			EBV receptor
CR_3	CD11b–CD18	iC3b > C3b > C3d factor X, others[a]	Mo-1, MAC-1
CR_4	CD11c–CD18	iC3b > C3b	gp150,95

[a] The existence of other ligands for CR_3 is controversial.

Interestingly CD11c expression is increased during differentiation of blood monocytes *in vivo* and *in vitro* (17, 136, 137).

5.1   Structure of complement receptors

CR_1 (CD35) binds C3b with high affinity. Native C3 and the product C3dg are not recognized by this receptor. CR_1 is a glycoprotein with a molecular weight that varies between 160 and 250 kDa. Four allelic variants that are expressed in a co-dominant fashion have been described (138). The CR_1 gene has been cloned (139, 140) and the predicted protein has a short cytoplasmic tail and a transmembrane-spanning domain of 25 residues. The extracellular portion is very large and consists of at least 30 repeated domains arranged in tandem. Each of these short consensus repeats (SCR) contains 60–70 amino acids with four conserved cysteines. The consensus sequence found in SCR is also present in several other proteins, including factor H, C4-binding protein, CR_2, factor B, C2, C1r, C1s, decay-accelerating factor (DAF), clotting factor XIIIb, IL-2 receptor, and in the selectins (141). The presence of the SCR in non-complement proteins indicates that the generic SCR must have other functions besides its capacity to bind C3/C4. Another conserved larger pattern of 450 amino acids is also observed in CR_1. Each of these long homologous repeats (LHR) contains seven SCR and are 70–99 per cent homologous to one another. It is thought that the different alleles of CR_1 are due to the expression of different numbers of LHR, so the 160 kDa receptor has four LHR, the 190 kDa five, etc. Binding sites for C3b and C4b have been identified on CR_1 (142). C4b is bound within the first two SCR of the most amino-terminal LHR (LHR-A). In contrast C3b is bound by the first two SCR within the following two LHR (LHR-B and LHR-C). Because C3b is a major opsonin, its receptor CR_1 is found on all phagocytic cells and some lymphocytes (143). Its presence on erythrocytes may aid phagocytosis and is important in clearance of circulating immune complexes.

CR_2 (CD21) is not found on phagocytic cells. It is a single chain glycoprotein with a similar structure to CR_1 comprising 16 SHR. It is the binding site for EBV and its complement ligand is C3dg or iC3b. It seems to be involved in activation of B cells, which is beyond the scope of this review.

CR_3 is the β_2 integrin MAC-1, which has been discussed in Section 3.2 in relation to its recognition of ICAM-1. As with all integrins recognition of iC3b requires the presence of divalent cations (Ca^{2+} and Mg^{2+}) for effective ligand binding.

5.2   Role of complement receptors in phagocytosis

The process of receptor-mediated ingestion involves two steps: binding and ingestion. During binding, the receptor must first interact with its ligand (opsonin) to bring the target particle in close contact with the phagocyte. For ingestion, the receptor has to deliver a signal to the cell to form pseudopods around the target particle (128). Experimental evidence exists that both binding of complement-opsonized targets and signalling by their receptors are regulated functions of phagocytes.

Resting PMN have a low capacity to bind C3b-opsonized particles, but it is rapidly upregulated by several cell activators including chemoattractants and PMA. A major effect of these compounds on phagocytes is to bring the large intracellular pool of CR_1 and CR_3 to the surface of the cell (144). The magnitude of this increase varies depending on the state of activation of the cells at the time of purification. Cell separation methods themselves cause increases in receptor expression (145), and the integrin complement receptor CR_3 can increase its ability to bind iC3b-coated particles independent of receptor number (40). TNF, IL-8, PMA, and FMLP can all increase CR_3-dependent adhesion even when upregulation of receptor number has been inhibited. In this ability, CR_3 is similar to other leukocyte integrins, which also undergo a process of affinity modulation. The molecular change which leads to this affinity modulation is unknown. Receptor phosphorylation has been proposed (41, 146), and phosphorylation of the CR_3 β chain correlates kinetically with enhancement of PMN binding to iC3b-coated particles (147). However, Hibbs *et al.* have demonstrated that receptor phosphorylation is independent of affinity modulation for the closely related integrin LFA-1 (42). This leads to some doubt about whether receptor phosphorylation explains the increased affinity of CR_3 for iC3b-coated erythrocytes upon PMN activation. Detmers *et al.* have proposed that CR_3 receptor clustering in the plasma membrane accounts for affinity modulation (148). The data in favour of this hypothesis are also only correlations of receptor clusters with function and are subject to the same criticisms as the phosphorylation data. Most recently, lipid modulation of CR_3 affinity has been proposed as a mechanism for the enhanced binding of iC3b by activated PMN (149). These data are consistent with the known interactions of lipids with integrins (150), the observation that a lipid milieu can affect integrin function (151), and with the defect in integrin functions found in essential fatty acid-deficient animals (152). An intriguing question is whether CR_1, which is not an integrin, also undergoes affinity modulation during cell activation. No data currently exist to address this question.

A second aspect of complement receptor regulation involves not only affinity modulation but phagocytic competence. C3b-coated particles will bind to resting phagocytes but will not be internalized until the receptors are turned 'competent' by activating the cell with PMA or Arg-Gly-Asp ligands (128, 153). PMA also causes a 30-fold increase in the capacity of CR_1 to promote phagocytosis (147). These results illustrate an important characteristic of complement receptor biology: the fact that activation is needed before full activity is expressed. Recent reviews of complement receptor biology (135) and the role of complement receptors in phagocytosis (154) have been published.

6   Modulation of neutrophil responses

Resting phagocytes have a reduced capacity for antimicrobial functions compared to cells at sites of inflammation. Here we present some of the inflammatory mechanisms that regulate phagocytes.

6.1   Cytokines

Many cytokines demonstrate a great multiplicity of effects on phagocyte function. Some of them like GM-CSF, INFγ, and TNF do not activate phagocytes on their own, but cause them to give enhanced responses to other stimuli, a phenomenon called 'priming'. TNFα is a cytokine secreted by monocytes and macrophages in response to LPS. It has several effects on phagocytes including increased INFγ-induced cytotoxicity (155) and killing of parasites (156), and priming of PMN for enhanced degranulation and production of oxygen products (157). Colony-stimulating factors are a group of cytokines that control production, proliferation, and differentiation of leukocytes. G-CSF enhances PMN chemotaxis to zymosan (158), GM-CSF enhances ADCC (159) and primes cells for chemotaxis and respiratory burst in response to FMLP (160). IFNγ causes upregulation of FcγRI in PMN (74, 161). PAF (1-alkyl-2(R)-acetyl-glycero-3-phospho-choline) has multiple pro-inflammatory effects. Chemical studies have shown that PAF is actually a mixture of different phospholipids whose composition varies with the stimulus and cell type that produces it (162). The several forms have different alkyl chains on position 1 of the glycerol backbone. The most abundant forms produced by human PMN contain hexadecyl or octadecyl alkyl chains (163). PAF induces many PMN responses including aggregation, superoxide anion production, degranulation, release of arachidonic acid (AA), and chemotaxis (162). Migration across the endothelium to a site of inflammation is one of the major responses of PMN to PAF. The 16-carbon, no double bond (C16:0) fatty acid is the most potent, followed in potency by the C18:0 and the C18:1 forms (164). PAF not only causes chemotaxis on its own, but also induces the release of AA which is metabolized by the 5-lipoxygenase pathway to produce LTB$_4$ (165), an even more potent stimulant of PMN aggregation and chemotaxis. Thus, PMN responses to PAF are in part mediated by autocrine production of LTB$_4$. Once phagocytes have been recruited into tissues, they need activated complement receptors for efficient phagocytosis. PAF, at nanomolar concentrations, is able to activate complement receptors for increased phagocytosis of C3b-coated erythrocytes and to stimuate the phosphorylation of CR_1 on monocytes (166). The effects of PAF are mediated by specific receptors on the plasma membrane of cells. However, more recently, a possible important role for intracellular PAF in regulation of phagocytic functions of PMN has been proposed, since the majority of newly synthesized PAF is retained intracellularly, and is localized to the phagolysosomal fraction in PMN exposed to opsonized zymosan (167).

Interleukin-1, made by monocytes and many other cell types is a potent inflammatory mediator with many effects on several cell types. In the case of phagocytes it has been shown to promote increased chemotaxis and thromboxane production by monocytes, enhanced demargination, and adhesion of PMN (168, 169), as well as priming for respiratory burst by FMLP (169). Other cytokines are able to regulate phagocyte responses mainly by regulating the expression of FcγR. IL-4 causes the downregulation of the three types of FcγR (170), while TGFβ increases FcγRIIIa on monocytes (171).

6.2   Extracellular matrix receptors

Once the PMN have left the circulation they encounter a complex array of molecules, the extracellular matrix (ECM) proteins, during emigration to the site of inflammation where phagocytosis is upregulated (66). It is not difficult to imagine that the various ECM proteins may have a significant effect on regulating PMN functions (172). When phagocytes are spread on surfaces coated with fibronectin (173, 174), serum amyloid P component (174), or laminin (175), their complement or IgG FcR are activated to achieve maximal phagocytosis.

Recent work has suggested that a member of the ECM protein group induces phagocytic activation through a single receptor which recognizes the Arg-Gly-Asp (RGD) sequence (10). Accordingly, we have characterized the RGD-binding proteins of human PMN and monocytes (176). Both types of phagocytes express a heterodimeric receptor that has immunological cross-reactivity with the integrin gpIIb/IIIa (β_3 subfamily of integrins) on platelets, and although it has structural similarity, is distinct from the LeuCAMs. Because this receptor mediated phagocytic responses to several RGD-containing proteins, we have named it the leukocyte-response integrin (LRI). Recently, we have identified the ligand specific for LRI on PMN. Peptides with the sequence KGAGDV, which is similar to the sequence KQAGDV found in the γ chain of fibrinogen, were the most potent in inhibiting LRI-dependent functions (177), suggesting that LRI is a unique integrin. After preparing polyclonal and monoclonal antibodies which inhibit RGD-dependent ligand binding, we found one mAb B6H12 that also inhibits the RGD-dependent enhancement of IgG-mediated phagocytosis by PMN (10). This mAB inhibited increased phagocytosis stimulated by fibronectin, collagen type IV, von Willebrand's factor, fibrinogen, and vitronectin, as well as by synthetic RGD-containing ligands; but did not affect laminin-enhanced ingestion. Because this antibody also immunoprecipitated a PMN receptor that in SDS–PAGE resembled the heterodimeric molecule previously purified on RGD–sepharose, we hypothesized that it recognized LRI. Our most recent work, however, indicates that this antibody does not recognize an integrin but a 50 kDa protein that is functionally and perhaps physically associated with LRI (178). This protein is widely expressed on cells, including erythrocytes, which do not have integrins. Using immunoprecipitation and affinity chromatography with B6H12, this 50 kDa protein was found associated with an integrin in platelets and placenta but not in red blood cells (178). Since this protein modulates LRI function in intact cells and may be physically associated with it, we have named it integrin-associated protein (IAP). Interestingly, cloning of IAP cDNA has shown that it predicts a structure which has several membrane-spanning domains, with homology to a sodium channel. We propose that IAP is part of the signal transduction mechanism of LRI. IAP may be a membrane ion channel gated by ligand binding to its associated integrin. The fact that IAP is also expressed on erythrocytes independently of integrins, suggests that this molecule might be involved in the signal transduction mechanism of other receptors (178).

7   Conclusion

While current pathologic studies reveal only simplistic information on processes like vasculitis, the new information presented in this chapter clearly offers the possibility of a deeper and more fundamental understanding of such diseases. Further investigations into the mechanisms of PMN activation are likely to provide both new insights into the pathophysiologic basis for these diseases and new opportunities for improved therapy.

References

1 Solbach, W., Moll, H., and Röllinghoff, M. (1991). Lymphocytes plays the music but the macrophage calls the tune. *Immunol. Today*, **12**, 4–6.
2 Unanue, E. R. and Cerottini, J. C. (1989). Antigen presentation. *FASEB J.*, **3**, 2496–502.
3 Harding, C. V. and Unanue, E. R. (1990). Cellular mechanisms of antigen processing and the function of class I and class II major histocompatibility complex molecules. *Cell Regul.*, **1**, 499–509.

4 Sprent, J. and Schaefer, M. (1990). Antigen-presenting cells for CD8$^+$ T cells. *Immunol. Rev.*, **117**, 213–34.

5 Springer, T. A. (1990). Adhesion receptors of the immune system. *Nature*, **346**, 425–34.

6 Hunkapillar, T. and Hood, L. (1989). Diversity of the immunoglobulin gene superfamily. *Adv. Immunol.*, **44**, 1–63.

7 Hynes, R. O. (1987). Integrins: a family of cell surface receptors. *Cell*, **48**, 549–54.

8 Hemler, M. E. (1988). Adhesive protein receptors on hematopoietic cells. *Immunol. Today*, **9**, 109–13.

9 Ruoslahti, E. (1991). Integrins. *J. Clin. Invest.*, **87**, 1–5.

10 Gresham, H. D., Googwin, J. L., Allen, P. M., Anderson, D. C., and Brown, E. J. (1989). A novel member of the integrin receptor family mediates Arg-Gly-Asp-stimulated neutrophil phagocytosis. *J. Cell Biol.*, **108**, 1935–43.

11 Phillips, D. R., Charo, I. F., and Scarborough, R. M. (1991). GPIIb-IIIa: The responsive integrin. *Cell*, **65**, 359–62.

12 Yoon, P. S., Boxer, L. A., Mayo, L. A., Yang A. Y., and Wicha, M. S. (1987). Human neutrophil laminin receptors: activation-dependent receptor expression. *J. Immunol.*, **138**, 259–65.

13 Bohnsack, J. F., Akiiyama, S. K., Damskky, C. H., Knape, W. A., and Zimmerman, G. A. (1990). Human neutrophil adherence to laminin in vitro: evidence for a distinct neutrophil receptor for laminin. *J. Exp. Med.*, **171**, 1221–37.

14 Arnaout, M. A. (1990). Leukocyte adhesion molecules deficiency: its structural basis, pathophysiology and implications for modulating the inflammatory response. *Immunol. Rev.*, **114**, 145–80.

15 Anderson, D. C. and Springer, T. A. (1987). Leukocyte adhesion deficiency: an inherited defect in the MAC-1, LFA-1, and gp150,95 glycoproteins. *Annu. Rev. Med.*, **38**, 175–94.

16 Diamond, M. S. (1991). Binding of the integrin Mac-1 (CD11b/CD18) to the third immunoglobulin-like domain of ICAM-1 (CD54) and its regulation by glycosylation. *Cell*, **65**, 961–71.

17 Myones, B. L., Dalzell, J. G., Hogg, N., and Ross, G. D. (1988). Neutrophil and monocyte cell surface p150,95 has iC3b-receptor (CR4) activity resembling CR3. *J. Clin. Invest.*, **82**, 640–51.

18 Kuijpers, T. W. and Ross, D. (1989). Leukocyte membrane adhesion proteins LFA-1, CR-3, and p150,95—a review of functional and regulatory aspects. *Res. Immunol.*, **140**, 461–86.

19 Bevilacqua, P. M., Stengelin, G., Gimbrone, M. A., Jr, and Seed, B. (1989). Endothelial leukocyte adhesion molecule 1: an inducible receptor for neutrophils related to complement regulatory proteins and lectines. *Science*, **243**, 1160–5.

20 Fokuda, M., Spooncer, E., Oates, J. A., Dell, A., and Klock, C. J.

(1984). Structure of sialylated fucosyl lactosaminoglycan isolated from human granulocytes. *J. Biol. Chem.,* **259,** 10925–35.

21 Symington, F. W., Hedges, D. L., and Hakomori, S.-I. (1985). Glyco-lipid antigens of human polymorphonuclear neutrophils and the in-ducible HL-60 myeloid leukemia line. *J. Immunol.,* **134,** 2498–506.

22 Bevilacqua, M., Butcher, E., Furie, B., *et al.* (1991). Selectins: a family of adhesion receptors. *Cell,* **67,** 233.

23 Hsu-Lin, S., Berman, C. L., Furie, B. C., August, D., and Furie, B. (1984). A platelet membrane protein expressed during platelet activa-tion and secretion. Studies using a monoclonal antibody specific for thrombin-activated platelets. *J. Biol. Chem.,* **259,** 9121–6.

24 Hattori, R., Hamilton, K. K., Fugate, R. D., McEver, R. P., and Sims, P. J. (1989). Stimulated secretion of endothelial von Willebrand factor is accompanied by rapid redistribution to the cell surface of the intracellular granule membrane protein GMP-140. *J. Biol. Chem.,* **264,** 7768–71.

25 Patel, K. D., Zimmerman, G. A., Prescott, S. M., McEver, R. P., and McIntyre, T. M. (1991). Oxygen radicals induce human endo-thelial cells to express GMP-140 and bind neutrophils. *J. Cell Biol.,* **112,** 749–59.

26 Picker, L. J., Kishimoto, T. K., Smith, C. W., Warnock, R. A., and Butcher, E. C. (1991). ELAM-1 is an adhesion molecule for skin-homing T cells. *Nature,* **349,** 796–9.

27 Yednock, T. A. and Rosen, S. D. (1989). Lymphocyte homing. *Adv. Immunol.,* **44,** 313–78.

28 Larsen, E., Palabrica, T., Sajer, S., Gilbert, G. E., Wagner, D. D., Furie, B. C., and Furie, B. (1990). PADGEM-dependent adhesion of platelets to monocytes and neutrophils is mediated by a lineage-specific carbohydrate, LNFIII (CD15). *Cell,* **63,** 467–74.

29 Siegelman, M. (1991). Sweetening the selectin pot. Identification of carbohydrate structures that act as ligands for the lectin-like domains of selectin proteins is helping to put cell–cell adhesion on a molecular basis. *Curr. Biol.,* **1,** 125–8.

30 Moore, K. L., Varki, A., and McEver, R. P. (1991). GMP-140 binds to a glycoprotein receptor on human neutrophils: Evidence for a lectin-like interaction. *J. Cell Biol.,* **112,** 491–9.

31 Aruffo, A., Kolanus, W., Walz, G., Fredman, P., and Seed, B. (1991). CD62/P-selectin recognition of myeloid and tumor cell sul-fatides. *Cell,* **67,** 35–44.

32 Phillips, M. L., Nudelman, E., Gaeta, F. C., Perez, M., Singhal, A. K., Hakomori, S., and Paulson, J. C. (1990). ELAM-1 mediates cell adhesion by recognition of a carbohydrate ligand, sialyl-Le$^\times$. *Science,* **250,** 1130–2.

33 Walz, G., Aruffo, A., Kolanus, W., Bevilacqua, M., and Seed, B.

(1990). Recognition by ELAM-1 of the sialyl-Le$^\times$ determinant on myeloid and tumor cells. *Science,* **250,** 1132–5.

34 Berg, E. L., Robinson, M. K., Mansson, O., Butcher, E. C., and Magnani, J. L. (1991). A carbohydrate domain common to both sialyl Le^a and sialyl Le$^\times$ is recognized by the endothelial cell leukocyte adhesion molecule ELAM-1. *J. Biol. Chem.,* **266,** 14869–72.

35 Lowe, J. B., Stoolman, L. M., Nair, R. P., Larsen, J. H., and Ginsburg, V. (1990). ELAM-1-dependent cell adhesion to vascular endothelium determined by transfected human fucosyltransferase cDNA. *Cell,* **63,** 475–84.

36 Goelz, S. E., Hession, C., Goff, D., Griffiths, B., Tizard, R., Newman, B., *et al.* (1990). ELFT: A gene that directs the expression of an ELAM-1 ligand. *Cell,* **63,** 1349–56.

37 Osborn, L. (1990). Leukocyte adhesion to endothelium in inflammation. *Cell,* **62,** 3–6.

38 Lo, S. K., VanSeventer, G. A., Levin, S. A., and Wright, S. D. (1989). Two leukocyte receptors (CD11a/CD18 and CD11b/CD18) mediate transient adhesion to endothelium by binding to different ligands. *J. Immunol.,* **143,** 3325–9.

39 Kuijpers, T. W., Hakkert, B. C., van Mourik, J. A., and Ross, D. (1990). Distinct adhesive properties of granulocytes and monocytes to endothelial cells under static and stirred conditions. *J. Immunol.,* **145,** 2588–94.

40 Vedder, N. B. and Harlan, J. M. (1988). Increased surface expression of CD11b/CD18 (Mac-1) is not required for stimulated neutrophil adherence to cultured endothelium. *J. Clin. Invest.,* **81,** 676–82.

41 Buyon, J. P., Slade, S. G., Reibman, J., Abramson, S. B., Philips, M. R., Weissmann, G., and Winchester, R. (1990). Constitutive and induced phosphorylation of the alfa- and beta-chains of the CD11b/CD18 leukocyte integrin family. Relationship to adhesion-dependent functions. *J. Immunol.,* **144,** 191–7.

42 Hibbs, M. L., Jakes, S., Styacker, S. A., Wallace, R. W., and Springer, T. A. (1991). The cytoplasmic domain of the integrin lymphocyte function-associated antigen 1 β subunit: sites required for binding to intercellular adhesion molecule 1 and the phorbol ester-stimulated phosphorylation site. *J. Exp. Med.,* **174,** 1227–38.

43 Geng, J.-G., Bevilacqua, M. P., Moore, K. L., McIntyre, T. M., Prescott, S. M., Kim, J. M., *et al.* (1990). Rapid neutrophil adhesion to activated endothelium mediated by GMP-140. *Nature,* **343,** 757–60.

44 Gamble, J. R., Skinner, M. P., Berndt, M. C., and Vadas, M. A. (1990). Prevention of activated neutrophil adhesion to endothelium by soluble adhesion protein GMP-140. *Science,* **249,** 414–17.

45 Lorant, D. E., Patel, K. D., McIntyre, T. M., McEver, R. P.,

Prescott, S. M., and Zymmerman, G. A. (1991). Coexpression of GMP-140 and PAF by endothelium stimulated by histamine or thrombin: a juxtacrine system for adhesion and activation of neutrophils. *J. Cell Biol.*, **115**, 223–34.

46 Staunton, D. E., Dustin, M. L., Erickson, H. P., and Springer, T. A. (1990). The arrangement of the immunoglobulin-like domains of ICAM-1 and the binding sites for LFA-1 and rhinovirus. *Cell*, **61**, 243–54.

47 Berendt, A. R., McDowall, A., Craig, A. G., Bates, P. A., Sternberg, M. J. E., Marsh, K., *et al.* (1992). The binding site on ICAM-1 for *Plasmodium falciparum*-infected erythrocytes overlaps, but is distinct from, the LFA-1-binding site. *Cell*, **68**, 71–81.

48 Luscinskas, F. W., Cybulsky, M. I., Kiely, J.-M., Peckins, C. S., Davis, V. M., and Gimbrone, M. A., Jr (1991). Cytokine-activated human endothelial monolayers support enhanced neutrophil transmigration via a mechanism involving both endothelial–leukocyte adhesion molecule-1 and intercellular adhesion molecule-1. *J. Immunol.*, **146**, 1617–25.

49 Lo, S. K., Lee, S., Ramos, R. A., Lobb, R., Rosa, M., Chi-Rosso, G., and Wright, S. D. (1991). Endothelial–leukocyte adhesion molecule 1 stimulates the adhesive activity of leukocyte integrin CR3 (CD11b/CD18, Mac-1, $a_m b_2$) on human neutrophils. *J. Exp. Med.*, **173**, 1493–500.

50 Lawrence, M. B., Smith, C. W., Eskin, S. G., and McIntyre, L. V. (1990). Effect of venous shear stress on CD18-mediated neutrophil adhesion to cultured endothelium. *Blood*, **75**, 227–37.

51 Lawrence, M. B. and Springer, T. A. (1991). Leukocytes roll on a selectin at physiologic flow rates: Distinction from a prerequisite for adhesion through integrins. *Cell*, **65**, 859–73.

52 Smith, W. C., Kishimoto, T. K., Abbass, O., Hughes, B., Rothlein, R., McIntyre, L. V., *et al.* (1991). Chemotactic factors regulate lectin adhesion molecule 1 (LECAM-1)-dependent neutrophil adhesion to cytokine-stimulated endothelial cells in vitro. *J. Clin. Invest.*, **87**, 609–18.

53 Abbassi, O., Lane, C. L., Krater, S., Kishimoto, T. K., Anderson, D. C., McIntyre, L. V., and Smith, W. C. (1991). Canine neutrophil margination mediated by lectin adhesion molecule-1 in vitro. *J. Immunol.*, **147**, 2107–25.

54 Jutila, M. A., Kishimoto, T. K., and Butcher, E. C. (1990). Regulation and lectin activity of the human neutrophil peripheral lymph node homing receptor. *Blood*, **75**, 1–5.

55 Williams, A. F. (1991). Out of equilibrium. *Nature*, **353**, 473–4.

56 Foote, J. and Milstein, C. (1991). Kinetic maturation of an immune response. *Nature*, **353**, 530–2.

57 Haynes, B. F., Telen, M. J., Hale, L. P., and Denning, S. M. (1989). CD44. A molecule involved in leukocyte adhesion and T-cell activation. *Immunol. Today*, **10**, 423–8.

58 Zhou, D. F., Ding, J. F., Picker, L. J., Bargatze, R. F., Butcher, E. C., and Goeddel, D. V. (1989). Molecular cloning and expression of Pgp-1. The mouse homolog of the human H-CAM (Hermes) lymphocyte homing receptor. *J. Immunol.*, **143**, 3390–5.

59 Dougherty, G. J., Landorp. P. M., Cooper, D. L., and Humpries, R. K. (1991). Molecular cloning of CD44R1 and CD44R2, two novel isoforms of the human CD44 lymphocyte 'homing' receptor expressed by hemopoietic cells. *J. Exp. Med.*, **174**, 1–5.

60 Aruffo, A., Stamenkovic, I., Melnick, M., Underhill, C. B., and Seed, B. (1990). CD44 is the principal cell surface receptor for hyaluronate. *Cell*, **61**, 1303–13.

61 Murakami, S., Miyake, K., Kincade, P. W., and Hodes, R. J. (1991). Functional role of CD44 (Pgp-1) on activated B cells. *Immunol. Res.*, **10**, 15–27.

62 Shimizu, Y., Van Seventer, G. A., Siraganian, R., Wahl, L., and Shaw, S. (1989). Dual role of the CD44 molecule in T cell adhesion and activation. *J. Immunol.*, **143**, 2457–63.

63 Huet, S., Groux, H., Caillou, B., Valentin, H., Prieur, A. M., and Bernard, A. (1989). CD44 contributes to T cell activation. *J. Immunol.*, **143**, 798–801.

64 Michl, J., Unkeless, J. C., Pieczonka, M. M., and Silverstein, S. C. (1983). Modulation of Fc receptors of mononuclear phagocytes by immobilized antigen–antibody complexes. Quantitative analysis of the relationship between ligand number and Fc receptor response. *J. Exp. Med.*, **157**, 1746–57.

65 Finbloom, D. S. (1985). Binding, endocytosis, and degradation of model immune complexes by murine macrophages at various levels of activation. *Clin. Immunol. Immunopathol.*, **36**, 275–88.

66 Gresham, H. D., McGarr, J. A., Shackelford, P. G., and Brown, E. J. (1988). Studies on the molecular mechanisms of human Fc receptor-mediated phagocytosis. Amplification of ingestion is dependent on the generation of reactive oxygen metabolites and is deficient in polymorphonuclear leukocytes from patients with chronic granulomatous disease. *J. Clin. Invest.*, **82**, 1192–201.

67 Pawlowski, N. A., Kaplan, G., Hamill, A. L., Cohn, A. L., and Scott, W. A. (1983). Arachidonic acid metabolism by human monocytes. Studies with platelet-depleted cultures. *J. Exp. Med.*, **158**, 393–412.

68 Graziano, R. F. and Fanger, M. W. (1987). Human monocyte-mediated cytotoxicity: the use of Ig-bearing hybridomas as target cells to detect trigger molecules on the monocyte cell surface. *J. Immunol.*, **138**, 945–50.

69 Karpovsky, B., Titus, J. A., Stephany, D. A., and Segal, D. M. (1984). Production of target specific effector cells using heterocross-linked aggregates containing anti-target cell and anti-Fcγ receptor antibodies. *J. Exp. Med.*, **160**, 1686–701.

70 Gresham, H. D., Clement L. T., Lehmeyer, J. E., Griffin, F. M., Jr, and Volanakis, J. E. (1986). Stimulation of human neutrophil Fc receptor-mediated phagocytosis by a low molecular weight cytokine. *J. Immunol.*, **137**, 868–75.

71 Unkeless, J. C. (1989). Human Fcγ receptors. *Curr. Opin. Immunol.*, **2**, 63–7.

72 Ravetch, J. V. and Kinet, J.-P. (1991). Fc receptors. *Annu. Rev. Immunol.*, **9**, 457–92.

73 Fridman, W. H. (1991). Fc receptors and immunoglobulin binding factors. *FASEB J.*, **5**, 2684–90.

74 Perussia, B., Dayton, E. T., Lazarus, R., Fanning, V., and Trinchieri, G. (1983). Immune interferon induces the receptor for monomeric IgG1 on human monocytic and myeloid cells. *J. Exp. Med.*, **158**, 1092–113.

75 Qiu, W. Q., de Bruin, D., Brownstein, B. H., Pearse, R., and Ravetch, J. V. (1990). Organization of the human and mouse low-affinity FcqR genes: duplication and recombination. *Science*, **248**, 732–5.

76 Van de Winkel, J. G. J. and Anderson, C. L. (1991). Biology of human immunoglobulin G Fc receptors. *J. Leukoc. Biol.*, **49**, 511–24.

77 Tax, W. J. M., Willems, H. W., Reekers, P. P. M., Capel, P. J. A., and Koene, R. A. P. (1983). Polymorphism in mitogenic effect of IgG1 monoclonal antibodies against T3 antigen on human T cells. *Nature*, **304**, 445–7.

78 Clark, M. R., Clarkson, S. B., Ory, P. A., Stollman, N., and Gold-stein, I. M. (1989). Molecular basis for a polymorphism involving Fc receptor II on human monocytes. *J. Immunol.*, **143**, 1731–4.

79 Warmerdam, P. A. M., van de Winkel, J. G. J., Gosselin, E. J., and Capel, P. A. J. (1990). Molecular basis for a polymorphism of human Fcγ receptor II (CD32). *J. Exp. Med.*, **172**, 19–25.

80 Miettinen, H. M., Rose, J. K., and Mellman, I. (1989). Fc receptor isoforms exhibit distinct abilities for coated pit localization as a result of cytoplasmic domain heterogeneity. *Cell*, **58**, 317–27.

81 Engelhardt, W., Gorczytza, H., Butterweek, A., Mönkemann, H., and Frey, J. (1991). Structural requirements of the cytoplasmic domains of the human macrophage Fc gamma receptor IIa and B-cell Fc gamma receptor IIb2 for the endocytosis of immune complexes. *Eur. J. Immunol.*, **21**, 2227–38.

82 Odin, J. A., Edberg, J. C., Painter, C. J., Kimberly, R. P., and Unkeless, J. C. (1991). Regulation of phagocytosis and $[Ca^{+2}]i$ flux by distinct regions of an Fc receptor. *Science*, **254**, 1785–8.

83 Selvaraj, P., Carpen, O., Hibbs, M. L., and Springer, T. A. (1989). Natural killer cell and granulocyte Fcγ receptor III (CD16) differ in membrane anchor and signal transduction. *J. Immunol.*, **143**, 3283–8.

84 Scallon, B. J., Scigliano, E., Freedman, V. H., Miedel, M. C., Pan, Y.-C. E., Unkeless, J. C., and Schlondorff, D. A. (1989). A human immunoglobulin G receptor exists in both polypeptide-anchored and phosphatidylinositol-glycan-anchored forms. *Proc. Natl Acad. Sci. USA*, **86**, 5079–83.

85 Kurosaki, T. and Ravetch, J. V. (1989). A single amino acid in the glycosyl phosphatidylinositol attachment domain determines the membrane topology of FcγRIII. *Nature*, **342**, 805–7.

86 Lanier, L. L., Cwirla, S., Yu, G., Testi, R., and Phillips, J. H. (1989). Membrane anchoring of a human IgG Fc receptor (CD16) determined by a single amino acid. *Science*, **246**, 1611–13.

87 Ory, P. A., Clark, M. R., Kwoh, E. E., Clarkson, S. B., and Goldstein, I. M. (1989). Sequences of complementary DNAs that encode the NA1 and NA2 forms of Fc receptor III on human neutrophils. *J. Clin. Invest.*, **84**, 1688–91.

88 Ory, P. A., Clark, M. R., Talhouk, A. S., and Goldstein, I. M. (1991). Transfected NA1 and NA2 forms of human neutrophil Fc receptor III exhibit antigenic and structural heterogeneity. *Blood*, **77**, 2682–7.

89 Chisei, R., Jouvin, M.-H. E., Blank, U., and Kinet, J.-P. (1989). A macrophage Fcγ receptor and the mast cell receptor for IgE share an identical subunit. *Nature*, **341**, 752–4.

90 Anderson, P., Caligiuri, M., Ritz, J., and Schlossman, S. F. (1989). CD3-negative natural killer cells express ζ TCR as part of a novel molecular complex. *Nature*, **341**, 159–62.

91 Anderson, P., Caligiuri, M., O'Brien, C., Manley, T., Ritz, J., and Schlossman, S. F. (1990). Fcγ receptor type III (CD16) is included in the ζ NK receptor complex expressed by human natural killer cells. *Proc. Natl Acad. Sci. USA*, **87**, 2274–8.

92 Orloff, D. G., Ra, C., Frank, S., Klausner, R. D., and Kinet, J.-P. (1990). Family of disulphide-linked dimers containing the ζ and η chains of the T-cell receptor and the γ chain of Fc receptors. *Nature*, **347**, 189–91.

93 Huizinga, T. W. J., De Haas, M., Kleijer, M., Nuijens, J. H., Roos, D., and Von dem Borne, A. E. G. K. (1990). Soluble Fcγ receptor III in human plasma originates from release by neutrophils. *J. Clin. Invest.*, **86**, 416–23.

94 Ravetch, J. V., Luster, A. D., Weinshank, R., Kochan, J., Pavlovec, A., Portnoy, D. A., Hulmes, J., Pan, Y. C., and Unkeless, J. C. (1986). Structural heterogeneity and functional domains of murine immunoglobulin G Fc receptors. *Science*, **234**, 718–25.

95 Amigorena, S., Bonnerot, C., Choquet, D., Fridman, W. H., and Teillaud, J. L. (1989). FcRγII expression in resting and activated B lymphocytes. *Eur. J. Immunol.*, **19**, 1379–85.

96 Pfefferkorn, L. C. and Fanger, M. W. (1989). Cross-linking of the high affinity Fc receptor for human immunoglobulin G1 triggers transient activation of NADPH oxidase activity. *J. Biol. Chem.*, **264**, 14112–20.

97 Willis, H. E., Browder, B., Feister, A. J., Mohanakumar, T., and Ruddy, S. (1988). Monoclonal antibody to human IgG Fc receptors. Cross-linking of receptors induces lysosomal enzyme release and superoxide generation by neutrophils. *J. Immunol.*, **140**, 234–9.

98 Huizinga, T. W. J., Dolman, K. M., Van der Linden, N. J. M., Kleijer, M., Nuijens, J. H., Von dem Borne, A. E. G. K., and Roos, D. (1990). Phosphatidylinositol-linked FcRIII mediates exocytosis of neutrophil granule proteins, but does not mediate initiation of the respiratory burst. *J. Immunol.*, **144**, 1432–7.

99 Crockett-Torabi, E. and Fantone, J. C. (1990). Soluble and insoluble immune complexes activate human neutrophil NADPH oxidase by distinct Fcγ receptor-specific mechanisms. *J. Immunol.*, **145**, 3026–32.

100 Trezzini, C., Jungi, T. W., Spycher, M. O., Maly, F. E., and Rao, P. (1990). Human monocyte CD36 and CD16 are signalling molecules. *Immunology*, **71**, 29–37.

101 Fanger, M. W., Shen, L., Graziano, R. F., and Guyre, P. M. (1989). Cytotoxicity mediated by human Fc receptors for IgG. *Immunol. Today*, **10**, 92–9.

102 Lanier, L. L., Ruittenberg, J. J., and Phillips, J. H. (1988). Functional and biochemical analysis of CD16 antigen on natural killer cells and granulocytes. *J. Immunol.*, **141**, 3478–85.

103 Debets, J. M. H., van de Winkel, J. G. J., Ceuppens, J. L., Dieteren, I. E. M., and Buurman, W. A. (1990). Cross-linking of both FcγRI and FcγRII induces secretion of tumor necrosis factor by human monocytes, requiring high affinity Fc–FcγR interactions. *J. Immunol.*, **144**, 1304–10.

104 Krutmann, J., Kirnbauer, R., Kock, A., Schwarz, T., Schopf, E., May, L. T., Sehgal, P. B., and Luger, T. A. (1990). Cross-linking Fc receptors on monocytes triggers IL-6 production. *J. Immunol.*, **145**, 1337–42.

105 Anderson, C. L., Shen, L., Eicher, D. M., Wewers, M. D., and Gill, J. K. (1990). Phagocytosis mediated by three distinct Fcγ receptor classes on human leukocytes. *J. Exp. Med.*, **171**, 1333–45.

106 Salmon, J. E., Kapur, S., and Kimberly, R. P. (1987). Opsonin-independent ligation of Fc gamma receptors. The 3G8-bearing receptors on neutrophils mediate the phagocytosis of concanavalin A-treated erythrocytes and nonopsonized *Escherichia coli. J. Exp. Med.*, **166**, 1798–813.

107 Salmon, J. E., Edberg, J. C., and Kimberly, R. P. (1990). Fcγ receptor III on human neutrophils. Allelic variants have functionally distinct capacities. *J. Clin. Invest.*, **85**, 1287–95.

108 Huizinga, T. W. J., Van Kemenade, F., Koenderman, L., Dolman, K. M., Von Dem Borne, A. E. G. K., Tetteroo, P. A. T., and Roos, D. (1989). The 40-kDa Fcγ receptor (FcRII) on human neutrophils is essential for the IgG-induced respiratory burst and IgG-induced phagocytosis. *J. Immunol.*, **142**, 2365–9.

109 Rosales, C. and Brown, E. J. (1991). Two mechanisms for IgG Fc-receptor-mediated phagocytosis by human neutrophils. *J. Immunol.*, **146**, 3937–44.

110 Indik, Z., Chien, P., Levinson, A. I., and Schreiber, A. D. (1991). The high affinity macrophage Fcγ receptor: structural requirements for the binding of IgG-sensitized cells, phagocytosis and signal transduction. *Clin. Res.*, **39**, 209A.

111 Indik, Z., Kelly, C., Chien, P., Levinson, A. I., and Schreiber, A. D. (1991). Human FcγRII, in the absence of other Fcγ receptors mediates a phagocytic signal. *J. Clin. Invest.*, **88**, 1766–71.

112 Salmon, J. E., Browle, N. L., Edberg, J. C., and Kimberly, R. P. (1991). Fcγ receptor III induces actin polymerization in human neutrophils and primes phagocytosis mediated by Fcγ receptor II. *J. Immunol.*, **146**, 997–1004.

113 Hunziker, W., Koch, T., Whitney, J. A., and Mellman, I. (1990). Fc receptor phosphorylation during receptor-mediated control of B-cell activation. *Nature*, **345**, 628–32.

114 Clark, M. R., Liu, L., Clarkson, S. B., Ory, P. A., and Goldstein, I. M. (1990). An abnormality of the gene that encodes neutrophil Fc receptor III in a patient with systemic lupus erythematosus. *J. Clin. Invest.*, **86**, 341–6.

115 Huizinga, T. W. J., Kuijpers, R. W. A. M., Kleijer, M., Schulpen, T. W. J., Cuypers, H. T. M., Roos, D., and Von dem Borne, A. E. G. K. (1990). Maternal genomic neutrophil FcRIII deficiency leading to neonatal isoimmune neutropenia. *Blood*, **76**, 1927–32.

116 Van de Winkel, J. G. J., Tax, W. J. M., Jacobs, C. W. M., Huizinga, T. W. J., and Willems, P. H. G. M. (1990). Cross-linking of both types of IgG Fc receptors, FcγRI and FcγRII, enhances intracellular Ca^{+2} in the monocytic cell line U937. *Scand. J. Immunol.*, **31**, 315–25.

117 Macintyre, E. A., Roberts, P. J., Abdul-Gaffar, R., O'Flynn, K., Pilkington, G. R., Farace, F., Morgan, J., and Linch, D. C. (1988). Mechanism of human monocyte activation via the 40-kDa Fc receptor for IgG. *J. Immunol.*, **141**, 4333–43.

118 Cassatella, M. A., Anegón, I., Cuturi, M. C., Griskey, P., Trinchieri, G., and Perussia, B. (1989). FcγR(CD16) interaction with ligand

induces Ca^{+2} mobilization and phosphoinositide turnover in human natural killer cells. *J. Exp. Med.,* **169,** 549–67.

119 Kimberly, R. P., Ahlstrom, J. W., Click, M. E., and Edberg, J. C. (1990). The glycosyl phosphatidylinositol-linked FcγRIII$_{PMN}$ mediates transmembrane signaling events distinct from FcγRII. *J. Exp. Med.,* **171,** 1239–55.

120 Sawyer, D. W., Sullivan, J. A., and Mandell, G. L. (1985). Intracellular free calcium localization in neutrophils during phagocytosis. *Science,* **230,** 663–6.

121 McNeil, P. L., Swanson, J. A., Wright, S. D., Silverstein, S. C., and Taylor, D. L. (1986). Fc-receptor-mediated phagocytosis occurs in macrophages without an increase in average $[Ca^{++}]i$. *J. Cell Biol.,* **102,** 1586–92.

122 Di Virgilio, F., Meyer, B. C., Greenberg, S., and Silverstein, S. C. (1988). Fc receptor-mediated phagocytosis occurs in macrophages at exceedingly low cytosolic Ca^{+2} levels. *J. Cell Biol.,* **106,** 657–66.

123 Young, J. D., Ko, S. S., and Cohn, Z. A. (1984). The increase in intracellular free calcium associated with IgG gamma 2b/ gamma 1 Fc receptor-ligand interactions: Role in phagocytosis. *Proc. Natl Acad. Sci. USA,* **81,** 5430–4.

124 Lew, D. P., Andersson, T., Hed, J., Di Virgilio, F., Pozzan, T., and Stendahl, O. (1985). Ca^{+2}-dependent and Ca^{+2}-independent phagocytosis in human neutrophils. *Nature,* **315,** 509–11.

125 Walker, B. A. M., Hagenlocker, B. E., Stubbs, E. B., Jr, Sandborg, R. R., Agranoff, B. W., and Ward, P. A. (1991). Signal transduction events and FcγR engagement in human neutrophils stimulated with immune complexes. *J. Immunol.,* **146,** 735–41.

126 Rosales, C. and Brown, E. J. (1992). Signal transduction by neutrophil IgG Fc receptors: Dissociation of $[Ca^{+2}]$ rise from IP$_3$. *J. Biol. Chem.,* **267,** 5265–71.

127 Brennan, P. J., Zigmond, S. H., Schreiber, A. D., and Southwick, F. S. (1988). IgG immune complex binding to the Fc receptor 2 induces actin filament assembly in human polymorphonuclear leukocytes (PMN). *J. Cell Biol.,* **107,** 452a.

128 Silverstein, S. C., Greenberg, S., Di Virgilio, F., and Steinberg, T. H. (1989). Phagocytosis. In *Fundamental immunology* (ed. W. E. Paul), pp. 703–20. Raven Press, New York.

129 Brown, E. J., Newell, A. M., and Gresham, H. D. (1987). Molecular regulation of phagocyte function. Evidence for involvement of guanosine triphosphate-binding protein in opsonin-mediated phagocytosis by monocytes. *J. Immunol.,* **139,** 3777–82.

130 Gresham, H. D., Clement, L. T., Volanakis, J. E., and Brown, E. J. (1987). Cholera toxin and pertussis toxin regulate the Fc-receptor-mediated phagocytic response of human neutrophils in a manner

analogous to regulation by monoclonal antibody 1C2. *J. Immunol.*, **139**, 4159–66.

131 Feister, A. J., Browder, B., Willis, H. E., Mohanakumar, T., and Ruddy, S. (1988). Pertussis toxin inhibits human neutrophil responses mediated by the 42-kilodalton IgG receptor. *J. Immunol.*, **141**, 228–33.

132 Paolini, R., Jouvin, M.-H., and Kinet, J.-P. (1991). Phosphorylation and dephosphorylation of the high-affinity receptor for immunoglobulin E immediately after receptor engagement and disengagement. *Nature*, **353**, 855–8.

133 Brozna, P. J., Hauff, N. F., Phillips, W. A., and Johnston, R. B. J. (1988). Activation of the respiratory burst in macrophages. Phosphorylation specifically associated with Fc receptor-mediated stimulation. *J. Immunol.*, **141**, 1642–7.

134 Zheleznyak, A. and Brown, E. J. (1992). IgG-mediated phagocytosis by human monocytes requires protein kinase C activation: Evidence for protein kinase C translocation to phagosomes. *J. Biol. Chem.*, **267**, 12042–8.

135 Ross, G. D. (1989). Complement and complement receptors. *Curr. Opin. Immunol.*, **2**, 50–62.

136 Keizer, G. D., te Velde, A. A., Schwarting, R., Figdor, C. G., and Vries, J. E. (1987). Role of p150,95 in adhesion, migration, chemotaxis and phagocytosis of human monocytes. *Eur. J. Immunol.*, **17**, 1317–22.

137 Hogg, N., Takacs, L., Palmer, D. G., Selvendran, Y., and Allen, C. (1986). The p150,95 molecule is a marker of human mononuclear phagocytes: comparison with expression of class II molecules. *Eur. J. Immunol.*, **16**, 240–8.

138 Dykman, T. R., Hatch, J. A., Aqua, M. S., and Atkinson, J. P. (1985). Polymorphism of the C3b/C4b receptor (CR1): characterization of a four allele. *J. Immunol.*, **134**, 1787–9.

139 Klickstein, L. B., Wong, W. W., Smith, J. A., Weis, H. J., Wilson, J. G., and Fearon D. T. (1987). Human C3b/C4b receptor (CR1): demonstration of long homologous repeating domains that are composed of the short consensus repeats characteristic of C3/C4 binding proteins. *J. Exp. Med.*, **165**, 1095–112.

140 Holers, V. M., Chaplin, D. D., Leykam, J. F., Gruner, B. A., Kumar, V., and Atkinson, J. P. (1987). Human complement C3b/C4b receptor (CR1) mRNA polymorphism that correlates with the CR1 allelic molecular weight polymorphism. *Proc. Natl Acad. Sci. USA*, **84**, 2459–63.

141 Reid, K. B. M., Bentley, D. R., Campbell, D. R., Cheng, L. P., Sim, R. B., Kristensen, T., and Tack, B. F. (1986). Complement system proteins which interact with C3b or C4b: a superfamily of structurally related proteins. *Immunol. Today*, **7**, 230–4.

142 Klickstein, L. B., Bartow, T. J., Miletic, V., Rabson, L. D., Smith, J. A., and Fearon, D. T. (1988). Identification of distinct C3b and C4b recognition sites in the human C3b/C4b receptor (CR1, CD35) by deletion mutagenesis. *J. Exp. Med.*, **168**, 1699–717.

143 Fearon, D. T. (1980). Identification of the membrane glycoprotein that is the C3b receptor of the human erythrocyte, polymorphonuclear leukocyte, B lymphocyte, and monocyte. *J. Exp. Med.*, **152**, 20–30.

144 O'Shea, J., Brown, E. J., Seligmann, B. E., Metcalf, J. A., Frank, M. M., and Gallin, J. I. (1985). Evidence for distinct intracellular pools of receptors for C3b and C3bi in human neutrophils. *J. Immunol.*, **134**, 2580–7.

145 Fearon, D. T. and Collins, L. A. (1983). Increased expression of C3b receptors on polymorphonuclear leukocytes induced by chemotactic factors and by purification procedures. *J. Immunol.*, **130**, 370–5.

146 Chatila, T. A., Geha, R. S., and Arnaout, M. A. (1989). Constitutive and stimulus-induced phosphorylation of CD11b/CD18 leukocyte adhesion molecules. *J. Cell Biol.*, **109**, 3435–44.

147 Wright, S. D. and Meyer, B. C. (1986). Phorbol esters cause sequential activation and deactivation of complement receptors on polymorphonuclear leukocytes. *J. Immunol.*, **136**, 1759–64.

148 Detmers, P. A., Wright, S. D., Olsen, E., Kimball, B., and Cohn, Z. A. (1987). Aggregation of complement receptors on human neutrophils in the absence of ligand. *J. Cell Biol.*, **105**, 1137–45.

149 Hermanowski-Vosatka, A., Van Strijp, J. A. G., Swiggard, W. J., and Wright, S. D. (1992). Integrin modulating factor-1: A lipid that alters the function of leukocyte integrins. *Cell,* **68**, 341–52.

150 Cheresh, D. A., Pytela, R., Pierschbacker, M. D., Klier, F. G., Rouslahti, E., and Reisfield, R. A. (1987). An Arg-Gly-Asp-directed receptor on the surface of human melanoma cells exists in a divalent cation-dependent functional complex with the disialoganglioside GD2. *J. Cell Biol.*, **165**, 1163–73.

151 Conforti, G., Zanetti, A., Pasquali-Ronchetti, I., Quaglino, D. J., Neyroz, P., and Dejana, E. (1990). Modulation of vitronectin receptor binding by membrane lipid composition. *J. Biol. Chem.*, **265**, 4011–19.

152 Lefkowith, J. B., Rogers, M., Lennartz, M. R., and Brown, E. J. (1991). Essential fatty acid deficiency impairs macrophage spreading and adherence. Role of arachidonate in cell adhesion. *J. Biol. Chem.*, **266**, 1971–6.

153 Wright, S. D. and Silverstein, S. C. (1982). Tumor-promoting phorbol esters stimulate C3b and C3b' receptor-mediated phagocytosis in cultured human monocytes. *J. Exp. Med.*, **156**, 1149–64.

154 Brown, E. J. (1991). Complement receptors and phagocytosis. *Curr. Opin. Immunol.*, **3**, 76–82.

155 Philip, R. and Epstein, L. B. (1986). Tumor necrosis factor as immunomodulator and mediator of monocyte cytotoxicity induced by itself, γ-interferon, and interleukin-1. *Nature, 323,* 86–9.

156 De Titto, E. H., Catterall, J. R., and Remington, J. S. (1986). Activity of human recombinant tumor necrosis factor on *Toxoplasma gondi* and *Trypanosoma cruzi. J. Immunol., 137,* 1342–5.

157 Klebanoff, S. J., Vadas, M. A., Harlam, J. M., Sparks, L. H., Gamble, J. R., Agosti, J. M., and Waltersdorph, A. M. (1986). Stimulation of neutrophils by tumor necrosis factor. *J. Immunol., 136,* 4220–5.

158 Donahue, R. E., Wang, E. A., Stone, D. K., Kamen, R., Wong, G. G., Sehgal, P. K., *et al.* (1986). Stimulation of haematopoiesis in primates by continuous infusion of recombinant human GM-CSF. *Nature, 321,* 872–5.

159 Lopez, A. F., Williamson, D. J., and Gambie, J. R. (1986). Recombinant human granulocyte-macrophage colony-stimulating factor stimulates in vitro mature human neutrophil and eosinophil function, surface receptor expression, and survival. *J. Clin. Invest., 78,* 1220–8.

160 Weisbart, R. H., Golde, D. W., and Gasson, J. C. (1986). Biosynthetic human GM-CSF modulates the number and affinity of neutrophil f-Met-Leu-Phe receptors. *J. Immunol., 137,* 3584–7.

161 Petroni, K. C., Shen, L., and Guyre, P. M. (1988). Modulation of human polymorphonuclear leukocytes IgG Fc receptors and Fc receptor-mediated function by INF-γ and glucocorticoids. *J. Immunol., 140,* 3467–72.

162 Pinckard, R. N., Ludwig, J. C., and McManus, L. M. (1988). Platelet-activating factors. In *Inflammation* (ed. J. I. Gallin, I. M. Goldstein, and R. Snyderman), pp. 139–67. Raven Press Ltd, New York.

163 Braquet, P., Touqui, L., Shen, T. Y., and Vargaftig, B. B. (1987). Perspectives in platelet-activating factor research. *Pharmacol. Rev., 39,* 97–145.

164 Carolan, E. J. and Casale, T. B. (1990). Degree of platelet activating factor-induced neutrophil migration is dependent upon the molecular species. *J. Immunol., 145,* 2561–5.

165 Lin, A. H., Morton, D. R., and Gorman, R. R. (1982). Acetyl-glyceryl ether phosphocholine stimulates leukotriene B_4 synthesis in human polymorphonuclear leukocytes. *J. Clin. Invest., 70,* 1058–65.

166 Bussolino, F., Fisher, E., Turrini, F., Kazatchkine, M. D., and Arese, P. (1989). Platelet-activating factor enhances complement-dependent phagocytosis of diamide-treated erythrocytes by human monocytes through activation of protein kinase C and phosphorylation of complement receptor type one (CR1). *J. Biol. Chem., 264,* 21711–19.

167 Riches, D. W. H., Young, S. K., Seccombe, J. F., Henson, J. E., Clay, K. L., and Henson, P. M. (1990). The subcellular distribution of

platelet-activating factor in stimulated human neutrophils. *J. Immunol.*, **145**, 3062–70.

168 Schleimer, R. P. and Rutledge, B. K. (1986). Cultured human vascular endothelial cells acquire adhesiveness for neutrophils after stimulation with interleukin 1, endotoxin, and tumor-promoting phorbol diesters. *J. Immunol.*, **136**, 649–54.

169 Sullivan, G. W., Carper, H. T., Sullivan, J. A., and Mandell, G. L. (1987). Interleukin-1 primes neutrophils. *Clin. Res.*, **35**, 657A.

170 Te Velde, A. A., Huijbens, R. J. F., De Vries, J. A., and Figdor, C. G. (1990). IL-4 decreases FcγR membrane expression and FcγR-mediated cytotoxic activity of human monocytes. *J. Immunol.*, **144**, 3046–51.

171 Welch, G. R., Wong, H. L., and Wahl, S. M. (1990). Selective induction of FcγRIII on human monocytes by transforming growth factor β. *J. Immunol.*, **144**, 3444–8.

172 Brown, E. J. (1986). The role of extracellular matrix proteins in the control of phagocytosis. *J. Leuk. Biol.*, **39**, 579–91.

173 Pommier, C. G., Inada, S., Fries, L. F., Takahashi, T., Frank, M. M., and Brown, E. J. (1983). Plasma fibronectin enhances phagocytosis of opsonized particles by human peripheral blood monocytes. *J. Exp. Med.*, **157**, 1844–54.

174 Wright, S. D., Craigmyle, L., and Silverstein, S. (1983). Fibronectin and serum amyloid P component stimulate C3b and C3bi-mediated phagocytosis in cultured human monocytes. *J. Exp. Med.*, **158**, 1338–43.

175 Bohnsack, J. F., Kleinman, H., Takahashi, T., O'Shea, J., and Brown, E. J. (1985). Connective tissue proteins and phagocytic cell function: laminin enhances complement and Fc-mediated phagocytosis by cultured human macrophages. *J. Exp. Med.*, **161**, 912–23.

176 Brown, E. J. and Goodwin, J. L. (1988). Fibronectin receptors of phagocytes. Characterization of the Arg-Gly-Asp binding proteins of human monocytes and polymorphonuclear leukocytes. *J. Exp. Med.*, **167**, 777–93.

177 Gresham, H. D., Adams, S. P., and Brown, E. J. (1992). Ligand binding specificity of the leukocyte response integrin expressed by human neutrophils. *J. Biol. Chem.*, **267**, 13895–902.

178 Brown, E., Hooper, L., Ho, T., and Gresham, H. (1990). Integrin-associated protein: a 50-kd plasma membrane antigen physically and functionally associated with integrins. *J. Cell Biol.*, **111**, 2785–94.

3 Signal transduction in neutrophil oxidative metabolism and chemotaxis

L. C. McPHAIL and L. HARVATH

1 Clinical case: chronic granulomatous disease (CGD)

A white male infant was referred in 1966 to a university medical centre for immunologic evaluation because of recurrent pneumonias and cervical adenitis. A diagnosis of chronic granulomatous disease (CGD) was made based on an abnormal neutrophil oxidative response as measured by the NBT (nitroblue tetrazolium) test (no reduction of NBT was noted) and absence of luminol-enhanced chemiluminescence in cells stimulated with opsonized zymosan or phorbol myristate acetate (PMA). His CGD appeared to be inherited in an X-linked manner based on the family history and the finding that the mother's neutrophil oxidative burst was 30 per cent of control while the father's was normal.

During the next few years he was hospitalized on various occasions for cervical adenitis, bacterial and fungal pneumonias, and abdominal abscesses due to *Staphylococcus aureus*. In 1980 he was admitted for a liver abscess in the right anterior lobe which was diagnosed by liver scan and ultrasound. Multiple abscesses were drained surgically. *S. aureus* sensitive to all antibiotics except penicillin was cultured from the liver. Nafcillin and gentamicin were administered intravenously. Fever continued unabated and rifampin was added to his antimicrobial therapy. He continued to have spiking temperatures despite a serum bactericidal titre of 1:64. Repeat radiologic studies showed persistence of the large right lobe defect together with several new defects. He was returned to surgery and multiple abscesses were drained. Cultures obtained during this surgery were negative. Vancomycin and gentamicin were given post-operatively. However, in spite of an adequate serum bactericidal titre, the temperature spikes continued, and he was therefore begun on daily granulocyte transfusions. There was a prompt temperature response and the patient soon became afebrile. Granulocyte and i.v. antibiotic therapies were discontinued after 2 weeks. He continued to improve on oral antibiotics, and repeat radiologic studies showed a decrease in the size and number of involved areas. Despite prophylaxis with trimethoprim-sulphamethoxazole, he was subsequently hospitalized for treatment of bacterial pneumonias and abdominal abscesses. In 1985 he was hospitalized for treatment of pneumonia due to *Aspergillus fumigatus*, but died despite aggressive antifungal therapy. Further discussion of the clinical manifestations of CGD and newer therapies can be found in Chapters 6 and 8, respectively.

When this patient died, the molecular basis of CGD was not known. However, it is now clear that defects in any of at least four genes can cause CGD (1–3). These genes code for four proteins that are thought to comprise NADPH oxidase, the enzyme responsible for the respiratory burst. Two of these proteins are subunits of a unique membrane-associated cytochrome, cytochrome b_{558}, while the other two are cytosolic proteins termed p47-*phox* and p67-*phox* (see Table 3.1). The cytosolic components appear to assemble with cytochrome b_{558} in the membrane upon activation of the respiratory burst (4, reviewed in 3). The two subunits of the cytochrome consist of a 22 kDa protein, termed p22-*phox*, and a 91 kDa glycoprotein, termed gp91-*phox* (reviewed in 1–3). The gene for gp91-*phox* is on the X chromosome (5, reviewed in 1–3), and is therefore likely to have been defective in the patient reported above. The genes for the other NADPH oxidase components (p22-*phox*, p47-*phox*, and p67-*phox*) are autosomal, located on chromosomes 16, 7, and 1, respectively (6, reviewed in 3). The relative prevalence of defects in these four genes in CGD has been determined in a group of 94 patients (7) and is summarized in Table 3.1. The most common defect is in the gene for gp91-*phox*, with a frequency of 56 per cent. The second most common defect is in the gene for p47-*phox*, accounting for 33 per cent of patients in the study. Defects in the genes for p22-*phox* and p67-*phox* occur much less frequently, with incidences of 5 per cent each. In a study reported by Smith and Curnutte (3), all patients with CGD had defects in one of these four genes. However, it is possible that defects in genes for other cytosolic proteins may cause CGD in rare cases (3).

Table 3.1   Molecular defects in CGD[a]

Protein	Inheritance	Gene locus	Frequency (%)
gp91-*phox*	X[b]	*CYBB* Xp21.1	56
p22-*phox*	AR	*CYBA* 16q24	5
p47-*phox*	AR	*NCF1* 7q11.23	33
p67-*phox*	AR	*NCF2* 1q25	5

[a] See text for references.
[b] Abbreviations: X, X-linked; AR, autosomal recessive.

2   Introduction

Neutrophils play a major role in host defence because they rapidly migrate to sites of infection and destroy invading micro-organisms. Specific signal molecules (chemoattractants), released by bacteria or endogenously generated by the host, can elicit directed neutrophil migration (chemotaxis) to the inflammatory site. Micro-organism destruction may involve oxidative and nonoxidative mechanisms. Nonoxidative killing involves the secretion of lysosomal enzymes (degranulation). Oxidative-dependent killing is mediated by oxygen metabolites generated upon activation of the neutrophil enzyme NADPH oxidase (the respiratory burst). Many chemoattractants provoke activation of NADPH oxidase.

The directed movement of neutrophils from the peripheral circulation to their destination is initiated by the specific interaction of chemoattractants with neutrophil plasma membrane receptors. The signal is then transmitted to the interior of the cell by a cascade of reactions that are collectively referred to as signal transduction. Biochemical events, including coupling of guanine nucleotide regulatory proteins (G proteins; also called GTPases) to chemoattractant receptors, activation of phospholipases, generation of second messengers, and activation of protein kinases, occur during the signal transduction cascade. In this chapter, we summarize the role of these biochemical events in triggering chemotaxis and the respiratory burst. We begin by providing a brief overview of each of these processes. Since several comprehensive reviews of neutrophil activation have been published within the last few years, we focus our discussion on the most recent observations and refer readers to detailed reviews that appear elsewhere.

2.1   Chemotaxis

Neutrophil chemotaxis requires chemoattractant binding to specific plasma membrane receptors, cell adherence to a substratum, and reversible assembly of critical cytoskeletal elements. Chemoattractant-stimulated neutrophils undergo rapid morphological changes from rounded, relatively smooth cells to elongated, ruffled cells with pseudopodia. When stimulated neutrophils are attached to a substratum, their pseudopodia form broad, thin lamellepodia that are extended anteriorly in the direction of an increasing chemoattractant concentration gradient (reviewed in 8, 9). A contractile uropod is formed posteriorly, which results in a polarized cell morphology. Neutrophil polarity is required for efficient directed migration. Neutrophils migrate by repetitive, complex events in which they extend lamellepodia in the direction of the gradient and retract their uropodia toward the cell body (9). During migration, the cells reversibly adhere to a substratum. A model of cell motility has been proposed which incorporates the hypothesis that regulated cell adhesions may enhance lamellepodial attachment and facilitate release of uropodial attachment (9). The mechanisms controlling these events remain unknown.

Actin, a 43 kDa globular protein of the microfilamentous cytoskeleton, is involved in cell migration (reviewed in 10). The polymerization of globular actin (G-actin) monomers into actin filaments (F-actin) occurs within seconds after neutrophils are stimulated with chemoattractants (reviewed in 11; discussed in Section 6 of this chapter). Dynamic alterations in F-actin polymerization correlate closely with chemoattractant-elicited neutrophil shape changes and migration rates (12, 13). Actin assembly is regulated by a variety of actin-binding proteins that control the reversible gelation and solation of a three-dimensional actin network (reviewed in 11, 14, 15). Agents that block actin polymerization, such as cytochalasins and botulinum C2 toxin, inhibit neutrophil migration *in vitro* (16, 17). Neutrophils from patients who have actin dysfunction or abnormal concentrations of microfilamentous cytoskeletal proteins that affect actin polymerization have severe motility defects (18–20). These findings demonstrate that actin is an essential protein for cell motility. Current models of cell migration propose that actin is involved in the force generation for cell movement (9, 10). The precise mechanisms of leukocyte force generation remain unknown.

Neutrophil motility may be random, chemokinetic, or chemotactic, and is classified by *in vitro* assays which quantify the directional migration response. Random migration (unstimulated motility) and chemokinetic migration (i.e. stimulated speed of cells) are motile responses which do not have consistent directionality. In contrast, chemotactic responses are directional. Although the relative importance of random, chemokinetic, and chemotactic migration *in vivo* has not been determined, it is likely that all three types of motility are involved in mobilization of neutrophils to inflammatory sites.

2.2   The respiratory burst

The enzyme (NADPH oxidase) responsible for the respiratory burst is inactive until the neutrophil is stimulated by engagement of receptors for chemoattractants or receptors mediating phagocytosis or responses to various cytokines. The signalling processes induced result in the rapid appearance of NADPH oxidase activity. The active enzyme catalyses the following reaction:

$$NADPH + 2O_2 \rightarrow NADP^+ + 2O_2^- + H^+$$

The activation of NADPH oxidase thus accounts for the burst of O_2 consumption by neutrophils during cell stimulation. Increased levels of

NADP$^+$ activate the pentose phosphate pathway (hexose monophosphate shunt) and NADPH is regenerated. The O_2^- formed by NADPH oxidase activity can be rapidly converted to H_2O_2 and other toxic species and these are responsible for injury to micro-organisms and surrounding tissue (21, 22, Chapter 4).

Active NADPH oxidase appears to be a multi-component enzyme system, consisting of four proteins (see Table 3.1): the heterodimeric cytochrome b_{558} and the two cytosolic proteins, p47-*phox* and p67-*phox* (1–3). The active enzyme complex is membrane-associated and appears oriented to interact with NADPH on one side of the membrane and O_2 on the other (23, reviewed in 3, 21). Cytochrome b_{558} is thought to be the terminal component in the presumed electron transport chain and transfers electrons directly to O_2 (reviewed in 1, 21). Although genes for the two subunits of cytochrome b_{558} have been cloned (reviewed in 1–3), the structural properties of the heterodimer responsible for its functional activity are not yet understood. Genes for the two cytosolic components have also been cloned (24; reviewed in 2, 3) and neither predicted sequence reveals a possible electron transfer function (i.e. NADPH- and/or flavin-binding sites). Therefore, the contribution of these proteins to the structure and function of the assembled oxidase is not clear. Possible roles of the four NADPH oxidase components are discussed further in Section 6 of this chapter.

The sequence of events leading to activation of NADPH oxidase by chemoattractants or other stimuli is still not clear. Unfortunately, approaches to link specific signalling events to NADPH oxidase activation primarily have been correlative in nature and, therefore, do not constitute final proof. In addition, it is likely that the biochemical pathways involved in signal transduction are complexly interrelated, complicating interpretation of inhibitor studies. One promising avenue of study is the use of a cell-free system for NADPH oxidase activation. This system was originally developed in the mid 1980s by Bromberg and Pick (25) in guinea-pig macrophages and by Heyneman and Vercauteren (26), Curnutte (27), and McPhail *et al.* (28) in neutrophils. The ability to achieve NADPH oxidase activation in a cell-free system should eventually allow reconstitution of a complete biochemical activation pathway. Results obtained using this system are summarized in Section 6 of this chapter.

This chapter summarizes the signal transductional mechanisms triggered by engagement of chemoattractant receptors and implicated in the activation of chemotaxis and the respiratory burst. Section 3 covers chemoattractant receptors and GTPases, Section 4 discusses phospholipases and the generation of second messengers, and Section 5 examines protein kinases and phosphorylation events. Sections 6 and 7 address the targets of the signalling pathways, Section 6 focuses on modifications of NADPH oxidase components and studies of the activation of NADPH oxidase in a cell-free system and Section 7 focuses on the cytoskeleton. The signalling pathways for the two functions also diverge at some point, even though the same ligand can trigger both events, and we conclude the chapter in Section 8 with a discussion of common and divergent pathways for activating chemotaxis and the respiratory burst.

3   Chemoattractant receptor–G protein interaction

3.1   Chemoattractants and their receptors

Neutrophils respond to a variety of chemoattractants, including *N*-formyl peptides, complement-derived C5a, leukotriene B_4 (LTB$_4$), interleukin-8 (IL-8), and platelet-activating factor (PAF) (recently reviewed in 29–31). Receptors for most of these attractants have recently been cloned (32–42). The chemoattractant receptors have been identified as members of the GTPase-coupled receptor superfamily, which have seven transmembrane spanning domains (Fig. 3.1).

Human *N*-formyl peptide, C5a, and IL-8 receptors have 350 amino acids containing potential N-linked glycosylation sites near the N terminus. The human PAF receptor contains 342 amino acids and lacks sites for N-linked glycosylation at the N terminus (37). Two isoforms of human *N*-formyl peptide (33) and IL-8 (39, 40) receptors have been identified. The two *N*-formyl peptide receptors differ by two amino acids and exhibit similar binding affinities (33). The human IL-8 receptors share 77 per cent amino acid homology and have different binding affinities; one form exhibits high affinity binding (39), whereas, the other exhibits low affinity binding of IL-

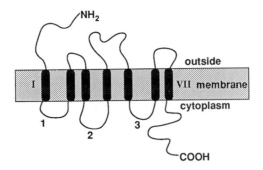

Fig. 3.1   A sketch of the human *N*-formyl peptide receptor adapted from the structure proposed by Boulay *et al.* (33). The proposed receptor structure predicts seven transmembrane domains (indicated by rods) and three intracellular loops. The third loop is a putative G protein-binding site and/or a PKA phosphorylation target.

8 (40). It is not known whether the isoforms of these receptors stimulate different functional neutrophil responses. The chemoattractant receptors cloned thus far have 29–34 per cent amino acid identity, with substantial homology occurring in the seven putative transmembrane domains (39). Predictions have been made for various regions of the receptors. The intracellular C-terminal region contains several serine and threonine residues that may be phosphorylated by specific kinases (33, 39). The third intracellular loop is postulated to be a G protein-binding domain (33, 39). The third intracellular loop of the C5a and *N*-formyl peptide receptors also contains a potential phosphorylation site for protein kinase A (35). Future studies with site-directed mutations of these receptors will clarify these predictions and permit direct exploration of the biochemical and molecular events that occur in specific regions of the receptor during chemoattractant–receptor binding.

3.2 G proteins

As mentioned above, chemoattractant receptors are predicted to couple to G proteins in order to transmit signals to the interior of the cell. These G proteins serve as intermediates between cell-surface receptors and effector enzymes responsible for generating second messengers. There are two separate classes of G proteins: heterotrimeric, consisting of α, β, and γ subunits, and monomeric, referred to as small G proteins, low molecular weight G proteins, or the *ras* superfamily (reviewed in 43). G proteins in both categories are likely to be involved in chemoattractant signalling (reviewed in 44).

All G proteins carry out a cycle of guanine nucleotide exchange and GTP hydrolysis, during which the protein undergoes several conformational changes (summarized in Fig. 3.2; reviewed in 43). The G protein is inactive for coupling to an effector enzyme in its GDP-bound form and becomes activated for effector binding when GDP is released and GTP binds to the empty site. Conversion back to the inactive state occurs once GTP is hydrolysed to form GDP. The rates of GDP release and GTP hydrolysis can be regulated by other proteins and this serves as the mechanism for controlling the participation of the G protein in the signalling process. Proteins that affect the rate of GDP release are termed guanine nucleotide release proteins (GNRPs), while proteins that increase the rate of GTP hydrolysis are termed GTPase-activating proteins (GAPs). For hetero-trimeric G proteins, ligand-bound receptor acts as a GNRP to enhance the rate of GDP release markedly. The site of guanine nucleotide binding to heterotrimeric G proteins is on the α subunit and receptor-induced re-placement of GDP with GTP results in dissociation of the α subunit from the βγ subunits. This permits the GTP-bound α subunit to couple to the

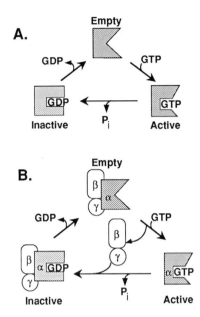

Fig. 3.2 The GTPase cycle carried out by G proteins. In the GTPase cycle of monomeric G proteins (panel A), the protein undergoes three conformational changes, depending on the guanine nucleotide bound. When GDP is bound, the protein is inactive. Upon the release of GDP, the protein changes conformation and is considered to be in an empty state. GTP then can bind and the protein converts to an active state, where it possesses GTPase activity and is also capable of interacting with an effector molecule. The hydrolysis of GTP converts the G protein back to the GDP-bound inactive form. The GTPase cycle of the heterotrimeric G proteins is shown in panel B. The cycle is similar to that of the monomeric G proteins, except that the βγ subunits dissociate from the α subunit in association with the binding of GTP to the empty state. The free α subunit possesses GTPase activity and interacts with effector molecules. The subunits reassociate once the α subunit hydrolyses GTP to GDP. Relative sizes of proteins are not to scale.

effector enzyme. Hydrolysis of GTP, which is not regulated by a GAP on heterotrimeric G proteins, allows the subunits to reassociate. The monomeric G proteins are regulated by both GNRPs and GAPs, as well as by proteins that inhibit GDP release (guanine nucleotide dissociation inhibitors or GDIs; reviewed in 45).

Each category (heterotrimeric and monomeric) of G proteins consists of several subclasses, distributed heterogeneously in different cell types (43–45). In neutrophils, studies thus far have identified at least three heterotrimeric G proteins—G_s, G_{i2}, and G_{i3}—and a multitude of monomeric G proteins, including *rap1A, rac1, rac2,* and proteins in the Rho family (46–

50, reviewed in 44). The functional roles of these multiple G proteins are not yet understood. The heterotrimeric G protein G_{i2} may couple directly to chemoattractant receptors, based on reports of co-purification with the *N*-formyl peptide (51) and C5a (52) receptors. It has also been shown that G proteins in the G_i class can directly couple the *N*-formyl peptide receptor to an effector (reviewed in 44). Based on these studies and on the inhibitory effects of pertussis toxin, described below, it is likely that chemoattractant receptors initiate signalling to the cell interior by coupling to G_{i2}, but it is not yet clear if G_{i3} has a similar role. G_s is likely to couple adrenergic and other receptors to adenylate cyclase, similar to its role in other cell types (43, 44).

The roles of the monomeric G proteins in neutrophils are much less clear. Co-purification of a subpopulation of *N*-formyl peptide receptors with monomeric G proteins of 24 and 26 kDa (51) suggests that monomeric G proteins may couple directly to chemoattractant receptors. However, recent observations suggest that these proteins will emerge as important regulators of the end-stage functional responses to chemoattractants. Most intriguing are reports (53–57) of association of *rac* and *rap1A* with the NADPH oxidase system (discussed in detail in Section 6 of this chapter).

Specific G proteins are targets for certain ADP-ribosylating bacterial toxins, including pertussis, cholera and botulinum C_3 (44). Pertussis and cholera toxins ADP-ribosylate heterotrimeric G proteins in the G_i and G_s subclasses, respectively, resulting in either inhibition (G_i) or activation (G_s) of the G protein. Botulinum C_3 toxin ADP-ribosylates monomeric G proteins in the Rho subclass but has not yet been found to inhibit their functional activity (44, 58). Pertussis toxin treatment inhibits most neutrophil responses to chemoattractants (59, 60, reviewed in 11, 31, 44). These studies were the first to suggest a role for a G protein in mediating signalling by chemoattractants. The pertussis toxin substrate has now been identified as most likely G_{i2} (47, reviewed in 44). Studies examining the effect of botulinum C_3 toxin on neutrophil responses have not been reported. However, an earlier study using botulinum D toxin contaminated with botulinum C_3 toxin found no effect on neutrophil responses to the *N*-formyl peptide fMet-Leu-Phe (FMLP) (61). In limited studies in certain other cell types, botulinum C_3 toxin treatment has been shown to alter microfilament function (62, reviewed in 63). Further studies in neutrophils with this toxin should be informative.

The effectors to which G proteins couple in neutrophils are under investigation. G_s couples to adenylate cyclase, as evidenced by the ability of cholera toxin to increase cAMP levels in these cells (reviewed in 44). The G proteins in the G_i class may couple to one or more phospholipases (discussed in Section 4). Effectors for the monomeric G proteins have not yet been identified in any cell type (43, 45).

3.3   Receptor affinity states

Neutrophil chemoattractant receptors exist in interconvertible high and low affinity states (reviewed in 64, 65). Receptor association with hetero-trimeric G proteins increases the receptor binding affinity (64). Sklar *et al.* propose that three states for the *N*-formyl peptide receptor exist on intact neutrophils: a ternary complex consisting of chemoattractant ligand, recep-tor, and G protein (LRG), a binary complex consisting of the ligand and receptor (LR), and a desensitized receptor state referred to as LRX which is slowly dissociating, irreversibly formed, and probably inactive (66). High affinity binding is attributed to the LRG ternary complex in which the ligand slowly dissociates from the receptor complex, and low affinity bind-ing is attributed to the binary complex in which the ligand rapidly dissoci-ates from the receptor. Recent evidence from real-time analysis of *N*-formyl peptide ligand, receptor, and G protein assembly in permeabilized human neutrophils demonstrates that the difference in binding affinities of the LR and LRG complexes is due to a change in the dissociation rate constant (67). The association rate constants for the LR and LRG com-plexes appear to be identical, whereas, the dissociation rate constants differ by approximately two orders of magnitude.

Receptor heterogeneity is implicated as an explanation for the physio-logic responses elicited by various concentrations of chemoattractants (68). Chemotaxis is typically initiated by chemoattractant concentrations that are one to two orders of magnitude lower than the concentrations required for the respiratory burst or degranulation. One explanation is that chemo-attractant binding to the high affinity receptors may activate chemotaxis, whereas, chemoattractant binding to the low affinity receptors may acti-vate the respiratory burst, degranulation, and other responses (68). A recent study indicates that neutrophil degranulation is stimulated by high affinity binding and offers an alternative model to explain functional recep-tor heterogeneity (69). Kermode *et al.* propose that ligand binding to the receptor causes conversion of the receptor to a high affinity state and triggers an immediate signal that is sufficient for degranulation. When the ligand has a high potency or binding affinity, the high affinity state is stabilized and signalling is sustained. The authors suggest that a stabilized high affinity state of sustained duration is necessary for signalling a chemo-tactic response. In contrast, when the ligand is less potent, the activated state is maintained for a short time and is not sufficient to sustain a chemotactic response. Therefore, transient high affinity states are suf-ficient for signalling activation of neutrophil degranulation, but not chemo-taxis.

The studies of Sklar *et al.* and Kermode *et al.* indicate that the residence time of a chemoattractant ligand in a receptor determines the ligand's potency in eliciting neutrophil responses. Heterotrimeric G proteins reversibly interact with chemoattractant receptors during receptor–ligand engagement and affect the dissociation rate of the ligand from the receptor (Fig. 3.3). Ligand residencies in receptors and subsequent interactions with G proteins are likely to be functions of the topological changes that occur in the proteins when the ligand is in the receptor-binding pocket. It remains to be determined whether the low molecular weight G proteins directly associate with the receptors.

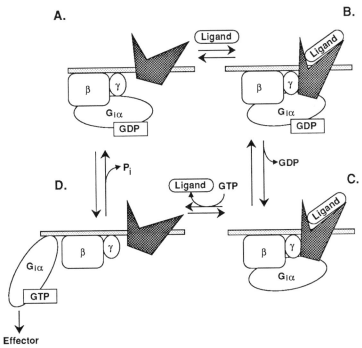

Fig. 3.3 A simplified scheme of potential chemoattractant receptor and heterotrimeric G protein interactions. Receptor (stippled structure dissociation from the G protein (panels A and D) results in a low binding affinity for the chemoattractant ligand, whereas receptor association with the G protein (panels B and C) confers a high binding affinity for the ligand. GTP binding to the α subunit results in dissociation of the complex and GTPase activity (panel D). GTPase activity occurs only when GTP is bound to the α subunit (panel D) and is absent in conditions represented in panels A, B, and C. During guanine nucleotide exchange, the complex may exist in a nucleotide-empty state (panel C). Several other receptor states, not illustrated in this figure, have been proposed. Kermode *et al.* (69) have postulated an additional activated state, occurring between panels C and D of this figure, in which the ligand–receptor and βγ subunits remain associated during the formation of GTPase activity. Sklar *et al.* (65, 66) have proposed that a ligand–receptor complex (LR) and a desensitized ligand–receptor complex (LRX) are formed after association with G protein.

4   Second messengers elicited by chemoattractants

4.1   Generation of second messengers

The levels of several second messengers increase dramatically in neutrophils in response to chemoattractant–receptor binding. These include cAMP, inositol triphosphate (IP_3), Ca^{2+}, diacylglycerol (DAG), phosphatidic acid (PA), and arachidonic acid (AA). The generation of these second messengers and their roles in modulation of neutrophil function have been reviewed previously (11, 30, 31, 70–73). These second messengers are generated, either directly or indirectly, as a consequence of the chemoattractant-mediated activation of phospholipases. The phospholipases that are activated include (see Fig. 3.4): phospholipase A_2 (PLA_2), which hydrolyses phosphatidylcholine (PC) and/or phosphatidylethanolamine (PE) to produce AA and lysoPC and/or lysoPE (reviewed in 30, 31); phospholipase C (PLC), which hydrolyses phosphatidylinositol-4,5-biphosphate (PIP_2) to produce DAG and IP_3 (reviewed in 30, 31, 72); and phospholipase D (PLD), which hydrolyses PC to produce PA and choline (74–78, reviewed in 30, 31). A PLD enzyme acting on phosphatidylinositol may also be present (79, 80). Phospholipase activation is mediated by the coupling of occupied chemoattractant receptors with a pertussis toxin-sensitive G protein (presumably G_{i2}, see Section 3.2), as evidenced by the ability of pertussis toxin treatment of neutrophils to inhibit the generation of second messengers (59, 60, 74, reviewed in 11, 30, 31, 44, 72, 73). However, it is not yet known whether the α subunit of G_i couples directly to each phospholipase or whether $G_{\alpha i}$ interaction with one phospholipase (e.g. PLC) leads to the second messenger-mediated activation of the others. Reconstitution studies with purified $G_{\alpha i}$ and each purified phospholipase will be needed to address this issue. The following paragraphs describe the mechanisms involved in the formation and metabolism of each of the second messengers formed by chemoattractant stimulation of neutrophils.

Chemoattractants stimulate a rapid and transient increase in cAMP levels that peaks at 10–20 s and declines to baseline by 2–3 min (reviewed in 73). The mechanism responsible for the increase in cAMP appears to be indirect, in that chemoattractant receptors do not couple to adenylyl cyclase via G_s in membrane preparations (82, reviewed in 73). The ability of FMLP to increase cAMP levels is pertussis toxin-sensitive (73) and shows a dependence on Ca^{2+} (82), further supporting an indirect mechanism. The Ca^{2+}-dependent mechanism responsible is still not clear, although the transient inhibition of a cAMP phosphodiesterase (82) or the generation of endogenous adenosine (83) have been suggested as possibilities.

An increase in the intracellular concentration of free Ca^{2+} ($[Ca^{2+}]_i$) induced by chemoattractants begins rapidly following agonist binding

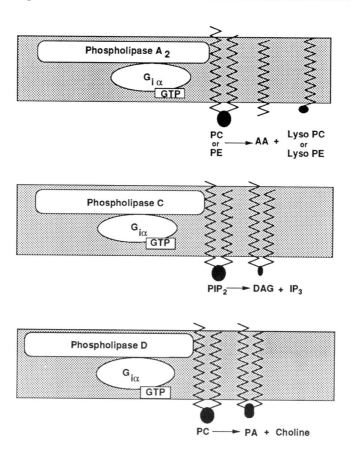

Fig. 3.4 Reactions carried out by phospholipases to generate second messengers. Each phospholipase may be activated by an α subunit in the G_i subclass of heterotrimeric G proteins ($G_{i\alpha}$). Phospholipid substrates are phosphatidylcholine (PC), phosphatidylethanolamine (PE), and phosphatidylinositol-4,5-bisphosphate (PIP$_2$). Second messengers generated are arachidonic acid (AA), diacylglycerol (DAG), inositol triphosphate (IP$_3$), and phosphatidic acid (PA).

(within 0.2–0.3 s) (84) and appears to involve at least two processes (reviewed in 71): (i) release from an intracellular storage compartment, the calciosome, mediated by the binding of IP$_3$ to its receptor on the calciosome; and (ii) an influx of Ca^{2+} from the extracellular medium. The mechanism responsible for the influx of Ca^{2+} is not yet clear, but may involve the participation of other second messengers, such as PA, Ca^{2+}, or the phosphorylated metabolite of IP$_3$, IP$_4$ (reviewed in 71). The increase in [Ca^{2+}]$_i$ induced by chemoattractants gradually returns to near baseline levels over 5–15 min (60, reviewed in 71) by mechanisms involving protein kinase C (PKC) and/or cAMP-dependent protein kinase (PKA). PKC can induce activation of the plasma membrane Ca^{2+}–ATPase, which pumps Ca^{2+} out of the cell, and both PKC and PKA can inhibit the generation of IP_3 (reviewed in 71, 72). The target(s) for PKC and PKA resulting in the decreased synthesis of IP_3 have not yet been identified, but could be at the level of chemoattractant receptors, the G protein, the PLC enzyme, or the enzymes that resynthesize PIP_2 (reviewed in 71, 72).

PLC consists of several isoforms divided into three classes termed β, γ, and δ (reviewed in 85). It has not yet been demonstrated that any isoform can couple to a pertussis toxin-sensitive G protein, such as G_{i2}, although direct coupling between a PLC-β isoform and a pertussis toxin-insensitive G protein, G_q, has been shown (86). The PLC-γ isoforms appear to be regulated by tyrosine kinases and not by G proteins (85). Activators of PLC-δ have not yet been discovered and it has been speculated that this class may be the target for pertussis toxin-sensitive G proteins (85, 86). It will be important to identify PLC isoforms present in neutrophils to help dissect the mechanisms involved in PLC activation by chemoattractants.

DAG formed in response to chemoattractants appears to be a product of both PLC and PLD activation. Several studies (87–91) demonstrated that FMLP induces two waves of DAG formation in neutrophils. One peak occurs at about 10–30 s and a second wave begins at about 30 s and continues for 5–10 min. These two waves can be pharmacologically dissociated (87, 89, 92), suggesting that two enzymatic pathways are responsible. The first peak coincides with PIP_2 hydrolysis and IP_3 formation (91, 92) and is presumably formed by activation of PLC. The mechanism responsible for the later accumulation of DAG appears to be activation of a PLD (74, 75, 91, 93, 94). The initial product of PLD activation is PA, which can be converted to DAG by the enzyme PA phosphohydrolase. Inhibition of this enzyme has been shown to reduce the levels of diradylglycerol (refers to all species of diglyceride, including DAG and alkylacylglycerol) and to increase PA levels formed in response to FMLP (95).

PA is currently receiving attention as a potential second messenger in neutrophils. PA can be formed by the enzyme DAG kinase, which phosphorylates DAG, as well as by PLD. The relative contributions of PLD and DAG kinase to the levels of PA in neutrophils are not yet clear. In addition to PA, the levels of other membrane phospholipids change following chemoattractant stimulation. Obviously, a transient decrease in levels of PC and PIP_2 occurs due to hydrolysis by phospholipases. Chemoattractants also stimulate the activity of at least two lipid kinases: phosphatidylinositol-4-phosphate kinase, which resynthesizes PIP_2 (96), and phosphatidylinositol-4,5-biphosphate-3 kinase, which synthesizes the novel polyphosphoinositide phosphatidylinositol-3,4,5-triphosphate (PIP_3) (72, 97). PIP_2 and PIP_3 may play a role in regulation of actin polymerization, as described in Section 4.2.

AA is formed via activation of PLA_2 and functions both directly as a second messenger and as a precursor for other lipid mediators. As a second messenger, AA is an activator of PKC (98). As a precursor, AA can be converted by lipoxygenases into hydroxyeicosatetraenoic acids (HETEs), lipoxins, and LTB_4 (99, 100). These lipids may have feedback regulatory roles on neutrophil function (99–101). A number of studies have shown that chemoattractants trigger only low levels of AA release in the absence of a second stimulus, such as a cytokine (102, reviewed in 31).

4.2   Role of second messengers in chemotaxis

Chemotaxis requires plasma membrane remodelling and phospholipid turnover (reviewed in 10, 103). Part of this requirement is to generate second messengers, although the precise mechanisms of action of second messengers for modulation of chemotaxis remain undefined. However, the modified levels of membrane phospholipids may have a direct effect on the regulation of chemotaxis. The polyphosphoinositide PIP_2 promotes actin polymerization through reactions that dissociate actin from profilin–actin complexes (104) and reactions that inhibit the severing activity of the actin-binding protein, gelsolin (105, 106). When profilin binds to PIP_2, PIP_2 hydrolysis by PLC is inhibited, indicating that profilin acts both as a negative regulator of the PLC signalling pathway and an inhibitor of actin polymerization (107). PIP_2 and elevated intracellular calcium levels occurring after chemoattractant receptor-mediated hydrolysis have been proposed as signals promoting F-actin assembly in chemoattractant-stimulated neutrophils (108). Recent evidence indicates that PIP_3 is also involved in regulating neutrophil F-actin polymerization (109). Since actin polymerization is required for neutrophil chemotaxis, it appears that phosphoinositides are involved in modulating chemotaxis through their effects on actin polymerization.

Exogenous calcium is not required for neutrophil orientation or initiation of chemotaxis (110); however, it may function in modulation of sustained directed motility. The depletion of intracellular calcium with the calcium chelator, quin 2, and removal of exogenous calcium partially inhibit, but do not abrogate, neutrophil chemotaxis (111). Chemoattractant-stimulated neutrophils exhibit rapid oscillations in $[Ca^{2+}]_i$ (112). Transient increases in $[Ca^{2+}]_i$ appear to be required for neutrophil migration on surfaces containing fibronectin, vitronectin, or poly-D-lysine (113, 114). Since fibronectin and vitronectin are extracellular matrix proteins that neutrophils encounter *in vivo*, neutrophils may modify their adhesive properties to these molecules through reactions requiring calcium. Subcellular localized increases in $[Ca^{2+}]_i$ have been observed in neutrophils undergoing chemotaxis and phagocytosis (115, 116), indicating that pseudopod formation may be regulated by increased cytoplasmic solation induced by calcium. Cytoskeletal protein modifications occur through calcium-mediated phosphorylation of actin-binding proteins (reviewed in 11). Several cytoskeletal proteins are phosphorylated in neutrophils during chemoattractant stimulation (reviewed in 11). It remains to be determined whether phosphorylation of these proteins is required for chemotaxis.

Agents that inhibit PLA_2 inhibit neutrophil chemotaxis (103). Although the specificity of the inhibitors used has been questioned (117, 118), some products of PLA_2 activation stimulate chemotaxis (reviewed in 29). The role of these lipoxygenase-generated intermediates in chemoattractant signalling remains unknown. It is possible that they amplify the chemotactic response elicited by external chemoattractants (priming) through interaction with their specific receptors or they may be inactivated or exert effects through incorporation into membrane phospholipids (100, 101, 103).

4.3   Role of second messengers in the respiratory burst

The second messengers generated by chemoattractant-mediated activation of phospholipases clearly participate in regulation of the respiratory burst. As with chemotaxis, the exact mechanisms involved are not yet clear. Cyclic AMP may have a down-modulatory role, since pharmacological means of elevating cAMP in neutrophils inhibit respiratory burst activation by chemoattractants (reviewed in 30, 31, 73). Cyclic AMP exerts its effects through activation of PKA and known targets of this enzyme are considered in Sections 5.3 and 6. Since both chemotaxis and the respiratory burst are inhibited by cAMP agonists (reviewed in 30, 31, 73), it is likely that PKA affects a very early step in the signalling process, perhaps at the level of receptor–G protein interactions. Consistent with this possibility is the demonstration that cAMP agonists inhibit activation of the various phospholipases by chemoattractants (77, 119, reviewed in 31, 72, 73).

Exogenous Ca^{2+} is not required for triggering of the respiratory burst by chemoattractants, but does increase the maximum response (120, reviewed in 71). Buffering of chemoattractant-induced $[Ca^{2+}]_i$ changes blocks activation of the respiratory burst, unless neutrophils have been previously exposed to an activator of PKC, such as PMA (121). Thus, Ca^{2+} may normally participate in the activation of PKC or the activation of PKC may bypass a Ca^{2+}-dependent step necessary for triggering of the respiratory burst.

When added exogenously to neutrophils, cell-permeable DAGs, AA, and certain forms of PA have each been shown to induce activation of the respiratory burst (reviewed in 30, 31), supporting their participation in NADPH oxidase activation by chemoattractants. The intracellular targets for these lipids are not yet clear, although phospholipases, PKC, and components of NADPH oxidase have been implicated (25–28, 98, 122, reviewed in 123, 124). Correlative studies implicate PA as the lipid most closely associated with activation of the respiratory burst (88, 125, 126, reviewed in 123, 124). However, modulatory roles for DAG and AA have also been suggested (88, 122, reviewed in 123, 124). It is likely that activation of NADPH oxidase involves a complex interplay between these lipid mediators and their targets.

5 Protein kinases

5.1 General overview of protein kinases in neutrophils

Neutrophils contain a variety of serine/threonine kinases and several tyrosine kinases (summarized in Table 3.2, reviewed in 127). Many of these are targets for specific second messengers and are likely to be important mediators for transducing the signals generated by chemoattractant–receptor interaction.

Cyclic AMP- and cGMP-dependent protein kinases have been identified in the cytosolic fraction of neutrophils (128, reviewed in 127). Cyclic AMP-dependent kinase substrates include *rap1A* in human neutrophils (129) and actin in rabbit neutrophils (reviewed in 127). Vimentin has been identified as a cGMP-dependent kinase substrate in human neutrophils (130). Immunocytochemical studies indicate that cyclic nucleotide-dependent kinases

Table 3.2 Protein kinases in neutrophils

Class	Activators	References
Serine/threonine		
Protein kinase A	cAMP	127, 128
Cyclic GMP dependent	cGMP	128
Protein kinase C	Diacylglycerol, calcium,	133–136
(isoforms α, β, ζ)	arachidonate, phosphatidic acid	
Calmodulin dependent	Calmodulin, calcium	127
Histone H4 kinase	?	127
Ecto-protein kinase	cAMP, ?	141
Others (e.g. MAP kinase)	?	127, 144, 145
Tyrosine		
p55^{fgr}	?	146
p59^{hck}	?	146
p60^{src}	?	147
Ecto-protein kinase	?	140, 142

appear in specific compartments during neutrophil activation (128). Chemoattractant-stimulated, adherent neutrophils exhibit transient focal changes in cGMP-dependent kinase that coincide with transient shape changes (128). Cyclic nucleotide-dependent kinases may participate in modifications to extracellular as well as intracellular substrates. Neutrophils release 20–50 per cent of the cAMP they generate into the extracellular environment (131).

Protein kinase C is a target for most of the known second messengers generated in neutrophils (e.g. Ca^{2+}, DAG, PA, AA) and thus has received much attention as a mediator of functional responses to chemoattractants. PKC is actually a family of six to eight isoforms that can be divided into two groups: Ca^{2+}-dependent, consisting of α, β_I, β_{II}, and γ; and Ca^{2+}-independent, consisting of δ, ϵ, ζ, and η (reviewed in 132). Recent studies suggest that neutrophils contain predominantly β_{II}, δ, and ζ isoforms, with lower amounts of α and β_I (133–136; McPhail, Sozzani, and Kent, unpublished data). Subcellular fractionation studies indicate that PKC activity is primarily cytosolic in unstimulated neutrophils (reviewed in 30, 31). Stimulation with chemoattractants causes a small and transient increase in membrane-associated PKC activity (133, reviewed in 30, 31); however, the isoform(s) undergoing translocation have not been unambiguously identified. It is likely that translocation of certain isoforms of PKC is necessary for activation by lipids, as well as for access to particular substrates. A few substrates for PKC in neutrophils have been identified, including the NADPH oxidase component p47-*phox*, lipocortins I and II (now known as annexins I and II), the myristoylated protein MARCKS (myristoylated, alanine-rich, C-kinase substrate), and vimentin (127, 137–139). The role that phosphorylation of these proteins by PKC has in regulating their functions is not yet understood.

Upon activation, human neutrophils exhibit at least three ecto-protein kinases (140, 141): one phosphorylates endogenous proteins, a second phosphorylates exogenous substrates in a cAMP-independent manner and is released in the presence of substrate, and a third phosphorylates the cAMP substrate, kemptide, in a cAMP-dependent manner (141). Substrates for neutrophil ecto-protein kinases include a phosphotyrosine-containing 180 kDa protein that is a member of the CD15 family, vitronectin, and basic fibroblast growth factor (141–143). The functional roles of these kinases remain unknown. The variety of endogenous and exogenous substrates for cyclic nucleotide-dependent kinases and ecto-protein kinases indicates that phosphorylation may be critical for cell–cell interactions, cell–matrix interactions, and intracellular regulatory events.

Other serine/threonine protein kinases are also present in neutrophils (reviewed in 127). These enzymes have not been well characterized in neutrophils and their functional roles are unclear. Huang has described an H4 kinase (named because of its preference for histone H4 as substrate) in rabbit neutrophils that is activated by FMLP. Other kinases reported to be present include Ca^{2+}/calmodulin-dependent protein kinase II, casein kinases, protamine kinases, and mitogen-associated protein kinase [MAP kinase, also known as microtubule-associated kinase or extracellular signal-regulated kinase (ERK)] (127, 144, 145).

Protein tyrosine kinases are emerging as important regulators of cell growth (reviewed in 146) and are divided into two families: cell–surface receptors (e.g. epidermal growth factor receptor) and intracellular tyrosine kinases, typified by the proto-oncogene c-*src*. Neutrophils contain three intracellular protein tyrosine kinases that are members of the *src* gene family including, p60^{src}, p59^{hck}, and p55^{fgr} (147, reviewed in 146). Expression of these kinases is substantially increased during myeloid differentiation (148). The *src* family of protein tyrosine kinases share common structural properties that probably determine their function. These properties include: (i) covalently linked myristate at their N termini, which may be partly responsible for their membrane associations; (ii) a central domain with structural homology (SH2 and SH3 regions) to an isoform of phosphatidylinositol (PI)-specific phospholipase C (PLC-γ), which may mediate interaction with growth factor receptors and/or the cytoskeleton; and (iii) ATP-binding motifs and two major tyrosine phosphorylation sites in the kinase domain that are involved in autophosphorylation (reviewed in 146, see also 85). Chemoattractant-stimulated neutrophils demonstrate a translocation of p55^{fgr} from secondary granules to the plasma membrane (147). The functional significance of this translocation and specific substrates for these kinases in neutrophils remains to be determined. Several studies have demonstrated that chemoattractant-stimulated neutrophils rapidly phosphorylate a variety of proteins on tyrosine residues (127, 144, 145, 149–154). Some of the substrates that have been identified include lipomodulin (lipocortin or annexins I and II) (127), *src*-like tyrosine kinase (149), and MAP kinase (145). The precise functional roles of most of these proteins and the effects of tyrosine phosphorylation on their activities remain unknown.

Neutrophils also contain protein phosphatases that dephosphorylate either tyrosine or serine/threonine residues (155–157). The plasma membrane protein tyrosine phosphatase CD45 may regulate chemotaxis and is discussed in Section 5.2. Serine/threonine phosphatases with specificity for the p47-*phox* component of NADPH oxidase have recently been described (157), but a functional role for this activity is not yet known.

5.2 Role of phosphorylation events in chemotaxis

Studies using pharmacologic inhibitors of protein kinases have provided indirect evidence that protein kinases are involved in neutrophil chemotaxis.

Neutrophil chemotaxis is inhibited in a concentration-dependent manner when cells are pre-treated with isoquinolinesulphonamides (158, 159), compounds that competitively bind to the ATP substrate site of mammalian protein kinases and inhibit phosphorylation by serine/threonine kinases. The inhibitory action is not due to an effect on adherence or chemoattractant–receptor binding (158). Erbstatin, a protein tyrosine kinase inhibitor, abolishes random and chemotactic migration and neutrophil adherence to serum-coated surfaces (160). These observations suggest that serine/threonine and tyrosine protein kinases are involved in neutrophil motility.

Neutrophils contain the abundant protein tyrosine phosphatase, leukocyte common antigen (CD45) (reviewed in 161). CD45 is expressed on the plasma membrane of all leukocytes. The cytoplasmic domain contains two tandem subdomains of 300 amino acids and has protein tyrosine phosphatase activity (162). CD45 is found on the plasma membranes of neutrophils and intracellularly is associated with tertiary and secondary granules (163). Monoclonal antibodies to selected CD45 epitopes significantly inhibit neutrophil chemotaxis to LTB_4 and C5a, but do not inhibit neutrophil superoxide production (164). These observations suggest that epitopes of neutrophil CD45 may interact with LTB_4 and C5a receptors or receptor-associated molecules and may regulate chemotactic responses. It remains to be determined whether the effects on chemotaxis are related to CD45 protein tyrosine phosphatase activity.

5.3   Role of phosphorylation events in the respiratory burst

A variety of studies indicate that protein kinases and protein phosphorylation events are important for activation of the respiratory burst by chemoattractants in neutrophils. In general, approaches have been correlative and have relied heavily on the use of pharmacological agents. These studies have been well reviewed recently (30, 31, 165, 166) and are summarized briefly here. Virtually all chemoattractants induce an increase in phosphorylation of many neutrophil proteins and the increase in several of these precedes activation of the respiratory burst, supporting a cause-and-effect relationship (30, 31, 165, 166). Several phosphoproteins that are either NADPH oxidase components or may regulate the activation mechanism have been identified. These include: (i) p47-*phox*, a substrate for PKC and PKA (137, 167); (ii) cytochrome b_{558} (168); and (iii) *rap1A*, a substrate for PKA (129). Phosphorylation of *rap1A* by PKA modifies the interaction of *rap1A* with cytochrome b_{558} (57); however, the functional effect of this interaction is not known. Effects of phosphorylation on the function of either p47-*phox* or cytochrome b_{558} are unknown.

Variable results have been obtained with protein kinase inhibitors (30,

31, 166, 167), indicating both the lack of specificity for a particular kinase of most inhibitors as well as the possibility of cross-talk between protein kinases. Thus, the observed effect of an inhibitor cannot be interpreted if more than one target for the inhibitor is present and/or if different inhibitor-sensitive kinases regulate the functional response measured. However, a variety of protein kinase inhibitors, with varying specificities, reduce activation of the respiratory burst by chemoattractants (30, 31, 166). This suggests that protein phosphorylation reactions mediate activation of NADPH oxidase, although the identity of the kinases involved cannot yet be ascertained. It is clear that new approaches for this problem are needed. A possibility is the use of newly described inhibitory synthetic peptides (pseudosubstrates), which compete at substrate-binding sites on specific protein kinases (169). A limitation of this approach is that the peptides are unable to cross the plasma membrane, requiring the use of permeabilized cells or microinjection. Genetic approaches are also possible; however, neutrophils *in vitro* are not amenable to such manipulations. A cell-free system for NADPH oxidase activation that is dependent on phosphorylation would be the most useful approach. Although PKC-dependent activation of NADPH oxidase in a cell-free system has been reported (166), activation does not require p47-*phox* and the level of oxidase activity achieved is too low for practical use.

6 Cell-free system for NADPH oxidase activation

The development of a cell-free system for achieving the activation of NADPH oxidase has led to major advances in identifying the components of the enzyme system and in understanding the mechanisms involved in the activation process. Cell-free activation was first reported in cell homogenates initiated by the addition of unsaturated fatty acids, such as AA (25–28). Bromberg and Pick (170) later reported that the anionic detergent sodium dodecyl sulphate (SDS) could substitute for AA. Of immediate interest was the observation that cytosolic proteins were necessary in order to achieve NADPH oxidase activation in the cell-free system (25–28). It was then discovered that certain patients with CGD were missing the cytosolic activity (171, 172). This directly led to the identification and subsequent cloning of two cytosolic proteins, p47-*phox* and p67-*phox*, each of which can cause CGD if absent (24, reviewed in 2, 3, 31).

Both cytosolic proteins partially translocate to membrane-containing fractions upon stimulation of intact cells (4, reviewed in 2, 3, 31) or in the cell-free system (124, 173, 174). Translocation of both proteins depends on the presence of p47-*phox* and does not occur in the absence of cytochrome b_{558} in the membrane (124, 174). This and other data (reviewed in 2, 3, 124) suggest that the two cytosolic proteins exist as a complex and that translocation involves stable binding between p47-*phox* and the C-terminal region of the large subunit of cytochrome b_{558}. It is not yet known whether the cytosolic proteins are part of the active NADPH oxidase complex.

The predicted primary sequence of both cytosolic proteins contains two repeats with similarity to a region known as SH3, found in the sequence for the protein tyrosine kinase $p60^{src}$, as well as that of a number of other proteins involved in cellular regulation (24, 85). Recent evidence suggests that this region may be involved in interaction of proteins with the cytoskeleton (85). Interestingly, p67-*phox* is reported to be cytoskeletal-associated in unstimulated neutrophils (175, 176) and activation of NADPH oxidase by chemoattractants is markedly enhanced by disruption of the cytoskeleton (17, 23). One can speculate that interaction of p67-*phox* with the cytoskeleton via SH3 regions prevents chemoattractant-triggered assembly of an active NADPH oxidase. However, stimulation of neutrophils with the PKC activator PMA results in association of the active NADPH oxidase with the cytoskeleton (175, 176). Thus, the roles of the cytoskeleton and the SH3 regions of the cytosolic components may vary with the stimulus used for NADPH oxidase activation.

The predicted sequence of p47-*phox* also contains a number of potential phosphorylation sites and is multiply phosphorylated during stimulation of neutrophils by FMLP (reviewed in 2, 3, 31). Inhibition of p47-*phox* phosphorylation does not prevent activation of the respiratory burst by chemoattractants (reviewed in 1, 31, 166), suggesting that phosphorylation of this protein is not required. However, it is possible that the inhibitor caused activation of a pathway that bypasses the requirement for phosphorylation of p47-*phox*. Phosphorylation of p47-*phox* occurs in the cell-free system during NADPH oxidase activation (172); however, enzyme activation can occur in the absence of ATP (177, 178, reviewed in 1–3, 31), suggesting that phosphorylation is not required for the activation process. Perhaps the pathway of activation utilized by chemoattractants in the presence of protein kinase inhibitors (reviewed in 1, 31, 166) operates in the cell-free system.

The cell-free system has also revealed a requirement for monomeric G proteins in the activation mechanism. Activation of NADPH oxidase in the cell-free system requires guanine nucleotides (177, 178, reviewed in 1–3, 31) and is inhibited by antibodies to the monomeric G protein *rap1A* (54). *Rap1A* co-purifies with cytochrome b_{558} (53), indicating it binds to this NADPH oxidase component. Binding can be disrupted by PKA-mediated phosphorylation of *rap1A* (57), although the functional consequences of the dissociation are unknown. In addition, another monomeric G protein has been implicated in the activation mechanism. Initial purification studies of cytosolic factor activity showed that a third component, other than p47-*phox* and p67-*phox*, was present (reviewed in 179). The third component has recently been identified by two laboratories (55, 56) as a monomeric G protein, *rac*. Each laboratory purified a different isoform of *rac—rac1* or *rac2*; however these two proteins share 92 per cent identity (48) and may be functionally interchangeable. One laboratory (55) also reported that a protein identical to *rho* GDI (guanine nucleotide dissociation inhibitor) co-purified with *rac*. *Rac* is in the Rho family, so it is possible that *rho* GDI will be effective on *rac*. These results suggest that a monomeric G protein may orchestrate the assembly and/or activation of NADPH oxidase.

The signal or signals that induces the assembly/activation process is still unknown. It is conceivable that lipids generated as second messengers in the cell are the direct signals. This is supported by the observations that either AA or PA triggers NADPH oxidase activation in the cell-free system (25–28, reviewed in 123) and that DAG can synergize with either SDS or PA (122, 124, reviewed in 123). The targets for these lipids in the cell-free system have not been identified and could be either *rap1A* or *rac* (or GDI), an NADPH oxidase component, or an unidentified intermediate. NADPH oxidase activation was recently achieved with SDS in a highly purified reconstitution system, using only cytochrome b_{558}, p47-*phox*, p67-*phox*, and *rac1* plus GDI (179). This makes it unlikely that an unidentified intermediate is the target for SDS; however, it is still possible that different lipids have separate targets. A speculative model summarizing the assembly/activation process is shown in Fig. 3.5.

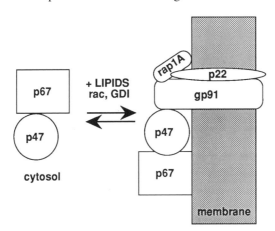

Fig. 3.5 Model for activation of NADPH oxidase. The phospholipase-mediated generation of second messenger lipids, such as PA, DAG, and AA, may directly initiate the assembly of an active NADPH oxidase enzyme in the membrane. Assembly requires the translocation of the cytosolic NADPH oxidase components, p47-*phox* and p67-*phox*, to the membrane-associated heterodimeric cytochrome b_{558} (p22 + gp91). Activation may require the participation of two additional proteins: *rac*, a 28 kDa monomeric G protein, and GDI, a 28 kDa inhibitor of GDP dissociation. Another monomeric G protein, *rap1A*, interacts with cytochrome b_{558}. The functions of the monomeric G proteins and GDI in the activation mechanism are unknown.

7   Cytoskeletal changes in actin during chemoattractant activation

The reversible assembly of G-actin into F-actin provides neutrophils with a dynamic architectural framework to explore the extracellular environment and shuttle receptors and their associated ligands to specific compartments. Rapid oscillations in actin polymerization and depolymerization have been observed during the initial seconds of neutrophil chemoattractant exposure (180, 181). Chemoattractant receptor–ligand complexes appear to rapidly associate with the neutrophil cytoskeleton through reactions requiring F-actin (182). The receptors translocate to actin- and fodrin-rich plasma membrane microdomains when they are in a high affinity state (183). This translocation is postulated to compartmentalize the receptors and regulate their interaction with G proteins.

Nucleation (the assembly of short actin polymers that support elongation) is the major rate-limiting step in actin polymerization (reviewed in 9, 108). The actin nuclei establish locations within the cell where actin polymerization proceeds by linear condensation reactions at ends of the filaments. The ends of actin filaments are structurally and kinetically distinct: the 'barbed' end has a higher affinity for G-actin and has a more rapid on-rate for actin monomers than the 'pointed' end. A variety of actin-binding proteins control the linear assembly of actin. Two of them, gelsolin and profilin, reversibly interact with actin and membrane phospholipids, and move between the cytoplasm and the cytoplasmic face of the plasma membrane (108). Profilin binds to actin monomers and inhibits their polymerization into actin filaments. Profilin is released from actin monomers within 10 s of neutrophil chemoattractant stimulation and reassociates with actin within 20 s after the stimulus is removed (184). The reversible association of profilin and actin is only partially responsible for the total change in F-actin content of chemoattractant-stimulated neutrophils (184). Gelsolin, a calcium-sensitive actin-binding protein, may promote actin assembly or disassembly, depending upon the calcium concentration and its interaction with polyphosphoinositides (reviewed in 185). In resting neutrophils, most of the gelsolin exists as a 1:1 gelsolin–actin monomer complex (185). The actin-complexed gelsolin is significantly decreased in neutrophils within 5 s after chemoattractant stimulation and corresponds with the appearance of barbed-end nucleating activity and an increase in F-actin content (185). These findings illustrate that gelsolin and profilin regulate neutrophil actin polymerization.

Migrating neutrophils, responding to chemoattractant while they are attached to a substratum, have multiple signals triggering actin polymerization. Actin polymerization is stimulated in neutrophils during their adherence to a surface (186). Adherence-elicited F-actin responses differ from chemoattractant-elicited actin polymerization in several ways. Adherence-induced responses are not sensitive to pertussis toxin inhibition, the adherence responses appear to be dependent upon extracellular calcium, and the kinetics of F-actin assembly proceed more slowly than chemoattractant-elicited actin polymerization (186). The chemoattractant-elicited F-actin responses are rapid, transient, pertussis toxin-sensitive, and do not require exogenous calcium (reviewed in 11). Chemoattractant-stimulated neutrophils contain two populations of F-actin: one population, found in the lamellipodia, is labile and turns over rapidly during stimulation, whereas, the second population, in the cortical region, is relatively stable (187). It is likely that neutrophil interaction with extracellular matrix proteins and adhesion molecules will also trigger neutrophil F-actin responses.

The actin filament system and its actin-binding proteins have been associated with phosphoinositide kinase, diacylglycerol kinase and PLC activities in human epidermoid A431 cells (188). Stimulation of the cells with epidermal growth factor significantly enhanced the association of these lipid kinases with the microfilamentous cytoskeleton. It is possible that similar associations will be found in chemoattractant-stimulated neutrophils.

8   Common and divergent pathways in chemotaxis and the respiratory burst

8.1   Common pathways

Chemotaxis and the respiratory burst clearly share portions of the signal transductional machinery. Initiation of both responses proceeds via chemoattractant binding to its receptor and subsequent participation of one or more pertussis toxin-sensitive G proteins. It is likely that both pathways involve the activation of phospholipases, the generation of second messengers, the mobilization of calcium and the activation of protein kinases. However, as summarized in the previous sections, most details of the mechanisms involved are still not clear.

8.2   Divergent pathways

A variety of studies indicate that differences exist in the signalling mechanisms that trigger chemotaxis and the respiratory burst. Certain pharmacologic agents differentially affect the two responses. General inhibitors of protein kinases, such as the isoquinolinesulphonamides, reversibly inhibit neutrophil chemotaxis to *N*-formyl peptides and C5a, but do not inhibit the respiratory burst under similar conditions (158). These results suggest that the kinases controlling migration and the respiratory burst are different.

Studies using agents that affect cytoskeletal function provide some of the clearest evidence for divergence of pathways regulating chemotaxis and the respiratory burst. Disruption of actin polymerization by cytochalasins or botulinum C_2 toxin enhances chemoattractant activation of the respiratory burst (17, 23, 189), but completely inhibits neutrophil migration (16, 17). Thus, actin polymerization is essential for migration of neutrophils, but is not required for activation of the respiratory burst. Possibly, actin polymerization downregulates NADPH oxidase assembly and/or induces disassembly.

Direct evidence for divergence of regulatory events required for neutrophil chemotaxis and the respiratory burst has come from studies using oxidized *N*-formyl peptide ligands (190). The sulphoxide and sulphone derivatives of FMLP bind to human neutrophils with lower affinity than parent, nonoxidized FMLP. The oxidized derivatives trigger the oxidative burst; however, neither activates neutrophil chemotaxis. Neutrophils exposed to saturating concentrations of the oxidized FMLP derivatives exhibit normal chemotactic responsiveness to C5a, indicating that the oxidized derivatives do not directly inhibit chemotaxis. The differences in the responses elicited by oxidized FMLP derivatives and the nonoxidized, parent FMLP suggest that binding affinity regulates the events occurring after receptor–ligand engagement.

8.3   Chemoattractant divergence

Chemoattractants are selective in their effectiveness for triggering chemotaxis and the respiratory burst. The relative chemoattractant effectiveness for neutrophil chemotaxis and the respiratory burst is summarized below (29, 59, 60, 84).

$$\text{Chemotaxis: IL-8} \geqslant \text{LTB}_4 \geqslant \text{C5a} \geqslant \text{FMLP} \gg \text{PAF}$$
$$\text{Respiratory burst: FMLP} > \text{C5a} \gg \text{PAF} \approx \text{IL-8} \approx \text{LTB}_4$$

IL-8 and LTB_4 are among the most potent and effective molecules for eliciting chemotaxis, but they are poor stimuli of the respiratory burst. FMLP, the most potent chemoattractant stimulus of the respiratory burst, is generated exogenously by invading bacteria, whereas the other chemoattractants are generated endogenously. This chemoattractant divergence suggests that endogenously generated chemoattractants effectively function to recruit neutrophils to inflammatory sites with minimal direct activation of the respiratory burst, possibly to prevent oxidative damage to host tissue and neutrophils during their migratory response (see Chapter 7 for discussion of neutrophil-induced tissue injury). In contrast, chemoattractants generated by invading micro-organisms, are potent stimuli of chemotaxis and oxidative metabolism, which are both required for effective neutrophil recruitment and microbicidal activity *in vivo*. Chemoattractant divergence may be related to the structural differences in chemoattractant receptors which contribute to the receptor's subsequent interactions with G proteins and cytoskeletal proteins and ultimately affect neutrophil physiologic responses.

Qualitative differences in neutrophil chemotactic responses to FMLP and LTB$_4$ have been observed. Neutrophils treated with isoquinoline-sulphonamide or forskolin do not migrate to FMLP, but do migrate to LTB$_4$ (131, 158). Monoclonal antibodies to selected epitopes of CD45 inhibit neutrophil chemotaxis to LTB$_4$, but have little or no effect on neutrophil chemotaxis to FMLP (164). These findings indicate that the activation pathways of neutrophil chemotaxis to FMLP and LTB$_4$ diverge. The second messenger responses of LTB$_4$-stimulated neutrophils are of lower magnitude and shorter duration than FMLP-stimulated neutrophils, possibly because *N*-formyl peptide receptors activate greater quantities of common G proteins than LTB$_4$ receptors in neutrophils (191). It remains to be determined whether structural differences in the *N*-formyl peptide and LTB$_4$ receptors will account for the quantitative and qualitative differences in G protein activation.

8.4 Interaction between chemotaxis and the respiratory burst

Although neutrophil chemotaxis and the respiratory burst are distinct functions, biochemical components of these processes may affect each other's activity. Normal neutrophils demonstrate deactivation (decrease) of their chemotactic response when exposed to high concentrations of chemotactic ligand (see Fig. 3.6, normal neutrophil response). Chemotactic deactivation typically occurs at chemotactic concentrations (10^{-7}–10^{-8} M) that maximally activate the respiratory burst. Some evidence suggests that products of the respiratory burst may be involved in chemotactic deactivation (192). Neutrophils from CGD patients are less sensitive to chemotactic deactivation (Fig. 3.6), suggesting that auto-oxidative neutrophil damage may be a component of chemotactic deactivation. Maximal stimulation of the respiratory burst, thus appears to downregulate neutrophil chemotaxis.

In contrast, prior exposure of neutrophils to chemotactic concentrations of chemoattractants enhances the magnitude of the respiratory burst in response to a second unrelated stimulus (193–196). This phenomenon is termed priming and the molecular basis for it is not yet clear. At least two mechanisms of priming have been proposed. The first focuses on an alteration in one or more signal transductional pathways. One feature of priming is that the onset of the respiratory burst in response to the second stimulus

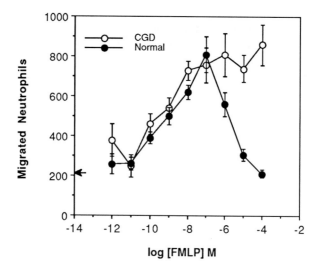

Fig. 3.6 Chemotactic responses of normal and CGD neutrophils to the *N*-formyl peptide, FMLP. Normal (●) and CGD (○) neutrophil migration through polycarbonate membrane was evaluated in a microwell chemotaxis assay chamber as previously described by Harvath *et al.* (190). The bars represent one SD of triplicate observations and the arrow indicates the random migration response to medium alone.

is more rapid (196), suggesting that a necessary step in the signalling pathway has already been accomplished by the priming stimulus. This step could be the translocation of PKC, based on studies indicating that chemoattractants increase the amount of membrane-associated PKC (197, 198). Another possible mechanism is an increase in the amount of NADPH oxidase components present in the cell due to chemoattractant-mediated enhancement of either transcription or translation. A recent report showed that FMLP enhances total mRNA and protein synthesis in human neutrophils (199). However, priming by FMLP occurs very rapidly (196), making it unlikely that effects on mRNA or protein synthesis are responsible. Further studies are needed to determine the mechanisms of priming.

9   Conclusions

In this chapter, we have summarized some of the signal transduction processes that occur in neutrophils in response to chemoattractants during triggering of oxidative metabolism and chemotaxis. The steps involved in the complex signalling process are becoming clearer, although much remains to be learned. An important recent development is the cloning of many of the chemoattractant receptors, which will allow structure–

function studies to be performed at the molecular level. Also, the development of a cell-free system for activation of the respiratory burst enzyme system has provided extraordinary insights into the molecular nature of the enzyme and how it may be activated. Finally, evidence has emerged that neutrophils release components of the signalling cascade, such as protein kinases and cAMP, to their exterior during chemoattractant stimulation. These released components may participate in biochemical modifications of membrane or extracellular matrix molecules which regulate subsequent neutrophil signalling and responses. Patients, such as the case described in this chapter, have contributed to our knowledge of the signal transduction process. As detailed in Chapter 8, these patients are also beginning to reap the benefits of this knowledge.

10 Acknowledgements

The authors appreciate the editorial comments of Drs J. Vostal and E. Bonvini. We thank the editors, Drs Gary Wheeler and Jon Abramson, for their helpful suggestions and, in particular, Jon, for the clinical description of CGD. Research by L.C.M. was supported by National Institutes of Health grant AI-22564.

References

1 Segal, A. W. (1989). The electron transport chain of the microbicidal oxidase of phagocytic cells and its involvement in the molecular pathology of chronic granulomatous disease. *J. Clin. Invest.*, **83**, 1785–93.

2 Clark, R. A. (1990). The human neutrophil respiratory burst oxidase. *J. Infect. Dis.*, **161**, 1140–7.

3 Smith, R. M. and Curnutte, J. T. (1991). Molecular basis of chronic granulomatous disease. *Blood*, **77**, 673–86.

4 Ambruso, D. R., Bolscher, B. G. J. M., Stokman, P. M., Verhoeven, A. J., and Roos, D. (1990). Assembly and activation of the NADPH:O_2 oxidoreductase in human neutrophils after stimulation with phorbol myristate acetate. *J. Biol. Chem.*, **265**, 924–30.

5 Francke, U., Ochs, H. D., deMartinville, B., Giacalone, J., Lindgren, V., Disteche, C., *et al.* (1985). Minor Xp21 chromosome deletion in a male associated with expression of Duchenne muscular dystrophy, chronic granulomatous disease, retinitis pigmentosa, and McLeod syndrome. *Am. J. Hum. Genet.*, **37**, 250–67.

6 Francke, U., Hsieh, C.-L., Foellmer, B. E., Lomax, K. J., Malech, H. L., and Leto, T. L. (1990). Genes for two autosomal recessive

forms of chronic granulomatous disease assigned to 1q25 (*NCF2*) and 7q11.23 (*NCF1*). *Am. J. Hum. Genet.*, **47**, 483–92.

7 Clark R. A., Malech, H. L., Gallin, J. I., Nunoi, H., Volpp, B. D., Pearson, D. W., *et al.* (1989). Genetic variants of chronic granulomatous disease: prevalence of deficiencies of two cytosolic components of the NADPH oxidase system. *N. Engl. J. Med.*, **321**, 647–52.

8 Devreotes, P. N. and Zigmond, S. H. (1988). Chemotaxis in eukaryotic cells: A focus on leukocytes and Dictyostelium. *Annu. Rev. Cell Biol.*, **4**, 649–86.

9 Cassimeris, L. and Zigmond, S. H. (1990). Chemoattractant stimulation of polymorphonuclear leukocyte locomotion. *Sem. Cell Biol.*, **1**, 125–34.

10 Singer, S. J. and Kupfer, A. (1986). The directed migration of eukaryotic cells. *Annu. Rev. Cell Biol.*, **2**, 337–65.

11 Omann, G. M., Allen, R. A., Bokach, G. M., Painter, R. G., Traynor, A. E., and Sklar, L. A. (1987). Signal transduction and cytoskeletal activation in the neutrophil. *Physiol. Rev.*, **67**, 285–322.

12 Howard, T. H. and Oresajo, C. O. (1985). The kinetics of chemotactic peptide-induced change in F-actin content, F-actin distribution, and the shape of neutrophil. *J. Cell Biol.*, **101**, 1078–85.

13 Watts, R. G., Crispens, M. A., and Howard, T. H. (1991). A quantitative study of the role of F-actin in producing neutrophil shape. *Cell Motil. Cytoskel.*, **19**, 159–68.

14 Southwick, F. S. and Stossel, T. P. (1983). Contractile proteins in leukocyte function. *Semin. Hematol.*, **20**, 305–21.

15 Stossel, T. P., Chaponnier, C., Ezzell, R. M., Hartwig, J. H., Janmey, P. A., Kwiathkowski, D. J., *et al.* (1985). Nonmuscle actin-binding proteins. *Annu. Rev. Cell Biol.*, **1**, 353–402.

16 Zigmond, S. H. and Hirsch, J. G. (1972). Effects of cytochalasin B on polymorphonuclear leukocyte locomotion, phagocytosis and glycolysis. *Exp. Cell Res.*, **73**, 383–93.

17 Norgauer, J., Kownatzki, E., Seifert, R., and Aktories, K. (1988). Botulinum C2 toxin ADP-ribosylates actin and enhances O_2^- production and secretion but inhibits migration of activated human neutrophils. *J. Clin. Invest.*, **82**, 1376–82.

18 Boxer, L. A., Hedley-Whyte, E. T., and Stossel, T. P. (1974). Neutrophil actin dysfunction and abnormal neutrophil behavior. *N. Engl. J. Med.*, **291**, 1093–9.

19 Southwick, F. S., Dabiri, G. A., and Stossel, T. P. (1988). Neutrophil actin dysfunction is a genetic disorder associated with partial impairment of neutrophil actin assembly in three family members. *J. Clin. Invest.*, **82**, 1525–31.

20 Coates, T. D., Torkildson, J. C., Torres, M., Church, J. A., and

Howard, T. H. (1991). An inherited defect of neutrophil motility and microfilamentous cytoskeleton associated with abnormalities in 47 kDa and 89 kDa proteins. *Blood*, **78**, 1338–46.

21 Curnutte, J. T. and Babior, B. M. (1987). Chronic granulomatous disease. In *Advances in human genetics* (ed. H. Harris and K. Hirchhorn), vol. 16, pp. 229–97. Plenum Press, New York.

22 Weiss, S. J. (1989). Tissue destruction by neutrophils. *N. Engl. J. Med.*, **320**, 365–76.

23 McPhail, L. C. and Snyderman, R. (1983). Activation of the respiratory burst enzyme in human polymorphonuclear leukocytes by chemoattractants and other soluble stimuli. *J. Clin. Invest.*, **72**, 192–200.

24 Leto, T. L., Lomax, K. G., Volpp, B.D., Nunoi, H., Sechler, J. M. B., Nauseef, W. M., *et al.* (1990). Cloning of a 67-kD neutrophil oxidase factor with similarity to a noncatalytic region of p60$^{c\text{-src}}$. *Science*, **248**, 727–30.

25 Bromberg, Y. and Pick, E. (1984). Unsaturated fatty acids stimulate NADPH-dependent superoxide production by cell-free system derived from macrophages. *Cell. Immunol.*, **88**, 213–21.

26 Heyneman, R. A. and Vercauteren, R. E. (1984). Activation of a NADPH oxidase from horse polymorphonuclear leukocytes in a cell-free system. *J. Leuk. Biol.*, **36**, 751–9.

27 Curnutte, J. T. (1985). Activation of human neutrophil nicotinamide adenine dinucleotide phosphate, reduced (triphosphopyridine nucleotide, reduced) oxidase by arachidonic acid in a cell-free system. *J. Clin. Invest.*, **75**, 1740–3.

28 McPhail, L. C., Shirley, P. S., Clayton, C. C., and Snyderman, R. (1985). Activation of the respiratory burst enzyme from human neutrophils in a cell-free system: evidence for a soluble cofactor. *J. Clin. Invest.*, **75**, 1735–9.

29 Harvath, L. (1991). Neutrophil chemotactic factors. In *Cell motility factors* (ed. I. D. Goldberg), pp. 35–52. Birkhauser Verlag, Basel, Switzerland.

30 Lambeth, J. D. (1988). Activation of the respiratory burst in neutrophils: on the role of membrane-derived second messengers, Ca^{++}, and protein kinase C. *J. Bioenerg. Biomembr.*, **20**, 709–33.

31 McPhail, L. C., Strum, S. L., Leone, P. A., and Sozzani, S. (1992). The neutrophil respiratory burst mechanism. In *Granulocyte responses to cytokines: basic and clinical research* (ed. R. Coffey), pp. 47–76. Marcel Dekker Inc., New York.

32 Boulay, F., Tardif, M., Brouchon, L., and Vignais, P. (1990). Synthesis and use of a novel N-formyl peptide derivative to isolate a human N-formyl peptide receptor cDNA. *Biochem. Biophys. Res. Commun.*, **168**, 1103–9.

33 Boulay, F., Tardif, M., Brouchon, L., and Vignais, P. (1990). The

human N-formyl peptide receptor. Characterization of two cDNA isolates and evidence for a new subfamily of G-protein-coupled receptors. *Biochemistry,* **29,** 11123–33.

34 Gerard, N. P. and Gerard, C. (1991). The chemotactic receptor for human C5a anaphylatoxin. *Nature,* **349,** 614–17.

35 Boulay, F., Mery, L., Tardif, M., Brouchon, L., and Vignais, P. (1991). Expression cloning of a receptor for C5a anaphylatoxin on differentiated HL-60 cells. *Biochemistry,* **30,** 2993–9.

36 Honda, Z.-i., Nakamura, M., Miki, I., Minami, M., Watanabe, T., Seyama, Y., *et al.* (1991). Cloning and functional expression of platelet-activating factor receptor from guinea-pig lung. *Nature,* **349,** 342–6.

37 Ye, R. D., Prossnitz, E. R., Zou, A., and Cochrane, C. G. (1991). Characterization of a human cDNA that encodes a functional receptor for platelet activating factor. *Biochem. Biophys. Res. Commun.,* **180,** 105–11.

38 Nakamura, M., Honda, Z.-i., Izumi, T., Sakanaka, C., Mutoh, H., Minami, M., *et al.* (1991). Molecular cloning and expression of platelet-activating factor receptor from human leukocytes. *J. Biol. Chem.,* **266,** 20400–5.

39 Holmes, W. E., Lee, J., Kuang, W.-J., Rice, G. C., Wood, W. I. (1991). Structure and functional expression of a human interleukin-8 receptor. *Science,* **253,** 1278–80.

40 Murphy, P. M. and Tiffany, H. L. (1991). Cloning of complementary DNA encoding a functional human interleukin-8 receptor. *Science,* **253,** 1280–3.

41 Thomas, K. M., Taylor, L., and Navarro, J. (1991). The interleukin-8 receptor is encoded by a neutrophil-specific cDNA clone, F3R. *J. Biol. Chem.,* **266,** 14839–41.

42 Beckmann, M. P., Munger, W. E., Kozlosky, C., VandenBos, T., Price, V., Lyman, S., *et al.* (1991). Molecular characterization of the interleukin-8 receptor. *Biochem. Biophys. Res. Commun.,* **179,** 784–9.

43 Bourne, H. R., Sanders, D. A., and McCormick, F. (1990). The GTPase superfamily: a conserved switch for diverse cell functions. *Nature,* **348,** 125–32.

44 Bokoch, G. M. (1990). Signal transduction by GTP binding proteins during leukocyte activation: phagocytic cells. *Curr. Top. Membr. Transp.,* **35,** 65–101.

45 Evans, T., Hart, M. J., and Cerione, R. A. (1991). The Ras super-families: regulatory proteins and post-translational modifications. *Curr. Opin. Cell Biol.,* **3,** 185–91.

46 Volpp, B. D., Nauseef, W. M., and Clark, R. A. (1989). Subcellular distribution and membrane association of human neutrophil sub-

strates for ADP-ribosylation by pertussis toxin and cholera toxin. *J. Immunol.*, **142**, 3206–12.

47 Rudolph, U., Koesling, D., Hinsch, K.-D., Seifert, R., Bigalke, M., Schultz, G., and Rosenthal, W. (1989). G-protein α-subunits in cytosolic and membranous fractions of human neutrophils. *Mol. Cell. Endocrinol.*, **63**, 143–53.

48 Didsbury, J., Weber, R. J., Bokoch, G. M., Evans, T., and Snyderman, R. (1989). *Rac,* a novel *ras*-related family of proteins that are botulinum toxin substrates. *J. Biol. Chem.*, **264**, 16378–82.

49 Dexter, D., Rubins, J. B., Manning, E. C., Khachatrian, L., and Dickey, B. F. (1990). Compartmentalization of low molecular mass GTP-binding proteins among neutrophil secretory granules. *J. Immunol.*, **145**, 1845–50.

50 Philips, M. R., Abramson, S. B., Kolasinski, S. L., Haines, K. A., Weissmann, G., and Rosenfeld, M. G. (1991). Low molecular weight GTP-binding proteins in human neutrophil granule membranes. *J. Biol. Chem.*, **266**, 1289–98.

51 Polakis, P. G., Evans, T., and Snyderman, R. (1989). Multiple chromatographic forms of the formyl peptide chemoattractant receptor and their relationship to GTP-binding proteins. *Biochem. Biophys. Res. Commun.*, **161**, 276–83.

52 Rollins, T. E., Siciliano, S., Kobayashi, S., Cianciarulo, D. N., Bonilla-Argudo, V., Collier, K., and Springer, M. S. (1991). Purification of the active C5a receptor from human polymorphonuclear leukocytes as a receptor-G_i complex. *Proc. Natl Acad. Sci. USA*, **88**, 971–5.

53 Quinn, M. T., Parkos, C. A., Walker, L., Orkin, S. H., Dinauer, M. C., and Jesaitis, A. J. (1989). Association of a ras-related protein with cytochrome b of human neutrophils. *Nature*, **342**, 198–200.

54 Eklund, E. A., Marshall, M., Gibbs, J. B., Crean, C. D., and Gabig, T. G. (1991). Resolution of a low molecular weight G protein in neutrophil cytosol required for NADPH oxidase activation and reconstitution by recombinant Krev-1 protein. *J. Biol. Chem.*, **266**, 13964–70.

55 Abo, A., Pick, E., Hall, A., Totty, N., Teahan, C. G., and Segal, A. W. (1991). Activation of the NADPH oxidase involves the small GTP-binding protein $p21^{rac1}$. *Nature*, **353**, 668–70.

56 Knaus, U. G., Heyworth, P. G., Evans, T., Curnutte, J. T., and Bokoch, G. M. (1991). Regulation of phagocyte oxygen radical production by the GTP-binding protein Rac 2. *Science*, **254**, 1512–15.

57 Bokoch, G. M., Quilliam, L. A., Bohl, B. P., Jesaitis, A. J., and Quinn, M. T. (1991). Inhibition of rap1A binding to cytochrome b_{558} of NADPH oxidase by phosphorylation of rap1A. *Science*, **254**, 1794–6.

58 Morii, N., Kawano, K., Sekine, A., Yamada, T., and Narumiya, S. (1991). Purification of GTPase activating protein specific for the *rho* gene products. *J. Biol. Chem.*, **266**, 7646–50.

59 Verghese, M. W., Charles, L., Jakoi, L., Dillon, S. B., and Snyderman, R. (1987). Role of a guanine nucleotide regulatory protein in the activation of phospholipase C by different chemoattractants. *J. Immunol.*, **138**, 4374–80.

60 Thelen, M., Peveri, P., Kernen, P., von Tscharner, V., Walz, A., and Baggiolini, M. (1988). Mechanism of neutrophil activation by NAF, a novel monocyte-derived peptide agonist. *FASEB J.*, **2**, 2702–6.

61 Mege, J. L., Volpi, M., Becker, E. L., and Sha'afi, R. I. (1988). Effect of botulinum D toxin on neutrophils. *Biochem. Biophys. Res. Commun.*, **152**, 926–32.

62 Wiegers, W., Just, I., Muller, H., Hellwig, A., Traub, P., and Aktories, K. (1991). Alteration of the cytoskeleton of mammalian cells cultured in vitro by *Clostridium* botulinum C2 toxin and C3 ADP-ribosyltransferase. *Eur. J. Cell Biol.*, **54**, 237–45.

63 Aktories, K. and Hall, A. (1989). Botulinum ADP-ribosyltransferase C_3: a new tool to study low molecular weight GTP-binding proteins. *Trends Pharmacol. Sci.*, **10**, 415–18.

64 Sklar, L. A. (1986). Ligand–receptor dynamics and signal amplification in the neutrophil. *Adv. Immunol.*, **39**, 95–143.

65 Sklar, L. A. and Omann, G. M. (1990). Kinetics and amplification in neutrophil activation and adaptation. *Semin. Cell Biol.*, **1**, 115–23.

66 Sklar, L. A., Mueller, H., Omann, G., and Oades, Z. (1989). Three states for the formyl peptide receptor on intact cells. *J. Biol. Chem.*, **264**, 8483–6.

67 Fay, S. P., Posner, R. G., Swann, W. N., and Sklar, L. A. (1991). Real-time analysis of the assembly of ligand, receptor, and G protein by quantitative fluorescence flow cytometry. *Biochemistry*, **30**, 5066–75.

68 Snyderman, R. and Pike, M. C. (1984). Chemoattractant receptors on phagocytic cells. *Annu. Rev. Immunol.*, **2**, 257–81.

69 Kermode, J. C., Freer, R. J., and Becker, E. L. (1991). The significance of functional receptor heterogeneity in the biological responses of the rabbit neutrophil to stimulation by chemotactic formyl peptides. *Biochem. J.*, **276**, 715–23.

70 McPhail, L. C. and Snyderman, R. (1984). Mechanisms of regulating the respiratory burst in leukocytes. In *Regulation of leukocyte function* (ed. R. Snyderman), pp. 247–81. Plenum Press, New York.

71 Di Virgilio, F., Stendahl, O., Pittet, D., Lew, P. D., and Pozzan, T. (1990). Cytoplasmic calcium in phagocyte activation. *Curr. Top. Membr. Transp.*, **35**, 180–205.

72 Traynor-Kaplan, A. E. (1990). Phosphoinositide metabolism during phagocytic cell activation. *Curr. Top. Membr. Transp.*, **35**, 303–32.

73 Reibman, J., Haines, K., and Weissmann, G. (1990). Alterations in cyclic nucleotides and the activation of neutrophils. *Curr. Top. Membr. Transp.*, **35**, 399–424.

74 Agwu, D. E., McPhail, L. C., Chabot, M. C., Daniel, L. W., Wykle, R. L., and McCall, C. E. (1989). Choline-linked phosphoglycerides. A source of phosphatidic acid and diglycerides in stimulated neutrophils. *J. Biol. Chem., 264*, 1405–13.

75 Gelas, P., Ribbes, G., Record, M., Terce, F., and Chap, H. (1989). Differential activation by fMet-Leu-Phe and phorbol ester of a plasma membrane phosphatidylcholine-specific phospholipase D in human neutrophils. *FEBS Lett., 251*, 213–18.

76 Mullmann, T. J., Siegel, M. I., Egan, R. W., and Billah, M. M. (1990). Complement C5a activation of phospholipase D in human neutrophils. A major route to the production of phosphatidates and diglycerides. *J. Immunol., 144*, 1901–8.

77 Agwu, D. E., McCall, C. E., and McPhail, L. C. (1991). Regulation of phospholipase D-induced hydrolysis of choline-containing phosphoglycerides by cyclic AMP in human neutrophils. *J. Immunol., 146*, 3895–903.

78 Kanaho, Y., Kanoh, H., Saitoh, K., and Nozawa, Y. (1991). Phospholipase D activation by platelet-activating factor, leukotriene B_4, and formyl-methionyl-leucyl-phenylalanine in rabbit neutrophils. Phospholipase D is involved in enzyme release. *J. Immunol., 146*, 3536–41.

79 Cockcroft, S. (1984). Ca^{++} dependent conversion of phosphatidylinositol to phosphatidic acid in neutrophils stimulated with f-met-leu-phe or ionophore A23187. *Biochim. Biophys. Acta, 795*, 37–46.

80 Balsinde, J., Diez, E., and Mollinedo, F. (1988). Phosphatidylinositol-specific phospholipase D, a pathway for generation of a second messenger. *Biochem. Biophys. Res. Commun., 154*, 502–8.

81 Marx, R. S., McCall, C. E., and Bass, D. A. (1980). Chemotaxin-induced changes in cyclic adenosine monophosphate levels in human neutrophils. *Infect. Immun., 29*, 284–6.

82 Verghese, M. W., Fox, K., McPhail, L. C., and Snyderman, R. (1985). Chemoattractant-elicited alterations of cAMP levels in human polymorphonuclear leukocytes require a Ca^{2+}-dependent mechanism which is independent of transmembrane activation of adenylate cyclase. *J. Biol. Chem., 260*, 6769–75.

83 Iannone, M. A., Wolberg, G., and Zimmerman, T. P. (1989). Chemotactic peptide induces cAMP elevation in human neutrophils by amplification of the adenylate cyclase response to endogenously produced adenosine. *J. Biol. Chem., 264*, 20177–80.

84 Wymann, M. P., von Tscharner, V., Deranleau, D. A., and Baggiolini, M. (1987). The onset of the respiratory burst in human neutrophils. Real time studies of H_2O_2 formation reveal a rapid agonist-induced transduction process. *J. Biol. Chem., 262*, 12048–53.

85 Rhee, S. G. (1991). Inositol phospholipid-specific phospholipase C:

interaction of the γ_1 isoform with tyrosine kinase. *Trends Biochem. Sci.,* **16,** 297–301.

86 Taylor, S. J., Chae, H. Z., Rhee, S. G., and Exton, J. H. (1991). Activation of the β1 isozyme of phospholipase C by α subunits of the G_q class of G proteins. *Nature,* **350,** 516–18.

87 Honeycutt, P. J. and Niedel, J. E. (1986). Cytochalasin B enhancement of the diacylglycerol response in formyl peptide-stimulated neutrophils. *J. Biol. Chem.,* **261,** 15900–5.

88 Korchak, H. M., Vosshall, L. B., Haines, K. A., Wilkenfeld, C., Lundquist, K. F., and Weissmann, G. (1988). Activation of the human neutrophil by calcium-mobilizing ligands. II. Correlation of calcium, diacyl glycerol, and phosphatidic acid generation with superoxide anion generation. *J. Biol. Chem.,* **263,** 11098–106.

89 Haines, K. A., Reibman, J., Vosshall, L., and Weissmann, G. (1988). Neutrophil activation: evidence for two sources of diacylglycerol distinguished by Protein I of *Neisseria gonorrhoeae. Trans. Assoc. Am. Phys.,* **101,** 163–72.

90 Agwu, D. E., McPhail, L. C., Wykle, R. L., and McCall, C. E. (1989). Mass determination of receptor-mediated accumulation of phosphatidate and diglycerides in human neutrophils measured by Coomassie blue staining and densitometry. *Biochem. Biophys. Res. Commun.,* **159,** 79–86.

91 Thompson, N. T., Tateson, J. E., Randall, R. W., Spacey, G. D., Bonser, R. W., and Garland, L. G. (1990). The temporal relationship between phospholipase activation, diradylglycerol formation and superoxide production in the human neutrophil. *Biochem. J.,* **271,** 209–13.

92 Truett, A. P., III, Verghese, M. W., Dillon, S. B., and Snyderman, R. (1988). Calcium influx stimulates a second pathway for sustained diacylglycerol production in leukocytes activated by chemoattractants. *Proc. Natl Acad. Sci. USA,* **85,** 1549–53.

93 Cockcroft, S. and Allan, D. (1984). The fatty acid composition of phosphatidylinositol, phosphatidate and 1,2-diacylglycerol in stimulated human neutrophils. *Biochem. J.,* **222,** 557–9.

94 Pai, J.-K., Siegel, M. I., Egan, R. W., and Billah, M. M. (1988). Activation of phospholipase D by chemotactic peptide in HL-60 granulocytes. *Biochem. Biophys. Res. Commun.,* **150,** 355–64.

95 Billah, M. M., Eckel, S., Mullmann, T. J., Egan, R. W., and Siegel, M. I. (1989). Phosphatidylcholine hydrolysis by phospholipase D determines phosphatidate and diglyceride levels in chemotactic peptide-stimulated human neutrophils. Involvement of phosphatidate phosphohydrolase in signal transduction. *J. Biol. Chem.,* **264,** 17069–77.

96 Pike, M. C., Bruck, M. E., Arndt, C., and Lee, C.-S. (1990). Chemo-

attractants stimulate phosphatidylinositol-4-phosphate kinase in human polymorphonuclear leukocytes. *J. Biol. Chem.*, **265**, 1866–73.

97 Stephens, L. R., Hughes, K. T., and Irvine, R. F. (1991). Pathway of phosphatidylinositol(3,4,5)-trisphosphate synthesis in activated neutrophils. *Nature*, **351**, 33–9.

98 McPhail, L. C., Clayton, C. C., and Snyderman, R. (1984). A potential second messenger role for unsaturated fatty acids: activation of Ca^{2+}-dependent protein kinase. *Science*, **224**, 622–5.

99 Nigam, S., Fiore, S., Luscinskas, F. W., and Serhan, C. N. (1990). Lipoxin A_4 and lipoxin B_4 stimulate the release but not the oxygenation of arachidonic acid in human neutrophils: dissociation between lipid remodeling and adhesion. *J. Cell. Physiol.*, **143**, 512–23.

100 Rossi, A. G. and O'Flaherty, J. T. (1991). Bioactions of 5-hydroxyicosatetraenoate and its interaction with platelet-activating factor. *Lipids*, **26**, 1184–8.

101 O'Flaherty, J. T., Redman, J. F., and Jacobson, D. P. (1990). Cyclical binding, processing, and functional interactions of neutrophils with leukotriene B_4. *J. Cell. Physiol.*, **142**, 299–308.

102 McColl, S. R., Drump, E., Naccache, P. H., Poubelle, P. E., Braquet, P., Braquet, M., and Borgeat, P. (1991). Granulocyte-macrophage colony-stimulating factor increases the synthesis of leukotriene B_4 by human neutrophils in response to platelet-activating factor. Enhancement of both arachidonic acid availability and 5-lipoxygenase activation. *J. Immunol.*, **146**, 1204–11.

103 Schiffmann, E. (1982). Leukocyte chemotaxis. *Annu. Rev. Physiol.*, **44**, 553–68.

104 Lassing, I. and Lindberg, U. (1985). Specific interaction between phosphatidylinositol 4,5-bisphosphate and profilactin. *Nature*, **314**, 472–4.

105 Janmey, P. A. and Stossel, T. P. (1987). Modulation of gelsolin function by phosphatidylinositol 4,5-bisphosphate. *Nature*, **325**, 362–4.

106 Janmey, P. A. and Stossel, T. P. (1989). Gelsolin–polyphosphoinositide interaction. Full expression of gelsolin-inhibiting function by polyphosphoinositides in vesicular form and inactivation by dilution, aggregation, or masking of the inositol head group. *J. Biol. Chem.*, **264**, 4825–831.

107 Goldschmidt-Clermont, P. J., Machesky, L. M., Baldassare, J. J., and Pollard, T. D. (1990). The actin-binding protein profilin binds to PIP_2 and inhibits its hydrolysis by phospholipase C. *Science*, **247**, 1575–8.

108 Stossel, T. P. (1989). From signal to pseudopod. How cells control cytoplasmic actin assembly. *J. Biol. Chem.*, **264**, 18261–4.

109 Eberle, M., Traynor-Kaplan, A. E., Sklar, L. A., and Norgauer, J. (1990). Is there a relationship between phosphatidylinositol trisphos-

phate and F-actin polymerization in human neutrophils. *J. Biol. Chem.*, **265**, 16725–8.

110 Marasco, W. A., Becker, E. L., and Oliver, J. M. (1980). The ionic basis of chemotaxis. *Am. J. Pathol.*, **98**, 749–68.

111 Meshulam, T., Proto, P., Diamond, R. D., and Melnick, D. A. (1986). Calcium modulation and chemotactic response divergent stimulation of neutrophil chemotaxis and cytosolic calcium response by the chemotactic peptide receptor. *J. Immunol.*, **137**, 1954–60.

112 Jaconi, M. E. E., Rivest, R. W., Schlegel, W., Wollheim, C. B., Pittet, D., and Lew, D. P. (1988). Spontaneous and chemoattractant-induced oscillations of cytosolic free calcium in single adherent human neutrophils. *J. Biol. Chem.*, **263**, 10557–60.

113 Marks, P. W. and Maxfield, F. R. (1990). Transient increases in cytosolic free calcium appear to be required for migration of adherent human neutrophils. *J. Cell Biol.*, **110**, 43–52.

114 Marks, P. W., Hendley, B., and Maxfield, F. R. (1991). Attachment to fibronectin or vitronectin makes human neutrophil migration sensitive to alterations in cytosolic free calcium concentration. *J. Cell Biol.*, **112**, 149–58.

115 Sawyer, D. W., Sullivan, J. A., and Mandell, G. L. (1985). Intracellular free calcium location in neutrophils during phagocytosis. *Science*, **230**, 663–6.

116 Marks, P. W. and Maxfield, F. R. (1990). Local and global changes in cytosolic free calcium in neutrophils during chemotaxis and phagocytosis. *Cell Calcium*, **11**, 181–90.

117 Hofmann, S. L., Prescott, S. M., and Majerus, P. W. (1982). The effects of mepacrine and p-bromophenacyl bromide on arachidonic acid release in human platelets. *Arch. Biochem. Biophys.*, **215**, 237–44.

118 Kyger, E. M. and Franson, R. C. (1984). Nonspecific inhibition of enzymes by p-bromophenacyl bromide. Inhibition of human platelet phospholipase C and modification of sulfhydryl groups. *Biochim. Biophys. Acta*, **794**, 96–103.

119 Tyagi, S. R., Olson, S. C., Burnham, D. N., and Lambeth, J. D. (1991). Cyclic AMP-elevating agents block chemoattractant activation of diradylglycerol generation by inhibiting phospholipase D activation. *J. Biol. Chem.*, **266**, 3498–504.

120 O'Flaherty, J. T., Rossi, A. G., Jacobson, D. P., and Redman, J. F. (1991). Roles of Ca^{2+} in human neutrophils responses to receptor agonists. *Biochem. J.*, **278**, 705–11.

121 Grzeskowiak, M., Della Bianca, V., Cassatella, M. A., and Rossi, F. (1986). Complete dissociation between activation of phosphoinositide turnover and of NADPH oxidase by formyl-methionyl-leucyl-phenyl-alanine in human neutrophils depleted of Ca^{2+} and primed by sub-

threshold doses of phorbol 12, myristate 13, acetate. *Biochem. Biophys. Res. Commun.,* **135**, 785–94.

122 McPhail, L. C., McCall, C. E., Agwu, D. E., and Qualliotine-Mann, D. (1991). Synergism with phosphatidic acid and diacylglycerol for cell-free activation of neutrophil NADPH oxidase. *J. Cell Biol.,* **115**, 362a.

123 Agwu, D. E., McPhail, L. C., Sozzani, S., Bass, D. A., and McCall, C. E. (1991). Phosphatidic acid as a second messenger in human polymorphonuclear leukocytes. Effects on activation of NADPH oxidase. *J. Clin. Invest.,* **88**, 531–9.

124 McPhail, L. C., Ellenburg, M. D., Leone, P. A., Agwu, D. E., McCall, C. E., Qualliotine-Mann, D., and Strum, S. L. (1992). Molecular mechanism of activation of leukocyte superoxide production. In *The molecular basis of oxidative damage by leukocytes* (ed. A. J. Jesaitis and E. A. Dratz), pp. 11–24. CRC Press Inc., Boca Raton.

125 Bonser, R. W., Thompson, N. T., Randall, R. W., and Garland, L. G. (1989). Phospholipase D activation is functionally linked to superoxide generation in the human neutrophil. *Biochem. J.,* **264**, 617–20.

126 Bauldry, S. A., Bass, D. A., Cousart, S. L., and McCall, C. E. (1991). Tumor necrosis factor α priming of phospholipase D in human neutrophils. Correlation between phosphatidic acid production and superoxide generation. *J. Biol. Chem.,* **266**, 4173–9.

127 Huang, C.-K. (1989). Protein kinases in neutrophils: A review. *Membr. Biochem.,* **8**, 61–79.

128 Pryzwansky, K. B., Wyatt, T. A., Nichols, H., and Lincoln, T. M. (1990). Compartmentalization of cyclic GMP-dependent protein kinase in formyl-peptide stimulated neutrophils. *Blood,* **76**, 612–18.

129 Quilliam, L. A., Mueller, H., Bohl, B. P., Prossnitz, V., Sklar, L. A., Der, C. J., and Bokoch, G. M. (1991). Rap1A is a substrate for cyclic AMP-dependent protein kinase in human neutrophils. *J. Immunol.,* **147**, 1628–35.

130 Wyatt, T. A., Lincoln, T. M., and Pryzwansky, K. B. (1991). Vimentin is transiently co-localized with and phosphorylated by cyclic GMP-dependent protein kinase in formyl-peptide stimulated neutrophils. *J. Biol. Chem.,* **266**, 21274–80.

131 Harvath, L., Robbins, J. D., Russell, A. A., and Seamon, K. B. (1991). Cyclic AMP and human neutrophil chemotaxis: Elevation of cyclic AMP differentially affects chemotactic responsiveness. *J. Immunol.,* **146**, 224–32.

132 Bell, R. M. and Burns, D. J. (1991). Lipid activation of protein kinase C. *J. Biol. Chem.,* **266**, 4661–4.

133 Pontremoli, S., Melloni, E., Sparatore, B., Michetti, M., Salamino, F., and Horecker, B. L. (1990). Isozymes of protein kinase C in

human neutrophils and their modification by two endogenous proteinases. *J. Biol. Chem.*, **265**, 706–12.

134 Stasia, M. J., Strulovici, B., Daniel-Issakani, S., Pilosin, J. M., Dianoux, A. C., Chambaz, E., and Vignais, P. V. (1990). Immunocharacterization of β- and ζ-subspecies of protein kinase C in bovine neutrophils. *FEBS Lett.*, **274**, 61–4.

135 Majumdar, S., Rossi, M. W., Fujiki, T., Phillips, W. A., Queen, C. F., Johnston, R. B., Jr, *et al.* (1991). Protein kinase C isotypes and signaling in neutrophils. Differential substrate specificities of a translocatable, calcium- and phospholipid-dependent β-protein kinase C and a novel calcium-independent phospholipid-dependent protein kinase which is inhibited by long chain fatty acyl coenzyme A. *J. Biol. Chem.*, **266**, 9285–94.

136 Smallwood, J. I. and Malawista, S. E. (1992). Protein kinase C isoforms in human neutrophil cytoplasts. *J. Leuk. Biol.*, **51**, 84–92.

137 Kramer, I. M., Verhoeven, A. J., van der Bend, R. L., Weening, R. S., and Roos, D. (1988). Purified protein kinase C phosphorylates a 47-kDa protein in control neutrophil cytoplasts but not in neutrophil cytoplasts from patients with the autosomal form of chronic granulomatous disease. *J. Biol. Chem.*, **263**, 2352–7.

138 Stoehr, S. J., Smolen, J. E., and Suchard, S. J. (1990). Lipocortins are major substrates for protein kinase C in extracts of human neutrophils. *J. Immunol.*, **144**, 3936–45.

139 Thelen, M., Rosen, A., Nairn, A. C., and Aderem, A. (1990). Tumor necrosis factor α modifies agonist-dependent responses in human neutrophils by inducing the synthesis and myristoylation of a specific protein kinase C substrate. *Proc. Natl Acad. Sci. USA*, **87**, 5603–7.

140 Dusenbery, K. E., Mendiola, J. R., and Skubitz, K. M. (1988). Evidence for ecto-protein kinase activity on the surface of human neutrophils. *Biochem. Biophys. Res. Commun.*, **153**, 7–13.

141 Skubitz, K. M., Ehresmann, D. D., and Ducker, T. P. (1991). Characterization of human neutrophil ecto-protein kinase activity released by kinase substrates. *J. Immunol.*, **147**, 638–50.

142 Skubitz, K. M., Mendiola, J. R., and Collett, M. S. (1988). CD15 monoclonal antibodies react with a phosphotyrosine-containing protein on the surface of human neutrophils. *J. Immunol.*, **141**, 4318–23.

143 Skubitz, K. M. and Gouelli, S. A. (1991). Basic fibroblast growth factor is a substrate for phosphorylation by human neutrophil ecto-protein kinase activity. *Biochem. Biophys. Res. Commun.*, **174**, 49–55.

144 Gomez-Cambronero, J., Huang, C.-K., Becker, E. L., and Sha'afi, R. I. (1991). Tyrosine phosphorylation of a 41 kDa protein in human neutrophils stimulated with various agonists. *J. Cell Biol.*, **115**, 361a.

145 Torres, M., Hall, F. L., and O'Neill, R. A. (1991). Tyrosine phosphorylation of a MAP-kinase in human neutrophils stimulated with f-Met-Leu-Phe. *J. Cell Biol.,* **115,** 274a.

146 Perlmutter, R. M., Marth, J. D., Ziegler, S. F., Garvin, A. M., Pawar, S., Cooke, M. P., and Abraham, K. M. (1988). Specialized protein tyrosine kinase proto-oncogenes in hematopoietic cells. *Biochim. Biophys. Acta,* **948,** 245–62.

147 Gutkind, J. S. and Robbins, K. C. (1989). Translocation of the FGR protein tyrosine kinase as a consequence of neutrophil activation. *Proc. Natl Acad. Sci. USA,* **86,** 8783–7.

148 Notario, V., Gutkind, J. S., Imaizumi, M., Katamine, S., and Robbins, K. C. (1989). Expression of the *fgr* protooncogene product as a function of myelomonocytic cell maturation. *J. Cell Biol.,* **109,** 3129–36.

149 Huang, C.-K., Laramee, G., and Casnellie, J. E. (1988). Chemotactic factor induced tyrosine phosphorylation of membrane associated proteins in rabbit peritoneal neutrophils. *Biochem. Biophys. Res. Commun.,* **151,** 794–801.

150 Gomez-Cambronero, J., Huang, C.-K., Bonak, V. A., Wang, E., Casnellie, J. E., Shiraishi, T., and Sha'afi, R. I. (1989). Tyrosine phosphorylation in human neutrophils. *Biochem. Biophys. Res. Commun.,* **162,** 1478–85.

151 Huang, C.-K., Bonak, V., Laramee, G. R., and Casnellie, J. E. (1990). Protein tyrosine phosphorylation in rabbit peritoneal neutrophils. *Biochem. J.,* **269,** 431–6.

152 Berkow, R. L. and Dodson, R. W. (1990). Tyrosine-specific protein phosphorylation during activation of human neutrophils. *Blood,* **75,** 2445–52.

153 Berkow, R. L., Dodson, R. W., and Kraft, A. S. (1989). Human neutrophils contain distinct cytosolic and particulate tyrosine kinase activities: possible role in neutrophil activation. *Biochem. Biophys. Acta,* **997,** 292–301.

154 Gomez-Cambronero, J., Wang, E., Johnson, G., Huang, C.-K., and Sha'afi, R. I. (1991). Platelet-activating factor induces tyrosine phosphorylation in human neutrophils. *J. Biol. Chem.,* **266,** 6240–5.

155 Kraft, A. S. and Berkow, R. L. (1987). Tyrosine kinase and phosphotyrosine phosphatase activity in human promyelocytic leukemia cells and human polymorphonuclear leukocytes. *Blood,* **70,** 356–62.

156 Grinstein, S., Furuya, W., Lu, D. J., and Mills, G. B. (1990). Vanadate stimulates oxygen consumption and tyrosine phosphorylation in electropermeabilized human neutrophils. *J. Biol. Chem.,* **265,** 318–27.

157 Ding, J. and Badwey, J. A. (1992). Utility of immobilon-bound phosphoproteins as substrates for protein phosphatases from neutrophils. *Biochim. Biophys. Acta,* **1133,** 235–40.

158 Harvath, L., McCall, C. E., Bass, D. A., and McPhail, L. C. (1987). Inhibition of human neutrophil chemotaxis by the protein kinase inhibitor, 1-(5-isoquinolinesulfonyl) piperazine. *J. Immunol.*, **139**, 3055–61.

159 Gaudry, M., Perianin, A., Marquetty, C., and Hakim, J. (1988). Negative effect of a protein kinase C inhibitor (H-7) on human polymorphonuclear neutrophil locomotion. *Immunology*, **63**, 715–19.

160 Gaudry, M., Caon, A. C., Gilbert, C., Lille, S., and Naccache, P. H. (1991). Evidence for the involvement of tyrosine kinases in the locomotory responses of human neutrophils. *J. Leuk. Biol.*, **Suppl. 2**, 17.

161 Thomas, M. L. (1989). The leukocyte common antigen family. *Annu. Rev. Immunol.*, **7**, 339–69.

162 Tonks, N. K., Charbonneau, H., Diltz, C. D., Fischer, E. H., and Walsh, K. A. (1988). Demonstration that the leukocyte common antigen CD45 is a protein tyrosine phosphatase. *Biochemistry*, **27**, 8695–701.

163 Lacal, P., Pulido, R., Sanchez-Madrid, F., and Mollinedo, F. (1988). Intracellular location of T200 and Mo1 glycoproteins in human neutrophils. *J. Biol. Chem.*, **263**, 9946–51.

164 Harvath, L., Balke, J. A., Christiansen, N. P., Russell, A. A., and Skubitz, K. M. (1991). Selected antibodies to Leukocyte Common Antigen (CD45) inhibit human neutrophil chemotaxis. *J. Immunol.*, **146**, 949–57.

165 Badwey, J. A. (1991). Transmembrane signaling, then and now: the decade of the eighties. *J. Bioenerg. Biomembr.*, **23**, 1–5.

166 Tauber, A. I., Karnad, A. B., and Ginis, I. (1990). The role of phosphorylation in phagocyte activation. *Curr. Top. Membr. Transp.*, **35**, 469–94.

167 Kramer, I. M., van der Bend, R. L., Verhoeven, A. J., and Roos, D. (1988). The 47-kDa protein involved in the NADPH:O_2 oxidoreductase activity of human neutrophils is phosphorylated by cyclic AMP-dependent protein kinase without induction of a respiratory burst. *Biochim. Biophys. Acta*, **971**, 189–96.

168 Garcia, R. C. and Segal, A. W. (1988). Phosphorylation of the subunits of cytochrome b_{-245} upon triggering of the respiratory burst of human neutrophils and macrophages. *Biochem. J.*, **252**, 901–4.

169 Pears, C. J. and Parker, P. J. (1991). Domain interactions of protein kinase C. *J. Cell Sci.*, **100**, 683–6.

170 Bromberg, Y. and Pick, E. (1985). Activation of NADPH-dependent superoxide production in a cell-free system by sodium dodecyl sulfate. *J. Biol. Chem.*, **260**, 13539–45.

171 Curnutte, J. T., Berkow, R. L., Roberts, R. L., Shurin, S. B., and Scott, P. J. (1988). Chronic granulomatous disease due to a defect in

the cytosolic factor required for nicotinamide adenine dinucleotide phosphate oxidase activation. *J. Clin. Invest.,* **81,** 606–10.

172 Caldwell, S. E., McCall, C. E., Hendricks, C. L., Leone, P. A., Bass, D. A., and McPhail, L. C. (1988). Coregulation of NADPH oxidase activation and phosphorylation of a 48-kD protein(s) by a cytosolic factor defective in autosomal recessive chronic granulomatous disease. *J. Clin. Invest.,* **81,** 1485–96.

173 Strum, S. L., Hendricks, C. L., and McPhail, L. C. (1990). Cell-free activation of NADPH oxidase: mechanisms regulating translocation of the 47 kDa oxidase component. *FASEB J.,* **4,** A2181.

174 Smith, R. M. and Connor, J. (1992). Translocation of neutrophil respiratory burst oxidase components from cytosol to membrane in a cell-free system. *Clin. Res.,* **40,** 31A.

175 Nauseef, W. M., Volpp, B. D., McCormick, S., Leidal, K. G., and Clark, R. A. (1991). Assembly of the neutrophil respiratory burst oxidase. Protein kinase C promotes cytoskeletal and membrane association of cytosolic oxidase components. *J. Biol. Chem.,* **266,** 5911–17.

176 Woodman, R. C., Ruedi, J. M., Jesaitis, A. J., Okamura, N., Quinn, M. T., Smith, R. M., *et al.* (1991). Respiratory burst oxidase and three of four oxidase-related polypeptides are associated with the cytoskeleton of human neutrophils. *J. Clin. Invest.,* **87,** 1345–51.

177 Seifert, R. and Schultz, G. (1987). Fatty-acid-induced activation of NADPH oxidase in plasma membranes of human neutrophils depends on neutrophil cytosol and is potentiated by stable guanine nucleotides. *Eur. J. Biochem.,* **162,** 563–9.

178 Uhlinger, D. J., Burnham, D. N., and Lambeth, J. D. (1991). Nucleoside triphosphate requirements for superoxide generation and phosphorylation in a cell-free system from human neutrophils. Sodium dodecyl sulfate and diacylglycerol activate independently of protein kinase C. *J. Biol. Chem.,* **266,** 20990–7.

179 Abo, A. and Pick, E. (1991). Purification and characterization of a third cytosolic component of the superoxide-generating NADPH oxidase of macrophages. *J. Biol. Chem.,* **266,** 23577–85.

180 Omann, G. M., Porasik, M. M., and Sklar, L. A. (1989). Oscillating actin polymerization/depolymerization responses in human polymorphonuclear leukocytes. *J. Biol. Chem.,* **264,** 16355–8.

181 Wymann, M. P., Kernen, P., Bengtsson, T., Andersson, T., Baggiolini, M., and Deranleau, D. A. (1990). Corresponding oscillations in neutrophil shape and filamentous actin content. *J. Biol. Chem.,* **265,** 619–22.

182 Sarndahl, E., Lindroth, M., Bengtsson, T., Fallman, M., Gustavsson, J., Stendahl, O., and Andersson, T. (1989). Association of ligand–receptor complexes with actin filaments in human neutrophils: A possible regulatory role for a G-protein. *J. Cell Biol.,* **109,** 2791–9.

183 Jesaitis, A. J., Bokoch, G. M., Tolley, J. O., and Allen, R. A. (1988). Lateral segregation of neutrophil chemotactic receptors into actin- and fodrin-rich plasma membrane microdomains depleted in guanyl nucleotide regulatory proteins. *J. Cell Biol.*, **107**, 921–8.

184 Southwick, F. S. and Young, C. L. (1990). The actin released from profilin–actin complexes is insufficient to account for the increase in F-actin in chemoattractant-stimulated polymorphonuclear leukocytes. *J. Cell Biol.*, **110**, 1965–73.

185 Howard, T. H., Chaponnier, C., Yin, H., and Stossel, T. (1990). Gelsolin–actin interaction and actin polymerization in human neutrophils. *J. Cell Biol.*, **110**, 1983–91.

186 Southwick, F. S., Dabiri, G., Paschetto, M., and Zigmond, S. H. (1989). Polymorphonuclear leukocyte adherence induces actin polymerization by a transductional pathway which differs from that used by chemoattractants. *J. Cell Biol.*, **109**, 1561–9.

187 Cassimeris, L., McNeill, H., and Zigmond, S. H. (1990). Chemoattractant-stimulated polymorphonuclear leukocytes contain two populations of actin filaments that differ in their spatial distributions and relative stabilities. *J. Cell Biol.*, **110**, 1067–75.

188 Payrastre, B., van Bergen en Henegouwen, P. M. P., Breton, M., den Hartigh, J. C., Plantavid, M., Verkleij, A. J., and Boonstra, J. (1991). Phosphoinositide kinase, diacylglycerol kinase, and phospholipase C activities associated to the cytoskeleton: effect on epidermal growth factor. *J. Cell Biol.*, **115**, 121–8.

189 Lehmeyer, J. E., Snyderman, R., and Johnston, R. B., Jr (1979). Stimulation of neutrophil oxidative metabolism by chemotactic peptides: Influence of calcium ion concentration and cytochalasin B and comparison with stimulation by phorbol myristate acetate. *Blood*, **54**, 35–45.

190 Harvath, L. and Aksamit, R. R. (1984). Oxidized N-formylmethionyl-leucyl-phenylalanine: Effect on the activation of human monocyte and neutrophil chemotaxis and superoxide production. *J. Immunol.*, **133**, 1471–6.

191 Schepers, T. M., Brier, M. E., and McLeish, K. R. (1992). Quantitative and qualitative differences in guanine nucleotide binding protein activation by formyl peptide and leukotriene B4 receptors. *J. Biol. Chem.*, **267**, 159–65.

192 Nelson, R. D., McCormack, R. T., Fiegel, V. D., Herron, M., Simmons, R. L., and Quie, P. G. (1979). Chemotactic deactivation of human neutrophils: possible relationship to stimulation of oxidative metabolism. *Infect. Immun.*, **23**, 282–6.

193 Yuo, A., Kitagawa, S., Kasahara, T., Matsushima, K., Saito, M., and Takaku, F. (1991). Stimulation and priming of human neutrophils by

interleukin-8: cooperation with tumor necrosis factor and colony-stimulating factors. *Blood,* **78,** 2708–14.

194 McCall, C. E., Bass, D. A., DeChatelet, L. R., Link, A. S., Jr, and Mann, M. (1979). In vitro responses of human neutrophils to N-formyl-methionyl-leucyl-phenylalanine: correlation with effects of acute bacterial infection. *J. Infect. Dis.,* **140,** 147–56.

195 Van Epps, D. E. and Garcia, M. L. (1980). Enhancement of neutrophil function as a result of prior exposure to chemotactic factor. *J. Clin. Invest.,* **66,** 167–75.

196 McPhail, L. C., Clayton, C. C., and Snyderman, R. (1984). The NADPH oxidase of human polymorphonuclear leukocytes. Evidence for regulation by multiple signals. *J. Biol. Chem.,* **259,** 5768–75.

197 Gay, J. C. and Stitt, E. S. (1988). Platelet-activating factor induces protein kinase activity in the particulate fraction of human neutrophils. *Blood,* **71,** 159–65.

198 O'Flaherty, J. T., Jacobson, D. P., Redman, J. F., and Rossi, A. G. (1990). Translocation of protein kinase C in human polymorphonuclear neutrophils. Regulation by cytosolic Ca^{2+}-independent and Ca^{2+}-dependent mechanisms. *J. Biol. Chem.,* **265,** 9146–52.

199 Beaulieu, A. D., Paquin, R., Rathanaswami, P., and McColl, S. R. (1992). Nuclear signaling in human neutrophils. Stimulation of RNA synthesis is a response to a limited number of proinflammatory agonists. *J. Biol. Chem.,* **267,** 426–32.

4 Neutrophil phagocytosis and killing: normal function and microbial evasion

J. VERHOEF and M. R. VISSER

1 Clinical case: hypogammaglobulinaemia

A previously healthy 2-year-old boy was admitted to hospital with fever and a stiff neck. He had been well until 4 days before admission, when he complained about pain in his left ear. His clinical condition deteriorated a few hours before admission. Because at admission his temperature was 40 °C and he was lethargic, the boy was given ceftriaxone and a lumbar puncture was performed. Gram's stain of the cerebral spinal fluid (CSF) revealed many polymorphonuclear leukocytes (PMN) and Gram-negative coccobacilli. The next day *Haemophilus influenzae*, type b was grown from the culture. The strain was shown to be susceptible to amoxicillin and therapy was changed accordingly. The opsonic activity of the boy's serum was below the lower limit of the opsonic activity observed in a series of 26 healthy controls, indicating that serum factors responsible for adequate phagocytosis by PMN were lacking. The levels of antibodies to *H. influenzae* organisms and capsular polysaccharides (anti-PRP) were also decreased. A significant relationship between the low levels of these antibodies and the observed low opsonic activity was noted.

As discussed later in this chapter, phagocytic cells and opsonins are important host determinants in preventing disease such as in the case of invasive *H. influenzae* infection noted above. Without an adequate complement system and type-specific antibodies, the process of phagocytosis is inefficient and serious infections may occur (1).

2 Introduction

The outcome of the interaction between certain micro-organisms and PMN determines health or disease. Once the barriers of the skin and mucous membranes have been breached, the host's health depends on PMN and other host resistance factors to combat invading micro-organisms that can cause infection (2). PMN originate in the bone marrow and are continuously discharged in vast numbers into the bloodstream. They only live for a few

days and each day about 10^{11} cells disappear from the body, even in the
absence of infection (see Chapter 1 for further discussion of PMN maturation).

As soon as microbes invade the tissues, circulating PMN are activated,
leave the bloodstream, adhere to activated endothelial cells, and move
through the endothelial barrier to the site of the infection. This process of
migration under guidance is called chemotaxis and is defined as directed
cell movement in one direction in response to an agent which signals and
induces the cell to move. While PMN migration occurs, the microbes are
opsonized; that is, the microbial surface is coated with antibody and
complement factors for recognition by PMN. PMN have receptors specifically designed to bind to the Fc fragment of the IgG molecule present on
the surface of the opsonized bacteria and other receptors designed to bind
to the activated complement factors (see Chapter 2 for further discussion).
The complement factors and the antibody molecules are ligands that promote attachment of the microbe to the cell enhancing otherwise inefficient
microbe–phagocyte interactions. After this receptor-mediated attachment,
PMN engulf the microbes and ingestion takes place. Once a microbe is
phagocytosed by the PMN, it is usually rapidly killed and digested.

During the last decade, our understanding of the molecular basis of the
different steps involved in the process of phagocytosis and killing (shown in
Fig. 4.1) has greatly improved. The steps that occur prior to phagocytosis
and killing (e.g. receptor–ligand interaction, transmembrane signalling,
chemotaxis) are discussed in detail in Chapters 2 and 3. It is now known

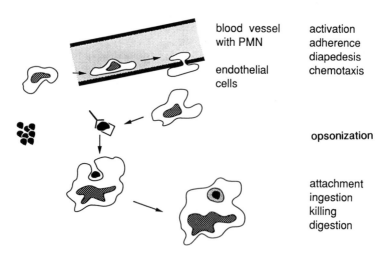

blood vessel   activation
with PMN   adherence
                    diapedesis
endothelial   chemotaxis
cells

                    opsonization

                    attachment
                    ingestion
                    killing
                    digestion

Fig. 4.1 Schematic representation of the different stages of PMN–microbial
interaction that occur upon invasion of the host by bacteria (activation, diapedese
and chemotaxis of PMN; opsonization of bacteria; ingestion and killing of the
microbes by the PMN). Y = antibody.

that the outcome of the interaction between PMN and microbes is determined not only by PMN but also by microbes. This chapter will concentrate on the actual process of PMN phagocytosis and killing and also detail some of the mechanisms by which microbes evade these cellular functions.

3 Opsonization

3.1 Opsonization in the presence of antibody and complement

Generally micro-organisms are only phagocytized after they have been properly opsonized; that is, loaded with activated C3 and IgG. Opsonization through activation of complement is primarily a function of C3b and iC3b. The PMN receptor that recognizes C3b is CR_1, while the receptor that recognizes iC3b is CR_3 (CD11b/CD18) (3). For most opsonized particles, especially encapsulated organisms, the iC3b–CR_3 interaction enhances attachment of the particle to PMN but not its ingestion. Ingestion only occurs in the presence of antibodies (3). Antibodies bind to specific antigens on the cell wall of bacteria; these antibody molecules also serve as ligands for the attachment of bacteria to PMN. Two receptors for IgG are present on the PMN cell membrane; FcRII and FcRIII. FcRII binds IgG1 and IgG3 equally well and does so better than IgG2 and IgG4. FcRIII binds only to monomeric IgG (4).

Many bacteria have developed a defence against opsonophagocytosis and are thus able to escape phagocytosis by PMN. The most important anti-phagocytic defence of bacteria is an enveloping capsule. These capsules protect the microbes against PMN by interfering with opsonization (5). For example, pathogens that cause pneumonia and meningitis, such as *H. influenzae, Neisseria meningitidis, Escherichia coli, Streptococcus pneumoniae, Klebsiella pneumoniae*, and group B streptococci, have polysaccharide capsules on their surface. Non-encapsulated derivatives of these organisms are less virulent. Although the chemical composition of these capsules can vary significantly between strains and species, most capsules are composed of polymers of repeated sugar residues. However, only a few types of capsules are commonly associated with disease. *H. influenzae* isolates can produce one of six different types of polysaccharide capsules, yet those organisms expressing type b capsules are predominantly isolated from serious infections. Capsules from bacterial pathogens prevent complement deposition on the bacterial surface, while capsules from non-virulent strains are less efficient at preventing this deposition. The capsules are only weakly immunogenic and mask the more immunogenic underlying bacterial surface structures that would directly activate complement. Thus, the capsule prevents opsonization of the organism, conferring resistance to phagocytosis (5).

Some other cell wall components that help micobes evade the phagocytic defence of the host are peptidoglycans, protein A (*Staphylococcus aureus*), and protein M (group A streptococci). The role of each of these cell wall components are discussed below in conjunction with the microbes on which they are found.

3.2   Opsonization in the absence of antibody and complement

Some bacteria are able to adhere to PMN in the absence of antibodies and/ or complement. *E. coli* adhesins, for example, are important components that they mediate adherence of *E. coli* directly to PMN without antibodies and complement. These adhesins can be divided into two groups: one where D-mannosides inhibit the adherence and one where they do not. The mannose-resistant (MR) phenotype is mediated by cell-bound adhesins or by specific protein fimbriae. Among the *E. coli* strains with MR haemagglutination, the P adhesins recognize the sequence α-D-Gal-(1-4)-β-D-Gal on the target cell receptors. P adhesin-expressing *E. coli* are frequently involved in human urinary tract infections.

E. coli possessing mannose-sensitive (MS) adhesins adhere avidly to urinary slime. In addition, a number of other adhesins have been detected (M, X, and S adhesins, type 1c and G fimbriae). MS fimbriae (type 1 adhesins) increase the susceptibility of *E. coli* to PMN phagocytosis in the absence of specific opsonins (6). MS adhesins recognize the mannose residues of three different membrane glycoproteins in the PMN: gp150, gp70–80, and gp100. gp150 (CD11C/CD18) is the major receptor for type 1 fimbriae (7). Adherence of *E. coli* to PMN via the interaction of type 1 fimbriae and mannose-containing receptors leads to phagocytosis and killing by PMN (6). In contrast, PMN lack receptors for P fimbriae, which block phagocytosis (8). S adhesins are widespread among *E. coli* isolates that cause sepsis or meningitis. These adhesins recognize a structure containing neuraminyl acid derivatives. In many strains these derivatives appear in the form of neuraminyl-α-(2-3)-galactoside.

A possible serum factor other than complement or antibody that functions as an opsonin are the lipopolysaccharide binding proteins (LBP). LBP is an acute-phase reactant that binds bacterial LPS. LBP can bind to the surface of Gram-negative bacilli and strongly enhances attachment of these particles to the CD14 molecule in the cell membrane of phagocytic cells. LBP bridges LPS-coated particles to PMN and macrophages by first binding to LPS and then to the CD14 receptor. This binding leads to enhanced phagocytosis (9).

Gonococci possess antigenically variable outer membrane proteins, termed PII proteins, that appear to mediate adherence to human PMN (10). These PIIs in the membrane of bacteria (outer membrane proteins) bind to carbohydrate moieties of glycoconjugates in a lectin-like manner. Anti-PII monoclonal antibodies abrogate adherence of non-piliated gonococci to human neutrophils. The neutrophil receptors for PII$^+$ gonococci appear to be stored in a subcellular granule population (10).

In plasma there is a high molecular weight glycoprotein, called fibronectin, that aids the reticuloendothelial system in clearing the cell of microorganisms and helps maintain vascular stability. Several bacteria, for example, *S. aureus* and groups A, B, C, and G streptococci, have receptors for fibronectin. Because PMN can also bind fibronectin, it is possible that this glycoprotein acts as a bridge between PMN and the bacteria and therefore facilitates phagocytosis in the absence of specific opsonins (11). It is also possible that fibronectin enhances the opsonic and protective activity of antibodies and complement (12).

3.3   Mechanisms for avoiding opsonization

3.3.1   Microbial adaptation to avoid opsonization

Many micro-organisms can escape from opsonization by varying their surface antigenic structure. Some bacteria are master chameleons. For example, *N. gonorrhoeae* possess at least two mechanisms for altering surface antigens.

1. They can change PII proteins. Most *N. gonorrhoeae* express several different PII proteins at any given time, and a given strain can potentially express up to seven different PII proteins. The genetic control of each PII gene appears unrelated to other PII genes, which results in many different combinations. The regulation of PII gene expression depends on the repeating five nucleotide CTCtt, which is located within the PII leader sequence. Variations in the number of repeats of this pentamer will vary the reading frame of the downstream PII gene.

2. They can change pilins. There are usually many silent pilin gene sequences. The gonococcus can undergo gene conversion by placing one of these incomplete sequences into the expression site, thus synthesizing a new antigenically distinct pilin molecule. Antigenic variation occurs in many other bacteria as well: e.g. group B streptococci, *H. influenzae, P. aeruginosa, Salmonella, Borrelia*, etc.

3.3.2   Interference of antibiotics with opsonization

Exposures of bacteria to antibiotics below the minimal inhibition concentration increases their susceptibility to the antimicrobial action of normal human PMN. Low concentrations of antibiotics influence cell wall composition. Clindamycin, for example, has an inhibitory effect on the M protein of streptococci and protein A of *S. aureus* and thereby facilitates opsonization and subsequent phagocytosis. Antibiotics may also interfere with K antigen synthesis and LPS assembly in *E. coli*. (During antimicrobial treatment K antigen synthesis may be inhibited.) Therefore, bacteria are more readily opsonized and subsequently phagocytosed. Thus, during infections antibiotics may act in different ways: they may either kill the microbe directly or change the cell wall composition in such a way that an increased number of receptors for IgG and C3b are produced, thereby enhancing opsonophagocytosis (13–15).

3.4 Normal opsonization and evasion of opsonization by specific microbes

3.4.1 Staphylococci

The major cell wall components of *S. aureus* are peptidoglycan, teichoic acids, and protein A. Peptidoglycan is a polysaccharidic polymer composed of B-linked (1, 2, 4, 16) chains containing alternating subunits of *N*-acetylmuramic acid and *N*-acetylglucosamine. Pentapeptide chains are linked to the muramic acid residue and are cross-linked by a pentaglycine bridge attached to L-lysine on one chain and D-alanine on the other (17). Teichoic acids are simple glycerol or ribitol phosphates in repeating units, while protein A is a 42 kDa protein with the capacity to bind human IgG subclasses (except IgG3) via their Fc terminals. Antibodies against peptidoglycan are opsonic (18). When antibodies against peptidoglycan were isolated from serum and incubated with staphylococci, these bacteria were readily phagocytosed. Peptidoglycan was also able to activate the complement system directly leading to deposition of C3b on the surface of the bacteria. However, more than 50 per cent of *S. aureus* isolates obtained from blood cultures of patients are encapsulated. These capsular polysaccharides may interfere with the effective opsonization by anti-peptidoglycan antibodies and hinder the interaction of complement with peptidoglycan (19–21). Anti-capsular antibodies are needed for the efficient phagocytosis of these encapsulated bacteria.

Four mechanisms of opsonization of unencapsulated *S. aureus* strains are described: the interaction of PMN with *S. aureus* through antibodies against peptidoglycan; the interaction through antibodies and C3b; the interaction through C3b generated by direct interaction of peptidoglycan with complement (classical pathway); and the interaction through direct activation via the alternative pathway (18–22). Antibodies against the *O*-acetyl group of capsular polysaccharide are most efficient in opsonization. While anti-peptidoglycan antibodies promote phagocytosis *in vitro*, their opsonic capacity *in vivo* is unclear, as most strains grown under *in vivo* conditions contain a capsule that shields the peptidoglycan from specific antibodies (Table 4.1). It would be of interest to test the protective capacity of both antibodies against peptidoglycan and capsules in an animal model.

Table 4.1   Opsonins for *Staphylococcus aureus*

Unencapsulated strains
  Antibodies against peptidoglycan.
  C3b and iC3b generated by antigen–antibody reaction via the classical complement pathway.
  C3b and iC3b generated by the classical and alternative pathway interaction with peptidoglycan.

Encapsulated strains
  Antibodies against the polysaccharide capsule.
  C3b and iC3b generated by the interaction of anti-capsular antibodies with the capsule.

During *S. aureus* infection of the host, antibodies against teichoic acid are also produced. Their role in opsonization is questionable and is probably indirect via activation of the complement cascade. In contrast, protein A probably plays a triple anti-phagocytic role in the bacterial–cell recognition process by virtue of its binding to the Fc portion of IgG: (i) extracellular soluble protein A can react with the Fc terminal of IgG molecules of human serum, thereby producing immune aggregates that consume complement; (ii) extracellular protein A can bind to the Fc portion of specific anti-staphylococcal antibodies coating the micro-organism with their Fab fragment, thereby preventing further interaction of the complex with the Fc receptor of phagocyte; and (iii) cell-bound protein A binds to the Fc fragment of any IgG molecule in its neighbour-hood, thereby eliminating non-specific and specific antibodies.

In recent years *Staphylococcus epidermidis*, and other coagulase-negative staphylococci have become major pathogens in hospitalized patients. Because of its ability to adhere to plastics, these organisms are formidable pathogens in the presence of foreign bodies. Principal adhesins that are responsible for the binding of *S. epidermidis* to catheters are a capsular polysaccharide and a protease-sensitive surface constituent from the slime-producing strains of *S. epidermidis*. In addition to promoting adherence to foreign bodies, these adhesins may also protect coagulase-negative staphylococci against phagocytosis. Antibodies to these adhesins may neutralize this shield and provide opsonization of the bacteria.

Monoclonal antibodies against *S. epidermidis* adhesins facilitate phagocytosis of homologous and heterologous *S. epidermidis* strains (24, 25).
The major PMN receptor for *S. epidermidis* opsonins is the FcRIII receptor (26). However, for strains that have a hydrophobic surface structure,
antibodies by themselves are not sufficient for opsonization. These strains
also need C3b or iC3b (27).

3.4.2   Streptococci

A major component of the *Streptococcus pyogenes* cell wall is M protein.
M proteins interfere with opsonization and therefore can be regarded as
important virulence factors. They form hair-like projections on the surface
of group A streptococci. About 80 per cent of M protein consists of blocks
of repeating amino acid sequences. The amino acids near the C terminus
bind M protein to the bacterial cytoplasmic membrane and, together with a
region rich in prolines and glycines, they anchor M protein in the cell wall.
This part of M protein is highly conserved and is also present in other cell
wall proteins of Gram-positive bacteria (e.g. staphylococcal protein A;
streptococcal protein G). The N-terminal end is the variable part of M
protein and has an excess of negatively charged amino acids. PMN also
exhibit a net negative charge on their surface. The negative charge of M
proteins may thus have evolved to hinder contact between streptococci and
phagocytic cells.

To add to this anti-phagocytic effect, M protein-positive streptococci do
not bind C3b efficiently and thus evade opsonization (Fig. 4.2). This
appears to be due to complement factor H binding to the M protein, which
prevents the deposition of C3b on the surface of *S. pyogenes*. In a sense,

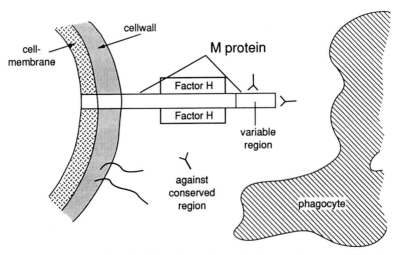

Fig. 4.2   Factor H inhibits binding of opsonic antibodies to the conserved region of
streptococcal M protein and thereby inhibits phagocytosis.

the M protein-bearing streptococcus cleverly disguises itself as a normal human cell to evade the complement system. During infection antibodies to the conserved and variable parts of the M proteins are made. Antibodies against the conserved part cannot bind when factor H is present and therefore do not have opsonic capacity. Antibodies against the variable region are opsonic and also neutralize the region's negative charge and thereby further assist phagocytosis [Fig. 4.2, (28)]. However, they are all type specific. Different streptococci with serologically different M proteins need different antibodies for efficient phagocytosis. One can thus be infected repeatedly with different group A streptococci.

Group B streptococci have cell wall components designed to evade the immature host defences of the neonate. These streptococci have polysaccharides and proteins in their cell walls which allow the strains to be differentiated into serotypes (Ia, Ib, Ic, II, and III). The capsular polysaccharide is type specific, while the C polysaccharide is group specific and common to all strains of group B streptococci. Surface proteins are additional antigenic markers (29).

Most late-onset infections (onset of infections 6 days to 3 months after birth) are caused by group B streptococci belonging to serotype III, while early onset of infection can be caused by serotypes I, II, or III. Infections with meningitis are almost always caused by serotype III strains. The classical complement pathway and heat-stable opsonins are required for maximal opsonic activity by human sera for type I, II, and III strains (30). For clinical isolates of type Ia group B streptococci, opsonization and phagocytosis may proceed via the classical complement pathway in an antibody-independent fashion, and C1 activation may be initiated by interactions with surface-bound capsular polysaccharides in these strains (29, 31, 32). Deficient opsonic activity of neonatal sera for clinical isolates of this serotype correlates with low levels of the classic pathway components C1q and C4. Since complement proteins in the neonate are not maternally derived and since levels of components in both the classical and alternative pathways are only 30–50 per cent of those in maternal or adult control sera at term, physiologically low levels of complement components or their receptors on phagocytes may provide a partial explanation for age-related susceptibility to group B streptococcal disease.

Direct activation of C_1 may paradoxically be an extra virulence factor of capsular polysaccharides. During infection large amounts of capsular material may be liberated from the bacteria. These fluid-phase macromolecules may then deplete complement by activating C_1. Complement components necessary for opsonization may then be absent.

Monoclonal antibodies (IgM and IgG) against type-specific antigens have been shown to be opsonic and to protect mice against lethal challenge with group B streptococci (33, 34). Interestingly, IgA monoclonal antibodies were also shown to be opsonic (35).

Opsonization is an important factor in host defence against *S. pneumoniae*. Again, a polysaccharide capsule is the important virulence factor that hampers opsonophagocytosis. Of the 83 different serotypes of *S. pneumoniae* 23 cause nearly 90 per cent of the pneumococcal infections. Like most bacteria, pneumococci are opsonized in the presence of complement through C3b and iC3b. Both activated complement factors are recognized by their specific receptors in the membrane of the PMN (CR_1 and CR_3). CR_1 can specifically recognize C3b, while CR_3 recognizes iC3b. It is possible to differentiate between the C3b–CR_1- and iC3b–CR_3-specific interactions with monoclonal antibodies (36). For example, the monoclonal antibody OKM10 is able to block CR_3-mediated phagocytosis of type 6A and 14 strains by 50–80 per cent. These strains almost exclusively bear iC3b. Blockade of the CR_1 receptor had no effect. For serotype III strains that bear C3b, iC3b, and C3d on the capsule, CR_3-mediated phagocytosis accounted for only 20 per cent of the uptake. Again, there was no evidence for CR_1-mediated phagocytosis. The iC3b ligand elicits more release of superoxide, myelperoxidase (MPO), and lactoferrin than C3b. The iC3b–CR_3 interaction is thus the primary trigger for phagocytosis of iC3b-bearing pneumococci and for stimulation of intracellular bactericidal processes (37). For comparison, it was shown that C3b, iC3b, and C3 make up 17, 64, and 19 per cent, respectively, on *S. aureus* and 53, 44, and 2 per cent, respectively, on *E. coli* (38). Even among capsulated pneumococci a diversity exists in opsonization. C3b and iC3b can be bound to the cell wall via a covalently linked thiolester-reactive binding or via an amide linkage. Interestingly, the C3b molecules are bound almost exclusively to the capsule via the thiolester-reactive site, while the amide linkage is used for unencapsulated surfaces. The amide-linked molecules are far more potent activators of phagocytosis than the thiolester-binding ones. This explains the ready phagocytosis of unencapsulated pneumococci and provides the capsule with another virulence mechanism.

Capsular polysaccharides may thus be regarded as virulence factors because they interfere with phagocytosis. This interference may be due to a variety of mechanisms preventing complement consumption (Fig. 4.3). For example, binding of inefficient opsonins such as C3b, or thiolester-active binding of the C3b or iC3b molecules makes opsonization less active by shielding or binding specific antibodies to cell wall antigens.

3.4.3   Haemophilus influenzae

Studies with *H. influenzae* have shown the crucial role for antibodies and complement in host defence. *H. influenzae* is the cause of respiratory tract infections in children and adults. In young children this micro-organism can also cause bacteraemia and meningitis. Although unencapsulated *H. influenzae* strains can cause serious infections, most invasive infections are caused by the encapsulated strains. The capsule of *H. influenzae* type b is a

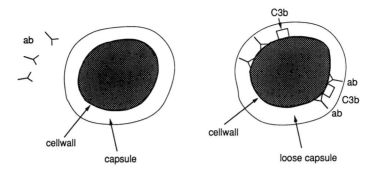

Fig. 4.3 Capsules of bacteria make bacteria resistant to phagocytosis by different processes: inhibition of complement activation by the encapsulated bacteria or by shielding of C3b by the capsule. ab = antibody.

polyribosyl-ribitol phosphate (PRP). Not only are antibodies against PRP necessary for opsonization and protection of the host against recurrent infections (1, 39), but classical complement components are also important for adequate opsonization. This was shown in experiments with C1q-deficient serum, which demonstrated that opsonization of *H. influenzae* type b may proceed through activation of the alternative pathway of complement, but that opsonization via the classical pathway is much more efficient (40). The addition of C1q to C1q-deficient serum greatly enhanced opsonic activity. Also, there is an increased risk for *H. influenzae* infections in patients with a deficiency of other early components of the classical pathway of complement. In contrast, serum from patients with factor D (alternative pathway component) deficiency show no impairment in opsonic activity for *H. influenzae*. This again underlines the predominant role of the classical pathway of complement in opsonization of *H. influenzae* type b.

The third complement component C3 assumes a central role in the complement system. It participates in both the classical and the alternative pathways as well as in the amplification loop and is one of the major opsonins. Patients with C3 deficiency suffer from recurrent and often severe respiratory tract and systemic infections, that are frequently due to *H. influenzae* type b (40).

3.4.4 Enterobacteriaceae

Enterobacteriaceae are able to evade host defence. This capacity is mainly determined by properties of the bacterial cell wall. As shown in Fig. 4.4, the Gram-negative bacterial cell wall consists of an inner cytoplasmic membrane, an intermediate murein or peptidoglycan layer, and an outer phospholipid–LPS bilayer in which proteins are inserted. LPS is anchored

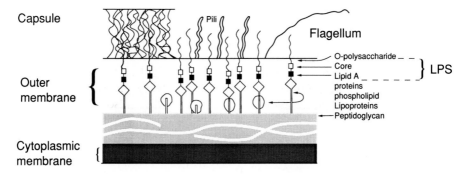

Fig. 4.4 Schematic representation of the Gram-negative bacteria cell wall (from Peterson, P. K. and Quie, P. G., *Annu. Rev. Med.* 1981; **32**, 29). Reproduced, with permission, from the *Annual Review of Medicine*, Vol. 32, © 1981 by Annual Reviews Inc.

by the lipid region (lipid A) in the outer leaflet of the outer membrane with a covalently bound core oligosaccharide structure directed outward. In addition, the outer part of the LPS of most strains that are present in nature (wild-type strains), contains a polysaccharide chain (O antigen) bound to the distal terminal of the core oligosaccharide. Some strains (e.g. many types of *E. coli* and *Klebsiella*) contain a surrounding capsular polysaccharide (K antigen). In addition, extruding protein structures, flagellae, pili, or fimbriae, may be present. These pili and fimbriae mediate the capacity of strains to adhere to and colonize mucosal surfaces.

Certain types of O and K antigens confer resistance to the bactericidal action of serum and phagocytosis by granulocytes. It has been suggested that the presence of large amounts of these polysaccharide structures may physically hinder the access of complement and/or antibodies to target structures on the bacterial surface, thereby either preventing activation of the complement pathways or causing formation of the membrane attack complex at a site too distant from the bacterial cytoplasmic membrane (41). Also, the anti-phagocytic effects of these structures may be related to interference with the hydrophobic nature of the bacterial surface.

Indeed, rough Gram-negative bacillary strains, defined by their lack of the polysaccharide side chain (O antigen), are sensitive to the bactericidal activity of the complement system and are readily ingested by granulocytes. Lipid A can bind the first complement factor (C1) directly, leading to an antibody-independent activation of the classical pathway. The polysaccharide region of LPS can activate the alternative pathway by a lipid A-independent, antibody-independent mechanism and has a modulating effect on the expression of lipid A binding and C1 activation. In addition to complement, specific antibodies to the surface structures are required for

killing encapsulated (K^+) and smooth (O^+) bacilli in serum and for phagocytosis of such bacilli by PMN (41). Thus, Gram-negative bacilli that
contain O and K antigens have an increased ability to survive in the
bloodstream. Indeed, most episodes of Gram-negative bacteraemia are
caused by smooth and/or encapsulated strains. Nevertheless, rough and
unencapsulated strains of Gram-negative bacilli may also cause bacteraemia and septic shock. This is, however, rare and is mostly seen in
patients with severely diminished host defence. Once the imbalance
between host defence and bacterial virulence has allowed the micro-
organisms to invade and survive in the bloodstream, the ensuing cascade of
events and ultimately the patient's outcome are dependent on the Gram-
negative bacillary strain. All Gram-negative bacillary strains possess
the capacity, upon invasion into the bloodstream, to cause septic shock
syndrome.

3.4.5   *Pseudomonas aeruginosa*

Studies on the opsonic requirements of *P. aeruginosa* have shown that
antibodies against mucoid exopolysaccharide (MEP; the primary constituent of the slime coat of mucoid strains) are important opsonins. These
mucoid strains are the primary pathogens in cystic fibrosis (CF) patients.
MEP promotes the adherence of *P. aeruginosa* strains to tracheal cells and
respiratory mucins.

The heteropolymeric nature of MEP is explained by the presence of both
common and type-specific epitopes; the common epitopes are divided into
those that bind opsonizing and those that bind non-opsonizing antibodies.
Most naturally occurring antibodies to MEP function poorly in *in vitro*
opsonophagocytosis assays with complement and are unable to protect
host animals. In contrast, antibodies that are highly opsonic protect host
animals against infection, and have been found in older CF patients who
are not colonized with *P. aeruginosa*. Opsonizing antibodies to MEP are
usually not found in younger non-colonized or chronically colonized CF
patients. These findings suggest a protective effect for the opsonizing
antibodies. MEP, therefore, has become a promising vaccine candidate for
the prevention of *P. aeruginosa* infection in CF patients. Unfortunately, in
humans MEP appears to be poorly immunogenic in inducing opsonic
antibodies (42, 43).

3.4.6   *Neisseria*

Specific antibodies and the complement system play key roles in host
defence against *N. meningitidis* and *N. gonorrhoea*. They can lyse bacteria,
enhance phagocytosis and neutralize the effects mediated by endotoxin
(44, 45). In *N. meningitidis* the presence of a bactericidal antibody, however, is of utmost importance. Anti-capsular polysaccharide antibodies and
anti-outer membrane protein antibodies in general facilitate phagocytosis

and killing. Antibodies against meningococcal LPS also appear to contribute to opsonophagocytosis. However, for optimal phagocytosis complement should also be present.

Although the alternative pathway is not able to halt meningococcal dissemination in susceptible infants (indicating the importance of antibodies and the classical complement pathway), the relative importance of the alternative pathway is shown in families with a sex-linked properdin (alternative pathway) deficiency. Individuals belonging to these families experience multiple, sometimes fatal, episodes of fulminant group B, C, and Y meningococcal infections (44). In contrast, individuals with a deficiency in early classical complement components show an unexpected lack of meningococcal disease. Some unknown compensatory mechanisms must be involved in the resistance against meningococci in these patients. Perhaps antibodies and the successful use of the alternative pathway may be responsible for this resistance mechanism.

3.4.7   Other micro-organisms

The opsonic requirements of many other micro-organisms (bacteria, fungi, parasites) have been studied. The general conclusion is that cell wall antigens may determine whether the micro-organisms are readily phagocytosed. In some micro-organisms the capsule is the determining factor, while in others proteins or lipopolysaccharides may be responsible for the resistance to opsonization. For example, the expression of plasmid-encoded proteins is associated with resistance to complement-mediated opsonization and neutrophil phagocytosis in the cell wall of *Yersinia enterocolitica*. PMN also play a role in eliminating virus particles (46, 47). For example, interaction of herpes virions through PMN-complement CR_1 and CR_3 results solely in binding to PMN, but not in internalization (46). For internalization, interaction with FcR is mandatory. Recently, it has been shown that some parasites (e.g. *Trypanosoma cruzi*, the causative agents of Chagas disease) produce a glycoprotein (gp160) that restricts complement activation by inhibiting C3 convertase formation. This glycoprotein is similar to a human complement regulatory protein, the decay-acceleration factor (48).

4   Phagocytosis

PMN takes up opsonized micro-organisms into phagosomes that fuse with secretory granules (lysosomes) to form phagolysosomes. Killing and digestion of micro-organisms take place within these phagolysosomes (49). Therefore, toxic events against the phagocytosed micro-organism can only occur when PMN granules fuse with the phagosome.

4.1   Normal phagocytosis

Phagocytosis is the process that leads to ingestion of the particle. It involves both attachment to receptors and subsequent engulfment.

Phagocytosis starts with receptor–ligand binding between PMN and the microbe. The receptor–ligand interaction activates the engine of the ingestion phase: actin, myosin, and actin-binding proteins. The actin microfilaments in the portion of the cytoplasm, which underlies the site of particle attachment undergoes polymerization. This polymerization leads to puckering of the plasma membrane at the site of contact, because the microfilaments attach to the membrane. The membrane envelops the particle and new particle–membrane contacts result. Pseudopodia (finger-like extensions of the plasma membrane) are produced, the particle becomes surrounded by these pseudopodia and a phagocytic vacuole (phagosome) occurs (4). While this is happening, granules in the cytoplasma fuse with the phagosome membrane, and a new phagolysosome is produced.

4.2   Microbial evasion of phagocytosis

Some bacteria are able to inhibit the fusion of the granules with the phagosome and thereby escape killing by PMN. These micro-organisms inhibit degranulation and are called intracellular pathogens (50). A strong correlation exists between inhibition of lysosome–phagosome fusion and impaired microbicidal function. For example, *Mycobacterium tuberculosis* is an obligate intracellular bacterium that survives by interfering with lysosome–phagosome fusion. When viable *M. tuberculosis* organisms are ingested, the azurophilic granules remain intact and do not fuse with the phagosomes containing *M. tuberculosis*. In contast, lysosomes do fuse with phagosomes containing non-viable *M. tuberculosis* (51). The reason for this apparent difference is that viable *M. tuberculosis* produce strongly acidic sulphatides that accumulate in azurophilic granules and prevent lysosome–phagosome fusion. Surface components of *Mycobacterium leprae* and *M. tuberculosis* are also responsible for the inhibition of fusion. For example, the cord factor, a cell wall glycolipid of mycobacteria, inhibits fusion between phospholipid vesicles in general and between phagosomes and lysosomes in particular. Therefore, metabolically active intracellular *M. tuberculosis* are able to avoid exposure to lysosomal contents by preventing degranulation (50).

Abnormalities in lysosome–phagosome fusion have also been demonstrated in neutrophils and macrophages that have phagocytosed other bacteria (such as *Salmonella* and gonococci), fungi (such as *Histoplasma capsulatum*), and live *Toxoplasma gondii*. This suggests that certain fungal and protozoal species also secrete factors that inhibit the disruption of lysosomes (50).

Virulent gonococci attach to PMN and stimulate an oxidative metabolic response. The azurophilic granules, however, do not release their contents into phagocytic vacuoles and the intracellular gonococci remain viable. Gonococci possess protein I as a major outer membrane protein. This protein is a porin, one of a class of specialized proteins used by bacteria to permit the passage of ions and nutrients through their otherwise impermeable outer membrane. Protein I possesses the unusual capacity to translocate from the gonococci into human cells (51). When inserted in membranes, the pore remains open unless a potential difference exceeding 60 mV is applied to the membrane in which the porin is inserted. Porin I can be translocated from the gonococcus into the phagolysosome membrane in an open state. This allows an influx of anions. As the potential difference increases, the porin closes. This leads to inhibition of degranulation but does not affect superoxide anion (O_2^-) generation, indicating that degranulation and superoxide anion generation have different ionic requirements (52). In the pathogenesis of *Y. enterocolitica*, infections of outer membrane proteins play a role. The presence of one of the outer membrane proteins is under the control of a virulence plasmid (extrachromosomal DNA). *Yersinia* strains containing these plasmids are more virulent than those without the plasmids. Strains with this outer membrane protein inhibit the PMN respiratory burst after phagocytosis (53). The reason for these effects is as yet unclear.

Opsonization may block the capacity of micro-organisms to inhibit phagosome–lysosome fusion. For example, live *Chlamydia* organisms are readily phagocytosed but little degranulation occurs and the organisms replicate within the phagosomes. However, when antibody-coated *Chlamydia* are phagocytosed, prompt lysosome–phagosome fusion is observed. Thus, many micro-organisms are able to protect themselves against exposure to toxic lysosomal contents; for example, viable *T. gondii*, *M. leprae*, *M. tuberculosis*, and *Salmonella typhimurium*. However, killed *T. gondii*, mycobacteria and, salmonella are unable to inhibit fusion. Also, opsonization may prevent inhibition of phagolysosome fusion in some cases, but not in others. For example, opsonization of *M. leprae* has no effect on inhibition of fusion, while opsonized *Salmonella* are more able to inhibit phagolysosome fusion than are non-opsonized *Salmonella* (49, 50, 54).

It is also possible that *de novo* synthesis of new bacterial proteins (stress proteins) in the intracellular environment of the PMN interfere with the phagosome membrane. These proteins are not produced when bacterial growth occurs under favourable circumstances.

Some bacteria are resistant to lysosomal enzymes. Capsular antigen lipopolysaccharides confer resistance of Gram-negative bacteria to lysosomal enzymes. Also, *Leishmania* are resistant and are able to replicate within the phagolysosome (50).

5 Killing

PMN are able to kill micro-organisms by two distinct mechanisms. One antimicrobial system is oxygen dependent, while the other can kill bacteria in the absence of oxygen.

5.1 Oxygen-dependent events

5.1.1 Normal function of the oxygen-dependent antimicrobial system

A detailed description of the activation of the oxidative burst can be found in Chapter 3. In this section the oxidative system will be described in relation to how various oxygen products participate in microbial killing. The oxygen-dependent antimicrobial mechanisms are set in motion when PMN undergo a 'respiratory burst'. NADPH oxidase in the phagolysosome membrane is activated and reduces O_2 to superoxide ($\cdot O_2^-$). O_2 reduction is the first step in a series of reactions that produces toxic oxygen species. For example, $\cdot O_2^-$ dismutates to H_2O_2 and the azurophil granule enzyme MPO catalyses the oxidation of Cl^- by H_2O_2 to yield HOCl. H_2O_2 is a powerful oxidant; however, it reacts sluggishly with biological materials. In addition, most micro-organisms contain enzymes that detoxify H_2O_2, such as catalase and/or NADH or sulphydryl-peroxidase, and therefore, are highly resistant to killing by H_2O_2 (49).

H_2O_2 and $\cdot O_2^-$ can give rise to more potent agents in the presence of ferric ion or Fe^{3+} chelates. $\cdot O_2^-$ reduces Fe^{3+} or Fe^{3+} chelates to Fe^{2+}. The reaction of H_2O_2 with Fe^{2+} chelates yields iron–oxygen complexes that react directly with microbial components or that release hydroxyl radicals ($\cdot OH$, Haber–Weiss reaction). Because $\cdot OH$ reacts rapidly with chemical bonds of all kinds, it causes damage near the site where it is produced. If $\cdot OH$ is produced in phagolysosomes, an enormous amount would be required for killing, because most of the $\cdot OH$ would be consumed in the oxidation of microbial surface components that are not essential to viability. Recent studies, therefore, cast doubts on the significance of $\cdot OH$ as an antimicrobial reactive oxygen species of PMN. *In vivo*, most of the extracellular iron is bound to transferrin or lactoferrin. Although some authors believe that transferrin and lactoferrin can catalyse the formation of $\cdot OH$ (55), there is also evidence that iron is bound in such a way that it is unable to catalyse the formation of $\cdot OH$ and other toxic oxygen species (56). However, it is still possible that transferrin (an iron-binding protein) shuttles iron from the outside to the inside of the PMN. Because of the low pH in the phagolysosome, iron is released and free iron can take part in the Haber–Weiss reaction (55). Some bacteria (e.g. *Pseudomonas aeruginosa*) produce proteases that can modify transferrin- and/or lactoferrin-forming iron complexes, yielding iron chelates that enhance ·OH formation (57). When the ·OH is produced outside PMN, increased tissue damage due to this toxic oxygen metabolite can occur.

HOCl is a potent microbicidal agent. However, it is unlikely that HOCl acts directly in phagolysosomes. This agent reacts rapidly with ammonia (NH_4^+) to yield monochloramine (NH_2Cl) and with amines to yield mono- and dichloramines ($RNHCl$ and $RNCl_2$). The concentration of nitrogen compounds is very high *in vivo*, so that HOCl has little opportunity to react directly with target cells. Instead, toxicity of the $MPO/H_2O_2/Cl^-$ system is mediated by chloramines (49).

5.1.2   *Microbial evasion of oxygen-dependent killing*

Micro-organisms differ greatly in their susceptibility to killing by oxidants. These differences are due in part to differing levels of intracellular protective enzymes produced by certain bacteria, such as superoxide dismutase (SOD), catalases, reductases, and peroxidases. However, it is not known whether any micro-organism has sufficiently high levels of such enzymes to escape killing by PMN oxidants *in vivo*. *E. coli*, *S. typhimurium*, and *Bacillus subtilis* exposed to sublethal concentrations of H_2O_2 adapt in such a way that they can survive subsequent exposures to considerably higher concentrations of this oxidant. Adaptation has been linked to the induction of antioxidant enzymes, competent DNA repair, and a variety of stress proteins. These proteins, resulting from oxidant stress, are similar to heat-shock proteins.

S. typhimurium becomes resistant to killing by H_2O_2 when pre-treated with non-lethal levels of this oxidant. This adaptation results in the transient accumulation of a distinct group of proteins. Most of these proteins are under the control of the so-called OXY R gene product. The expression of the kat G (catalase) gene also appears to be regulated by OXY R at the level of mRNA (58).

Candida albicans.   This fungus is a leading cause of opportunistic mycosis, and it undergoes reversible high-frequency phenotypic switching (59). This switching is a genetically programmed phenomenon. The phenotypic difference reflects changes in surface properties of blastoconidia and pseudohyphae and leads to differences in colony morphology (white and opaque phenotypes). Blastoconidia of the opaque phenotypes are more susceptible to killing by neutrophils or cell-free oxidants like H_2O_2 or the $MPO/H_2O_2/Cl^-$ system, than are those of the white phenotype. They are also more potent stimuli of the neutrophil superoxide generation system than are the white cells. In addition, both neutrophils and oxidants (re-agents H_2O_2 or NOCl as well as the $MPO/H_2O_2/Cl^-$ system) induce uni-directional increases in the spontaneous rates of switching from white to opaque phenotypes. Differences in expression of *C. albicans* phenotypes, therefore, may determine the relative susceptibility to neutrophil fungicidal mechanisms, and the neutrophils themselves appear capable of selectively augmenting the switching process.

Listeria monocytogenes.   This bacteria is the causative agent of listeriosis, and is able to avoid the lethal effects of oxygen metabolites. Interestingly, this resistance appears to be related to the growth phase of the bacteria. *In vitro* listeria in the logarithmic phase of multiplication are more resistant to toxic oxygen species than are listeria in the resting stage (60). This is because of a higher rate of catalase production during the logarithmic phase; thus, catalase is present in higher concentrations than when listeria are in a stationary phase.

Neisseria gonorrhoeae.   This bacteria has a habitat that is strictly limited to human hosts. This organism forms little or no SOD, even under redox stress. However, exposure of gonococci to sublethal concentrations of superoxide and H_2O_2 results in resistance to oxidant stress. This adapta-tion requires new protein synthesis but is not related to increased produc-tion of SOD or catalase. It appears that gonococci bound to human PMN use PMN-derived lactase. This leads to an increase in oxygen consumption and the creation of an anaerobic environment for the gonococcus. This could be important for the survival of bacteria exposed to phagocytes (61).

Legionella pneumophila.   This bacteria replicates intracellularly in macro-phages and fibroblasts, behaving like an obligate intracellular organism. Since *L. pneumophila* does not replicate extracellularly *in vivo*, some aspects of the metabolism of host monocytes and macrophages would appear to contribute to the bacterial replication. *L. pneumophila* produces a toxin that inhibits the oxidative response of macrophages during phago-cytosis. Since both virulent and avirulent strains are susceptible to products of the oxidative reaction of phagocytes, survival and replication of these organisms within macrophages are thus enhanced by inhibition of host–cell oxidative metabolism (62).

Iron also plays an important role in the survival of legionella in the phagosome. Iron is taken up by PMN and monocytes when it is bound to lactoferrin or transferrin. Lactoferrin, an iron-binding protein with a high degree of homology to transferrin, is found in specific granules of PMN. In its unsaturated form, lactoferrin has been found to have either a bacterio-static or bactericidal effect against a variety of extracellular bacteria *in vitro*. At sites of inflammation, such as occur at infected sites in the body, unsaturated lactoferrin is released by the specific granules of neutrophils into the extracellular environment. At the acidic pH often found at sites of inflammation, free iron is present because transferrin is unable to bind and hold iron under acidic conditions. Since lactoferrin has a high affinity for iron under acidic conditions, it can bind this free iron, rendering it unavailable to pathogenic micro-organisms. Iron–lactoferrin is then taken up by mononuclear phagocytes via receptors with a specificity for lactoferrin. By this mechanism, lactoferrin contributes to localized hypoferremia at sites of infection or inflammation, and may also contribute to systemic hypoferremia.

The release of iron from lactoferrin within the mononuclear phagocyte appears to involve a different mechanism than that from transferrin. In the case of transferrin, endocytosed iron–transferrin enters a distinct, mildly acidic endosomal compartment within the cell where it releases iron and is then recycled back to the cell surface. Iron–lactoferrin also cycles through a mildly acidic endosomal compartment, but does not release iron under this condition. Iron is released from lactoferrin when a portion of the endocytosed lactoferrin enters the lysosomal compartment and is degraded. Thus, there is a potential indirect role for PMN in host defence against legionella. PMN provide monocytes with lactoferrin and thereby enable the monocyte to inhibit *L. pneumophila* intracellular multiplication (62).

Aspergillus. The resting conidia stage of this fungus is resistant to killing. Despite their susceptibility to phagocytosis, resting conidia of *Aspergillus fumigatus* only marginally stimulate production of superoxide anion, hydrogen peroxide (H_2O_2), and hypochlorous acid (HOCl) and induce less MPO-dependent iodination by PMN than do metabolically active conidia. Metabolically active conidia were more readily killed by PMN than are resting conidia. However, PMN of patients with chronic granulomatous disease (CGD) do not kill these fungal elements, indicating the importance of toxic oxygen species in killing conidia. In a recent trial interferon-γ was shown to enhance killing of aspergillus by CGD cells (63). Certain group B streptococci are also readily ingested but not killed, presumably due to inhibition of the PMN respiratory burst by the bacteria. This may be due to presence of C protein in the cell wall of these bacteria (64).

5.2   Oxygen-independent events

5.2.1   *Normal function of the oxygen-independent system*

PMN cytoplasmic granules contain additional antimicrobial agents that are released into phagolysosomes and do not require the production of oxidants for activity. These agents include proteases, other hydrolytic enzymes, such as phospholipases, glycosidases, and lysozymes, and other proteins and peptides that disrupt microbial functions or structural components. It is likely that all of these agents must bind to the microbial cell surface to have antimicrobial activity. Therefore, the activity of each agent is limited to certain micro-organisms. Three well-characterized granule components known as B/PI (bactericidal/permeability-increasing protein), CLCP (chymotrypsin-like cationic protein; cathepsin G), and defensins, have microbicidal activity *in vitro* (4, 49).

B/PI. This 58 kDa protein of the primary (azurophil) granules may contribute to the ability of neutrophils to kill Gram-negative bacteria. Within 15 s after exposure to B/PI *E. coli* no longer form colonies (65). Loss of viability is caused by an increase in outer membrane permeability to hydrophobic molecules and by activation of enzymes that are able to degrade peptidoglycan and outer membrane phospholipids. The specificity of B/PI for Gram-negative bacteria is due to the interactions between B/PI and LPS. The interactions between cationic B/PI molecules and anionic phosphate or 2-keto-3-deoxy-D-mannooctulonic acid (KDO) residues disrupt the LPS layer. Binding of B/PI to the outer membrane of Gram-negative bacilli also leads to displacement of KDO- and phosphate-bound divalent cations that stabilize the outer membrane by hydrophobic binding of B/PI to the outer membrane. The displaced calcium ions then activate bacterial phospholipases.

Other investigators have also purified 55–58 kDa antimicrobial proteins from human PMN (65–68). Shafer *et al.* (66) referred to their material as CAP-57 (cationic antimicrobial protein-57) and described its activity against *S. typhimurium*, *E. coli*, and *N. gonorrhoeae*. Hovde and Gray (67) purified and characterized a 55 kDa protein, BP55, that is highly active against *P. aeruginosa*. The activity of BP55 is inhibited by LPS. It is likely that CAP-57 and BP55 are very similar to B/PI (69).

CLCP. Azurophil granules of human PMN contain three immunologically cross-reactive cationic proteins that have both antibacterial and chymotrypsin-like neutral protease activity *in vitro*. Exposure of *S. aureus* or *E. coli* to CLCP causes inhibition of multiplication due to inhibition of macromolecular (protein, RNA, and DNA) synthesis. The ability of CLCP to kill *S. aureus* and *E. coli in vitro* is markedly inhibited by altering the incubation conditions, for example, by adding millimolar concentrations of calcium or magnesium ions or by increasing ionic strength or acidity. The microbicidal activity of CLCP persists when protease activity is abolished by heat or by active-site inhibitors. Therefore, the microbicidal activity of CLCP does not depend on a primary proteolytic activity. CLCP has also been shown to sensitize Gram-negative bacteria *Acinetobacter* 199A to lysozyme and to act synergistically with PMN elastase against *E. coli* and *S. aureus* (49).

Defensins. The cytoplasmic granules of PMN contain a variety of anti-microbial cationic proteins with potent antimicrobial activity. Three structurally and functionally homologous peptides, called defensins, exist in human PMN. These peptides are small (3.5 kDa), cysteine-rich, only moderately cationic, and identical except at their N-terminal residues (49, 70, 71). They are also remarkably abundant—up to 5–7 per cent of the total protein of human PMN and 30–50 per cent of the total protein of the primary (azurophil) granules. These peptides have a broad spectrum of activity *in vitro* against Gram-positive and -negative bacteria, fungi (including *Candida* species and *Cryptococcus neoformans*), and certain enveloped viruses. Human PMN defensins only kill metabolically active bacteria and induce loss of outer and inner membrane integrity.

Other granular agents that contribute to bactericidal activity of the PMN are, for example, elastase and lactoferrin. Lactoferrin binds iron and produces an iron-free milieu in the PMN. It is bacteriostatic because most bacteria do not multiply in the absence of iron (72, 73). Lactoferrin also alters the cell wall of bacteria so that it becomes more accessible to lysozyme. Thus, lactoferrin and lysozyme act synergistically (74).

Chapter 7 contains additional information on the different types of enzymes found in the primary, secondary, and tertiary granules contained in PMN.

5.2.2   Evasion of nonoxidative mechanisms

In reality any alteration induced by a microbe in opsonization or phago-cytosis (including phagosome–lysosome fusion) will allow evasion of non-oxidative killing. Few examples of direct inhibition of lysosomal proteins are known.

6   Digestion

It is often assumed that most micro-organisms are digested after being killed and that bacterial components are rapidly degraded by the numerous granule-associated degradate enzymes. The degree of digestion of engulfed bacteria depends on the structure of the bacterial cell envelope and on the presence of digestive enzymes in the phagocyte. For example, non-encapsulated *E. coli* strains exhibit a rapid and extensive degradation of macromolecules such as proteins, RNA, and peptidoglycan by PMN. Intracellular killing of ingested bacteria takes place during the first few minutes of phagocytosis. In contrast to the rapid killing and extensive breakdown of non-encapsulated strains, strains with capsular K antigen are more resistant to killing and resist degradation by PMN (75, 76).

7 Conclusions

The phagocytic cell is the cornerstone in host defence. Without adequate numbers of PMN or properly functioning PMN, patients suffer from infections. The basic processes that are involved in eliminating invading micro-organisms are chemotaxis, opsonization, digestion, and killing. The case presented at the beginning of this chapter is an example of how a deficiency in antibody production results in decreased opsonization, phagocytosis and killing of *H. influenzae* by PMN.

Many micro-organisms have developed strategies to resist phagocytosis. Some produce substances that paralyse PMN and hinder the directional movement of PMN to the vicinity of the bacteria. Many virulent microbes are equipped with cell wall structures that enable them to resist opsonization (e.g. *H. influenzae*). Other bacteria have capsules, which are not very immunogenic. Therefore antibodies against these capsules are often absent. Capsules also prevent complement activation and reaction between IgG and cell wall epitopes. The capsule may also prevent the PMN from intracellular killing of bacteria. Once ingested, bacteria utilize a large armamentarium to escape toxic events in the phagolysosome. Some of these avoidance mechanisms impact on the host's immune response in such a way that secondary infections can occur (see Chapter 6).

Future work should be undertaken to enhance the killing capacity of phagocytic cells against intracellular bacterial survivors. Recombinant cytokines like the colony stimulating factors are likely candidates (as noted in Chapter 8). Also, vaccines that can lead to the development of antibodies against capsular epitopes are of importance. The dramatic decrease in the incidence of invasive *H. influenzae* type b disease associated with the introduction of *H. influenzae* type b vaccine is evidence of this point. The role of antibodies against cell wall components such as peptidoglycans, outer membrane proteins, and teichoic acid, in the host defence against certain bacteria is still largely unknown. The study of antigenic variations and regulation of genes that play a role in intracellular survival of microbes is still largely *terra incognita*.

References

1 Moxon, E. R. (1990). *Haemophilus influenzae*. In *Principles and practice of infectious diseases*, 3rd edition (ed. S. L. Mandell, R. G. Douglas, and J. E. Bennett), pp. 1722–33. Churchill Livingstone Inc., New York.

2 Densen, P. and Mandell, G. L. (1990). Granulocytic phagocytes. In *Principles and practice of infectious diseases*, 3rd edition (ed. S. L. Mandell, R. G. Douglas, and J. E. Bennett), pp. 81–101. Churchill Livingstone Inc., New York.

3 Metzger, H. (ed.) (1990). *Fc receptors and the action of antibodies.* ASM Publications, Washington DC.

4 Sawyer, D. W., Donowitz, G. R., and Mandell, G. L. (1989). Polymorphonuclear neutrophils: an effective antimicrobial force. *Rev. Infect. Dis.,* **2, suppl 7,** S1532–S44.

5 Finlay, B. B. and Falkow, S. (1989). Common themes in microbial pathogenicity. *Microbiol. Rev.,* **53,** 210–30.

6 Sobel, J. D. and Kaye, D. (1990). Urinary tract infection. In *Principles and practice of infectious diseases,* 3rd edition (ed. E. L. Mandell, R. G. Jr Douglas and J. E. Bennett), pp. 582–611. Churchill Livingstone Inc., New York.

7 Rodriguez-Ortega, M., Ofek, I., and Sharon, N. (1987). Membrane glycoproteins of human polymorphonuclear leukocytes that act as receptors for mannose-specific *Escherichia coli. Infect. Immun.,* **55,** 968–73.

8 Svanborg Eden, C., Bjursten, L. M., Hull, R., Hull, S., Magnusson, K. E., Moldovano, Z., and Leffler, H. (1984). Influence of adhesins on the interaction of *Escherichia coli* with human phagocytes. *Infect. Immun.,* **44,** 672–80.

9 Wright, S. D., Tobias, P. S., Ulevitch, R. J., and Ramos, R. A. (1989). Lipopolysaccharide (LPS) binding protein opsonizes LPS-bearing particles for recognition by a novel receptor on macrophages. *J. Exp. Med.,* **170,** 1231–41.

10 Farrell, C. F. and Rest, R. F. (1990). Up-regulation of human neutrophil receptors for *Neisseria gonorrhoeae* expressing PII outer membrane proteins. *Infect. Immun.,* **58,** 2777–84.

11 Proctor, R. A., Prendergast, E., and Mosher, D. F. (1984). Fibronectin mediates attachment of *Staphylococcus aureus* to human neutrophils. *Blood,* **59,** 681.

12 Hill, H. R., Shigeoka, A. O., Augustine, N. H., Pritchard, D., Lundblad, J. L., and Schwartz, R. S. (1984). Fibronectin enhances the opsonic and protective activity of monoclonal and polyclonal antibody against group B streptococci. *J. Exp. Med.,* **159,** 1618–28.

13 Gemmell, C. and O'Dowd, A. (1983). Regulation of protein A biosynthesis in *Staphylococcus aureus* by certain antibiotics: its effect on phagocytosis by leukocytes. *J. Antimicrob. Chemother.,* **12,** 587–97.

14 Milatovic, D. (1983). Antibiotics and phagocytosis. *Eur. J. Clin. Microbiol.,* **2,** 414–25.

15 Veringa, E. M. and Verhoef, J. (1987). Clindamycin at subinhibitory concentrations enhances antibody- and complement-dependent phagocytosis by human polymorphonuclear leukocytes of *Staphylococcus aureus. Chemotherapy,* **33,** 243–9.

16 Berridge, M. J. and Irvine, R. F. (1984). Inositol triphosphate, a novel second messenger in cellular signal transduction. *Nature,* **312,** 315–21.

17 Davis, B. D., Dulbecco, R., Eisen, H. N., Ginsberg, H. S., and Wood, W. B. Jr (eds) (1990). *Microbiology,* Harper & Row, Hagerstown, MD.

18 Verbrugh, H. A., Dijk, W. C. van, Peters, R., Erne, M. E., van, Daha, M. R., Peterson, P. K., and Verhoef, J. (1980). Opsonic recognition of staphylococci mediated by cell wall peptidoglycan: antibody-dependent activation of human complement and opsonic activity of peptidoglycan antibodies. *J. Immunol.,* **124,** 1167–73.

19 Wilkinson, B. J., Peterson, P. K., and Quie, P. G. (1979). Cryptic peptidoglycan and the antiphagocytic effect of the *Staphylococcus aureus* capsule: model for the antiphagocytic effect of bacterial cell surface polymers. *Infect. Immun.,* **23,** 502–8.

20 Verbrugh, H. A., Peterson, P. K., Nguyen, B. Y. T., Sisson, S. P., and Kim, Y. (1982). Opsonization of encapsulated *Staphylococcus aureus*: the role of specific antibody and complement. *J. Immunol.,* **129,** 1681–7.

21 Karakawa, W. W., Sutton, A., Schneerson, R., Karpas, A., and Finn, W. F. (1988). Capsular antibodies induce type-specific phagocytosis of capsulated *Staphylococcus aureus* by human polymorphonuclear leucocytes. *Infect. Immun.,* **56,** 1090–5.

22 Nelles, M. J., Niswander, C. A., Karakawa, W. W., Vann, W. F., and Arbeit, R. D. (1985). Reactivity of type-specific monoclonal antibodies with *Staphylococcus aureus* clinical isolates and purified capsular polysaccharide. *Infect. Immun.,* **49,** 14–18.

23 Verhoef, J. and Verbrugh, H. A. (1981). Host determinants in staphylococcal disease. In *Annual review of medicine,* vol. 32 (ed. W. P. Creger, C. H. Coggins, and E. W. Hancock), pp. 107–22. Annual Review Inc., Palo Alto, CA.

24 Kojima, Y., Tojo, M., Goldmann, D. A., Tosteson, T. D., and Pier, G. B. (1990). Antibody to the capsular polysaccharide/adhesin protects rabbits against catheter-related bacteremia due to coagulase-negative staphylococci. *J. Infect. Dis.,* **162,** 435–41.

25 Timmerman, C. P., Besnier, J. M., Graaf, L. de, Torensma, R., Verkley, A. J., Fleer, A., and Verhoef, J. (1991). Characterisation and functional aspects of monoclonal antibodies specific for surface proteins of coagulase-negative staphylococci. *J. Med. Microbiol.,* **35,** 65–71.

26 Schutze, G. E., Hall, M. A., Baker, C. J., and Edwards, M. S. (1991). Role of neutrophil receptors in opsonophagocytosis of coagulase-negative staphylococci. *Infect. Immun.,* **59,** 2573–8.

27 Pascual, A., Fleer, A., Westerdaal, N. A. C., Berghuis, M., and Verhoef, J. (1988). Surface hydrophobicity and opsonic requirements of coagulase-negative staphylococci in suspension and adhering to a polymer substratum. *Eur. J. Clin. Microbiol. Infect. Dis.,* **7,** 161–6.

28 Fischetti, V. A. (1991). Streptococcal M protein. *Sci. Am.,* **June,** 32–9.

29 Baker, C. J., Edwards, M. S., Webb, B. J., and Kasper, D. L. (1982).

Antibody-independent classical pathway-mediated opsonophagocytosis of type 1a, group B *Streptococcus. J. Clin. Invest.,* **69**, 394–404.

30 Baker, C. J., Webb, B. J., Kasper, D. L., and Edwards, M. S. (1986). The role of complement and antibody in opsonophagocytosis of type II group B streptococci. *J. Infect. Dis.,* **152**, 47–54.

31 Levy, N. J. and Kasper, D. L. (1986). Surface-bound capsular polysaccharide of type 1a group B *Streptococcus* mediates C1 binding and activation of the classic complement pathway. *J. Immunol.,* **136**, 4157–62.

32 Edwards, M. S., Kasper, D. L., Jennings, H. J., Baker, C. L., and Nicholson-Weller, A. (1982). Capsular sialic acid prevents activation of the alternative complement pathway by type III, group B streptococci. *J. Immunol.,* **128**, 1278–83.

33 Egan, M. L., Pritchard, D. G., Dillon, H. C., and Gray, B. M. (1983). Protection of mice from experimental infection with type III group B streptococcus using monoclonal antibodies. *J. Exp. Med.,* **156**, 1006.

34 Hill, H. R., Shigeoka, A. O., Augustine, N. H., Pritchard, D., Lundblad, J. L., and Schwartz, R. S. (1984). Fibronectin enhances the opsonic and protective activity of monoclonal and polyclonal antibody against group B streptococci. *J. Exp. Med.,* **159**, 1618.

35 Bonhsack, J. F., Hawley, M. M., Pritchard, D. G., Egan, M. L., Shigeoka, A. O., Yang, K. D., and Hill, H. R. (1989). An IgA monoclonal antibody directed against type III antigen on group B streptococci acts as an opsonin. *J. Immunol.,* **143**, 3338–42.

36 Gordon, D. L., Johnson, D. M., and Hostetter, M. K. (1986). Ligand–receptor interactions in the phagocytosis of virulent *Streptococcus pneumoniae* by polymorphonuclear leukocytes. *J. Infect. Dis.,* **154**, 619–26.

37 Hoostetter, M. K. (1986). Serotypic variations among virulent pneumococci in deposition and degradation of covalently bound C3b: implications for phagocytosis and antibody production. *J. Infect. Dis.,* **153**, 682–93.

38 Gordon, D. L., Rice, J., Finlay-Jones, J. J., McDonald, P. J., and Hostetter, M. K. (1988). Analysis of C3 deposition and degradation on bacterial surfaces after opsonization. *J. Infect. Dis.,* **157**, 697–704.

39 Cates, K. L., Marsh, K. H., and Granoff, D. M. (1985). Serum opsonic activity after immunization of adults with *Haemophilus influenzae* type-b-diphtheria toxoid conjugate vaccine. *Infect. Immun.,* **48**, 183–9.

40 Roord, J. J., Daha, M., Kuis, W., Verbrugh, H. A., and Verhoef, J. (1983). Inherited deficiency of the third component of complement associated with recurrent pyogenic infections, circulating immune complexes, and vasculitis in a Dutch family. *Pediatrics,* **71**, 81–7.

41 Vermeulen, C., Cross, A., Byrne, W. R., and Zollinger, W. (1988). Quantitative relationship between capsular content and killing of K1-encapsulated *Escherichia coli. Infect. Immun.*, **56**, 2723–30.

42 Schreiber, J. R., Pier, G. B., Grout, M., Nixon, K., and Patawaran, M. (1991). Induction of opsonic antibodies to *Pseudomonas aeruginosa* mucoid exopolysaccharide by an anti-idiotypic monoclonal antibody. *J. Infect. Dis.*, **164**, 507–14.

43 Garner, C. V., DesJardins, D., and Pier, G. B. (1990). Immunogenic properties of *Pseudomonas aeruginosa* mucoid exopolysaccharide. *Infect. Immun.*, **58**, 1835–42.

44 Jarvis, G. A. and Vedros, N. A. (1987). Sialic acid of group B *Neisseria meningitidis* regulates alternative complement pathway activation. *Infect. Immun.*, **55**, 174–80.

45 Ross, S. C., Rosenthal, P. J., Berberich, H. J., and Densen, P. (1987). Killing of *Neisseria meningitidis* by human neutrophils: implications for normal and complement-deficient individuals. *J. Infect. Dis.*, **155**, 1266–75.

46 Strijp, J. A. G. van, Kessel, K. P. M. van, Tol, M. E. van der, and Verhoef, J. (1989). Complement-mediated phagocytosis of herpes simplex virus by granulocyte binding or ingestion. *J. Clin. Invest.*, **84**, 107–12.

47 Turner, R. B. (1990). The role of neutrophils in the pathogenesis of rhinovirus infections. *Pediatr. Infect. Dis. J.*, **9**, 832–5.

48 Joiner, K. A., Dias daSilva, W., Rimoldi, M. T., Hammer, C. H., Sher, A., and Kipnis, T. L. (1988). Biochemical characterization of a factor produced by *Trypanosoma cruzei* that accelerates the decay of complement C3 convertases. *J. Biol. Chem.*, **23**, 11317–35.

49 Thomas, L. T. and Lehrer, R. I. (1988). Human neutrophil antimicrobial activity. *Rev. Infect. Dis.*, **10, suppl 2**, S450–56.

50 Quie, P. G. (1983). Perturbation of the normal mechanisms of intra-leukocytic killing bacteria. *J. Infect. Dis.*, **148**, 189–93.

51 Armstrong, J. A. and Hart, P. D. (1971). Response of cultured macrophages to *Mycobacterium tuberculosis* with observations on fusion of lysosomes with phagosomes. *J. Exp. Med.*, **134**, 713–40.

52 Haines, K. A., Yeh, L., Blake, M. S., Cristello, P., Korchak, H., and Weissmann, G. (1988). Protein I, a translocatable ion channel from *Neisseria gonorrhoeae*, selectively inhibits exocytosis from human neutrophils without inhibiting O_2^- generation. *J. Biol. Chem.*, **263**, 945–51.

53 Lian, C. J. and Pai, C. H. (1985). Inhibition of human neutrophil chemiluminescence by plasmid-mediated outer membrane proteins of *Yersinia enterocolitica. Infect. Immun.*, **49**, 145–51.

54 Buchmeier, N. A. and Heffron, F. (1991). Inhibition of macrophage phagosome–lysosome fusion by *Salmonella typhimurium. Infect. Immun.*, **59**, 2232–8.

55 Klebanoff, S. J. and Walterdorph, A. M. (1990). Prooxidant activity of transferrin and lactoferrin. *J. Exp. Med.*, **172**, 1293–303.

56 Cohen, M. S., Brigitan, B. E., Hasselt, D. J., and Rosen, G. M. (1988). Phagocytes O_2 reduction, and hydroxyl radical. *Rev. Infect. Dis.*, **10**, 1088–96.

57 Britigan, B. E. and Edeker, B. L. (1991). *Pseudomonas* and neutrophil products modify transferrin and lactoferrin to create conditions that favor hydroxyl radical formation. *J. Clin. Invest.*, **88**, 1092–102.

58 Morgan, R. W., Christman, M. F., Jacobson, F. S., Storz, G., and Ames, B. N. (1986). Hydrogen peroxide-inducible proteins in *Salmonella typhimurium* overlap with heat shock and other stress proteins. *Proc. Natl Acad. Sci. USA*, **83**, 8059–63.

59 Kolotila, M. P. and Diamond, R. D. (1990). Effects of neutrophils and in vitro oxidants on survival and phenotypic switching of *Candida albicans* WO-1. *Infect. Immun.*, **58**, 1174–9.

60 Bortolussi, R., Vandenbroucke-Grauls, C. M. J. E., Asbeck, van B. S., and Verhoef, J. (1987). Relationship of bacterial growth phase to killing of *Listeria monocytogenes* by oxidative agents generated by neutrophils and enzyme systems. *Infect. Immun.*, **55**, 3197–202.

61 Fu, K. S., Hassett, D. J., and Cohen, M. S. (1989). Oxidant stress in *Neisseria gonorrhoeae:* adaptation and affects on L-(+)-lactate dehydrogenase activity. *Infect. Immun.*, **57**, 2173–8.

62 Byrd, T. F. and Horwitz, M. A. (1991). Lactoferrin inhibits or promotes *Legionella pneumophila* intracellular multiplication in nonactivated and interferon gamma-activated human monocytes depending upon its degree of iron saturation: iron–lactoferrin and nonphysiologic iron chelates reverse monocyte activation against *Legionella pneumophila*. *J. Clin. Invest.*, **88**, 1103–12.

63 Rex, J. H., Bennett, J. E., Gallin, J. I., Malech, H. L., DeCarlo, E. S., and Melnick, D. A. (1991). In vivo interferon-γ therapy augments the in vitro ability of chronic granulomatous disease neutrophils to damage *Aspergillus hyphae*. *J. Infect. Dis.*, **163**, 849–52.

64 Payne, N. R., Kim, Y., and Ferrieri, P. (1987). Effect of differences in antibody and complement requirements on phagocytic uptake and intracellular killing of 'c' protein-positive and -negative strains of type II group B streptococci. *Infect. Immun.*, **55**, 1243–51.

65 Elsbach, P. and Weiss, J. (1985). Oxygen-dependent and oxygen-independent mechanisms of microbicidal activity of neutrophils. *Blood*, **11**, 159–63.

66 Shafer, W. M., Martin, L. E., and Spitznagel, J. K. (1984). Cationic antimicrobial proteins isolates from human neutrophil granulocytes in the presence of diisopropyl fluorophosphate. *Infect. Immun.*, **45**, 29–35.

67 Hovde, C. J. and Gray, B. H. (1986). Characterization of a protein

from normal human polymorphonuclear leukocytes with bactericidal activity against *Pseudomonas aeruginosa. Infect. Immun.,* **54,** 142–8.

68 Wasiluk, K. R., Skubitz, K. M., and Gray, B. H. (1991). Comparison of granule proteins from human polymorphonuclear leukocytes which are bactericidal toward *Pseudomonas aeruginosa. Infect. Immun.,* **59,** 4193–200.

69 Pereira, H. A., Spitznagel, J. K., Winton, E. F., Shafer, W. M., Martin, L. E., Guzman, G. S. *et al.* (1990). The ontogeny of a 57-Kd cationic antimicrobial protein of human polymorphonuclear leukocytes: localization to a novel granule population. *Blood,* **76,** 825–34.

70 Ganz, T., Selstedt, M. E., Szklarek, D., Harwig, S. S. L., Daher, K., Bainton, D. F., and Lehrer, R. I. (1985). Defensins: natural peptide antibiotics of human neutrophils. *J. Clin. Invest.,* **76,** 1427–35.

71 Selsted, M. E., Harwig, S. S. L., Ganz, T., Schilling, J. W., and Lehrer, R. I. (1985). Primary structures of three human neutrophil defensins. *J. Clin. Invest.,* **76,** 1436–9.

72 Bullen, J. J. (1981). The significance of iron in infection. *Rev. Infect. Dis.,* **3,** 1127–38.

73 Bullen, J. J., Ward, C. G., and Rogers, H. J. (1991). The critical role of iron in some clinical infections. *Eur. J. Microbiol. Infect. Dis.,* **10,** 613–17.

74 Ellison, R. T. and Giehl, T. J. (1991). Killing of Gram-negative bacteria by lactoferrin and lysozyme. *J. Clin. Invest.,* **88,** 1080–91.

75 Rozenberg-Arska, M., Salters, M. E. C., Strijp, J. A. G. van, Geuze, J. J., and Verhoef, J. (1985). Electron microscopic study of phagocytosis of *Escherichia coli* by human polymorphonuclear leukocytes. *Infect. Immun.,* **50,** 852–9.

76 Rozenberg-Arska, M., Strijp, J. A. G. van, Hoekstra, W. P. M., and Verhoef, J. (1984). Effect of human polymorphonuclear and mononuclear leukocytes on chromosomal and plasmid DNA of *Escherichia coli. J. Clin. Invest.,* **73,** 1254–62.

5 Microbial and pharmacological induction of neutrophil dysfunction

J. G. WHEELER and J. S. ABRAMSON

1 Clinical case: influenza and staphylococcal pneumonia

A previously healthy 14-year-old white female developed cough, coryza, malaise, and fever. After 3 days she clinically improved, but on the fifth day left lower chest pain and dyspnoea occurred. A chest roentgenogram revealed left lower lobe pneumonia and she was admitted for treatment with i.v. antibiotics (cefuroxime). The next day she had increasing dyspnoea and a repeat chest roentgenogram revealed a large left sided pleural effusion and extension of the pneumonia to the right lung. A chest tube was placed and 500 ml of cloudy fluid was removed. Laboratory study of this fluid showed 5950 white blood cells/mm^3 (99 per cent neutrophils), glucose of 6.7 mmol/l (serum glucose 12.2 mmol/l), protein of 41 g/l, lactate dehydrogenase of 3480 units/l, pH of 7.45 and pleural fluid culture grew *Staphylococcus aureus*. Other abnormal laboratory studies included a peripheral white cell count of 4.8 × 10^9/l with 48 per cent segmented neutrophils and 21 per cent bands, haemoglobin 115 g/l (normal:120–160 g/l), platelets 141 × 10^9/l (160 000–360 000); serum sodium of 131 mmol/l (136–143), calcium 1.9 mmol/l (2.2–2.58), phosphorous 0.58 mmol/l (1–2), protein 53 g/l (60–80), albumin 32 g/l (38–54) and lactate dehydrogenase 424 units/l (100–400). Sputum cultures grew both influenza B virus and *S. aureus*.

Over the next few days she became increasingly dyspnoeic in association with worsening arterial blood gases and hypotension. She required assisted ventilation and vasopressor therapy for her hypotension. During the next week she developed a left sided pneumothorax and a bronchopleural fistula. She had several chest tubes and a Swan–Ganz catheter fitted. The pneumothorax eventually resolved and ventilatory support was discontinued 2 weeks after initiation. She received a total of 3 weeks of i.v. antibiotics and at the time of discharge did not require supplemental oxygen. Three months after discharge she was clinically doing well. However, she continued to have residual necrotizing changes in the left lung on chest roentgenogram and her pulmonary function tests remained abnormal.

The patient described in the case report provides an excellent example of the severity of secondary infections that can occur as a consequence of influenza virus infection. While most people who die of these superinfections are at either end of the age spectrum (<1 or >65 years of age), the above case highlights the observation that influenza viruses can cause serious morbidity and mortality in all age groups. This chapter will focus on the pathogenic mechanisms by which various agents (microbes and drugs) cause secondary infections.

2   Introduction

Strategically positioned throughout the body, the cells of the phagocytic cell system (neutrophils, monocytes, and macrophages) are equipped for immediate and lethal action against invasion of the host by bacterial and fungal micro-organisms. The neutrophil is the first cell to emigrate to the site of microbial invasion and is the principal cell involved in the immune response to invasion of the host by most bacteria and some fungi. Decreased neutrophil counts (<1000 cells/mm^3) are known to increase the risk of the host developing bacterial and fungal diseases (1).

Qualitative abnormalities in neutrophil function can also result in increased risk of infection by decreasing the movement of cells to the site of infection and/or depressing bactericidal activities against the invading organism (2). The events that occur when a neutrophil is stimulated are described in detail in Chapters 1–4. Briefly, upon invasion of the host by a microbe, chemotactic stimuli (e.g. a bacterial peptide) are released and attach to specific receptors on the neutrophil outer membrane. Occupation of the receptor by the stimulus initiates signal transduction, a sequence of biochemical steps (collectively termed the activation pathway) which results in end-stage functions (i.e. chemotactic, phagocytic, oxidative, and secretory). The signal transduction steps include enhancement of G protein activity (G proteins link receptor to the initial enzymes which start the activation pathway), ionic fluxes, changes in cyclic nucleotide levels, release of lipid metabolites, phosphorylation/dephosphorylation of intracellular proteins, and alterations in the cytoskeleton structure. Chemotaxis is the initial end-stage function which occurs (within 1 min of receptor–ligand interaction). During the chemotactic process neutrophils in the blood adhere to vascular endothelium and then migrate through the endothelial cell junction to the site of infection. Once at the site of infection, microbes attach to the cell by binding to other specific receptors (e.g. Fc and CR$_3$ receptors); this receptor–ligand interaction initiates an activation pathway which is similar, although not identical, to the activation pathway induced by stimuli causing only chemotaxis. Thereafter the microbes are phagocytosed, a process where organisms are taken up in large intra-cellular vacuoles known as phagosomes (structures in which the microbe is surrounded by the plasma membrane of the neutrophil). Secretory activi-ties then occur in which lysosomal granules fuse with phagosomes and other cellular plasma membrane sites and release enzymes into intracellular and extracellular spaces thereby killing and degrading the microbes. Simul-taneously, the oxidative burst is activated, allowing for production of oxygen products which are also lethal to the organism.

Certain microbes and pharmacological compounds can alter neutrophil function by interfering with one or more of the above noted activation steps and thereby predispose animal and human hosts to superinfections. The evidence that microbes and pharmacological compounds can interfere with neutrophils is most compelling for the respiratory viruses, especially influenza virus. However, data are accumulating which suggest that other viruses [e.g. cytomegalovirus (CMV)], bacteria (e.g. *Bordetella pertussis*), fungi (e.g. *Aspergillus fumigatus*) and pharmacological agents (e.g. corti-costeroids) can also cause neutrophil dysfunction which leads to secondary infections. The aim of this chapter is to review what is known about the suppressive effect of various types of agents on neutrophils and the impact that these alterations have on predisposition of the host to superinfections.

3 Microbe-induced neutrophil dysfunction

Lists of the specific microbes known to be associated with secondary infections and the effect of these microbes on neutrophil function are noted in Tables 5.1 and 5.2, respectively (these tables contain only microbes which are known to be associated with human disease). The pathogenesis of microbial-induced superinfections is discussed in detail for one or two specific organisms for each class of microbes (i.e. viruses, bacteria and fungi). These specific organisms were chosen for discussion because our knowledge of how they induce secondary infections is the most extensive, rather than because the mechanism by which they cause their effect is representative of other microbes in the same family (indeed the evidence, to date, suggests that even within a class of microbes the mechanisms by which neutrophil dysfunction occurs and the pathogenesis of the superin-fections differs for individual organisms).

3.1 Viruses

The role of viruses in predisposing the host to secondary bacterial infec-tions was last reviewed in 1988 (85), and has been best documented for

Table 5.1 Agents associated with superinfections: types of infections and the potential role of neutrophil dysfunction in causing these secondary infections

Predisposing agent	Superinfecting organisms[a,b]	Superinfected organ	PMN dysfunction[d] important	Selected references[c]
Viruses				
Adenovirus	**BP, CT, HI, MC, MP, NM, SP**	Blood, CNS, ear, lung	?[e]	3–8
CMV	**AF, CS, CT, EC, HI, MN, NA, PA, PC, SA, SM**	Blood, bone, CNS, lung	Yes	4, 9–11
Epstein–Barr	**BC, CH, EC, FN, GAS, MS**	Blood, URT	?[e]	12, 13
Enterovirus	**CT, GBS, HI, NM, SA, SP**	CNS	Yes	14, 15
Hepatitis B	**EC, MP, PA, SP**	Blood, lung, renal	Yes	16
Herpes simplex	**CS, KP, PA, PM, SA**	Eye, skin/abscess	Yes	17, 18
Human herpes 6	**LP**	Lung	?[e]	19
HIV	**CN[f], EC, HI, MT, PA, PC, SA, SP, SS**	Blood, CNS, GI, lung, renal, skin/abscess	Yes	20–22
Influenza	**AF, GBS, HI, KP, LM, NM, MC, MT, SA[g], SP**	Blood, CNS, ear, lung	Yes	3–5, 7, 23–39
Parainfluenza	**HI, MC, MP, NM, SP**	CNS, ear, lung	Yes	4, 6, 7, 40–42
RSV	**BP, CT, HI, KP, NM, SA, SP**	CNS, ear, lung	Yes	3–5, 7, 39, 43

Rhinovirus	**HI, MC, SA, SP**	Ear, lung	?[e]	4, 44
Rotavirus	**EC**	GI	?[e]	45
Rubeola	**HI, KP, MP, NM, PA, SA, SP, SS**	Blood, ear, lung	Yes	46, 47
Varicella–Zoster	**GAS, SA**	Blood, lung, skin/abscess	?[e,h]	18, 48
Bacteria				
Mycoplasma	**HI, NM, SP**	CNS	?[e]	6

[a] Superinfecting organisms listed in bold type are those for which the neutrophil has an important role in the immune response to invasion of the host by that particular microbe (e.g. *Pneumocystis carinii* is not listed in bold type because neutrophils do not appear to be important in controlling disease due to this organism). In some of the reports it is not possible to distinguish co-infections from secondary infections.

[b] Abbreviations: *Aspergillus fumigatus* (AF), *Bacteroides capillosus* (BC), *Bordetella pertussis* (BP), *Candida* species (CS), *Chlamydia trachomatis* (CT), *Corynebacterium hemolyticum* (CH), *Cryptococcus neoformans* (CN), *Cytomegalovirus* (CMV), *Escherichia coli* (EC), *Fusibacterium necrophorium* (FN), group A streptococcus (GAS), group B streptococcus (GBS), *Haemophilus influenzae* (HI), human immunodeficiency virus (HIV), *Klebsiella pneumoniae* (KP), *Legionella pneumophilia* (LP), *Listeria monocytogenes* (LM), *Morexalla catarrhalis* (MC), *Morganella morganni* (MM), *Mucor* species (MS), *Mycobacteria tuberculosis* (MT), *Mycoplasma pneumoniae* (MP), *Neisseria meningiditis* (NM), *Nocardia asteroides* (NA), *Proteus mirabilis* (PM), *Pseudomonas aeruginosa* (PA), respiratory syncytial virus (RSV), *Salmonella* species (SS), *Serratia marcescens* (SM), *Staphylococcus aureus* (SA), *Streptococcus pneumoniae* (SP), *Streptococcus viridans* (SV).

[c] A more complete list of references can be found in reference 85.

[d] Data in the literature suggest that the particular agent causes neutrophil dysfunction and that this has an important role in predisposing the host to the associated superinfections (see Table 5.2 for the specific neutrophil abnormalities which a particular agent causes).

[e] Insufficient data exist to determine if the predisposing agent causes neutrophil dysfunction.

[f] The organisms that have been associated with secondary infections in patients with HIV are protean and therefore the superinfecting microbes contained in this table are limited to those which occur frequently.

[g] Includes patients with toxic shock syndrome.

[h] Superinfections due, at least in part, to breakdown of the skin.

Table 5.2 Agents associated with *in vivo* and/or *in vitro* neutrophil dysfunction: specific end-stage functions and signal transduction steps that are altered

Predisposing agent (viruses)	End-stage functions impaired[a]	Transduction steps altered	Agent attaches to and/or enters cell	Selected references
CMV[b]	ADH, BACT, CT[c], OX[c], PHAG[c]		Yes	11, 49–51
EBV	BACT, OX		?[d]	52
Enterovirus	BACT, CT, OX	Membrane fluidity	Yes	52, 53
Hepatitis B	BACT, CT, OX, PHAG, SEC			54–57
HIV	BACT, CT, SEC, PHAG[b]		?[e]	22, 58–61
Herpes simplex	CT, OX[c], SEC			62–64
Influenza	BACT, CT, SEC, OX[c], PHAG[f]	LYS–PHAG fusion, protein phosphorylation, intracellular [CA[++]][g], actin polymerization, G protein activity	Yes	26, 65–78
Mumps	PHAG		?[d]	78
Parainfluenza	BACT, SEC	LYS–PHAG fusion[h]	Yes	40, 79, 80
Rotavirus	ADH		?[d]	50
RSV	ADH, BACT, CT, OX		?[d]	81
Rubella	SEC		?[d]	82
Rubeola	CT, SEC		?[d]	82, 83
Varicella–Zoster	SEC		?[d]	82, 83

[a] Abbreviations: adherence (ADH), bactericidal (BACT), chemotaxis (CT), lysosome–phagosome (LYS–PHAG), oxidative (OX), phagocytosis (PHAG), secretory (SEC).

[b] Signal activation steps which lead to one or more end-stage functions.

[c] Most, but not all, studies have found depression of this particular function.

[d] Insufficient data exist to determine if the predisposing agent attaches to and/or enters the neutrophil.

[e] Very low levels of HIV nucleic acid material were found in 32% (8/25) patients with either asymptomatic HIV infection or AIDS (61).

[f] Most studies have shown that this particular function is not impaired (e.g. 28, 29).

[g] Conflicting results have been obtained in the two studies which examined the effect of influenza virus on intracellular calcium levels (73, 74).

[h] Decreased lysosome–phagosome fusion due to parainfluenza virus has been demonstrated in alveolar macrophages (40, 80), but similar studies have not been done in neutrophils.

influenza A virus. In humans, infection with influenza A virus caused approximately 20 000 excess deaths per year during each of the >20 epidemics that have occurred since 1957, and >40 000 excess deaths have occurred in several of the most recent epidemics (86, 87). Most of the mortality and morbidity is due to secondary infections with *S. pneumoniae* or *Staphylococcus aureus*, but other pathogens including *Escherichia coli, Haemophilus influenzae, Neisseria meningitidis* and *A. fumigatus* can also cause disease. For example, culture or serologic evidence of recent influenza illness has been noted in a large percentage of adults with pneumococcal pneumonia (26), and children with bacterial meningitis due to *H. influenzae, S. pneumoniae* and *N. meningitidis* (6). During an outbreak of meningococcal disease in the UK in the winter of 1989, the incidence of serologically confirmed recent influenza infection was 4-fold higher than in controls (27). These superinfections occur mainly in people at either end of the age spectrum and those with underlying illnesses (26). However, as highlighted by the patient presented at the beginning of this chapter, immunocompetent children and adults can also succumb to these secondary infections. The mortality due to influenza A virus infection continues to be high despite the availability of influenza vaccine, antiviral agents (i.e. amantadine), and antibacterial therapies (26, 86, 87).

In animal models, influenza A virus has been shown to increase the incidence of secondary local and systemic diseases caused by diverse bacteria, including *S. pneumoniae, S. aureus, Streptococcus pyogenes,* group B *Streptococcus, H. influenzae, Mycobacterium tuberculosis* and *Listeria monocytogenes*. When influenza A virus was inoculated into animals prior to or concomitant with bacteria, an increased incidence of bacterial pneumonia, otitis media, and sepsis and meningitis occurred compared to animals inoculated with bacteria alone (Table 5.1). While these human and animal studies provide a compelling argument that influenza A virus predisposes the host to secondary bacterial infections, they do not reveal the mechanism by which this occurs.

Many viruses, including influenza A virus, are known to cause immunosuppression. While the importance of the neutrophil in controlling viral infections is often minimal, compared to that of mononuclear cells, the neutrophil is the principal cell involved in the immune response to invasion of the host by most bacteria. A large number of *in vivo* and *in vitro* studies involving animals and humans indicate that influenza A virus has an immunosuppressive effect on neutrophils (Table 5.2). Neutrophil dysfunction precedes and predisposes to the development of secondary disease in animals infected with influenza A virus (28, 29). The specific neutrophil functions altered by influenza A virus vary in different reports suggesting that the exact nature of the cellular defect which occurs in response to the virus is a function of several factors; these include the specific strain of virus used, the host that is infected or from whom the cells were obtained, the route of inoculation of the host, the specific assay used to measure an end-stage function, and the ratio of virus to cells used *in vitro*. In general the studies have shown that influenza A virus decreases neutrophil oxidative, chemotactic, secretory, and bactericidal activities, while phagocytosis remains unaltered (see Table 5.2). These data support the concept that virus-induced neutrophil dysfunction has an important role in the development of superinfections.

Infection due to influenza virus starts in the upper respiratory tract. The route by which influenza A virus comes in contact with neutrophils and thereby causes alterations in cellular function is not clear. Studies suggest that neutrophil dysfunction can occur even in the absence of viremia which has only rarely been reported in influenza A virus infections. The virus can persist in pulmonary tissue for up to 2 weeks and thereby alter neutrophil function for prolonged periods at this site (88). We have shown that when intact virus attaches to the neutrophil membrane there is rapid (within 5 min) inhibition of cellular responses (68) to subsequent stimuli. Additionally, the haemagglutinin (HA) component of the virus, by itself, can cause neutrophil dysfunction within 2 min of incubation with neutrophils (69), and HA may be shed into the bloodstream even if the intact virus is not. Thus, even in the absence of viremia, there is an opportunity for the virus to interact with the neutrophil and cause cellular dysfunction.

The mechanism by which influenza A virus causes neutrophil dysfunction is currently the focus of investigation in several laboratories. The possibility that influenza A virus-induced neutrophil dysfunction could be due to 'exhaustion' of the cell's metabolic response or intrinsic damage to the cell from toxic oxygen products is raised by reports showing that opsonized and unopsonized influenza A virus can stimulate the cell's respiratory burst (70, 71, 89). However, data from several studies indicate that these are not the mechanisms for neutrophil dysfunction. Incubation of influenza A virus with neutrophils does not decrease cell viability (68). Additionally, there is no correlation between the capacity of influenza A virus to induce an oxidative response and its ability to cause neutrophil dysfunction (68), and the depressed oxidative response in neutrophils cannot be prevented by using oxygen scavengers (71).

The fact that virus-induced neutrophil depression occurs within a few minutes after exposure of cells to the virus (68), suggests that a virus envelope component(s), which mediate the early events in virus–cell interaction, causes neutrophil dysfunction. We had previously shown that the neuraminidase component of influenza A virus was not responsible for inhibition of cell function (66). Therefore, studies were done to examine the role of the purified HA component in altering neutrophil function. These experiments utilized the luminol-enhanced chemiluminescence assay which has been shown to be a sensitive and reliable indicator of oxidative and bactericidal activities of neutrophils (90, 91), and also a reliable screening test for monitoring influenza A virus-induced neutrophil depression (28, 29, 66–68). HA protein aggregates or HA incorporated into liposomes caused depression of the chemiluminescence response to phorbol myristate acetate (PMA), opsonized zymosan or n-formyl-methionyl-leucylphenylalanine (FMLP) within 2 min and this depressing effect lasted for more than 2 h (69). The percentage decrease in the chemiluminescence response, compared to control cells, was always more than 30 per cent and comparable to influenza A virus on an equimolar basis in simultaneously run experiments (Fig. 5.1).

Haemagglutinin is responsible for both receptor binding of influenza A virus to cells and the fusion of viral envelope with the host cell's plasma membrane resulting in the formation of the endocytic vesicle. To determine which of these two activities is involved in neutrophil depression, influenza A virus was grown in the absence of serum to obtain virions that contained uncleaved HA which could then be cleaved with trypsin. Cleavage of HA must occur before the sterically protected fusion sequence of the HA can be exposed. The viral envelope can then fuse with the host cell

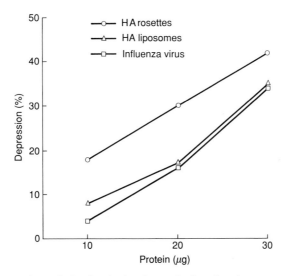

Fig. 5.1 Depression of the luminol-enhanced chemiluminescence response in neutrophils exposed to influenza virus, HA rosettes and HA incorporated into liposomes. These purified HA preparations were preincubated with neutrophils (2.5×10^4 cells/ml), at the indicated concentrations, for 20 min at 25 °C. Control samples were incubated with an equal amount of buffer solution. Peak chemiluminescence response was measured after the addition of PMA (100 ng/ml). The per cent depression represents the peak response of neutrophils preincubated with HA preparations, divided by the peak response of control cells ×100. The data shown are from a representative experiment. Similar results were obtained when opsonized zymosan or FMLP was used to stimulate the cells instead of PMA. The figure shown here is a modification of a figure in reference 69.

membrane. Cleavage of HA is not required for binding of the virus to receptors on the cell's outer plasma membrane. There was no difference in the ability of cleaved and uncleaved HA to depress the neutrophil chemiluminescence response, suggesting that the fusion event is not required for cell dysfunction. These data do not provide conclusive proof that fusion is unnecessary for neutrophil depression to occur, because neutrophil proteases could cleave HA. However, we performed other studies with sialic acid-specific binding lectins (i.e. lectins from *Limulus polyphemus* and *Limax flavus*) which cannot fuse with the cell membrane. When the cells were exposed to these lectins, depression of the cell's chemiluminescence response to secondary stimuli (i.e. FMLP or PMA) was similar to that seen with influenza A virus and HA (69).

To test the hypothesis further that it is the binding of influenza A virus (via its HA component) to one or more types of neutrophil receptors which contain sialic acid that causes cell dysfunction, the effect on neutrophil function was measured for three other lectins: wheat germ agglutinin (WGA; this compound interacts with terminally located sialic acid residues and internally located *N*-acetylglucosamine residues of cell-surface glycoproteins and glycolipids), succinylated WGA (succinylation decreases WGA interaction with sialic acid but not with *N*-acetylglucosamine) and Concanavalin A (Con A; binds to mannose-containing receptors). WGA, but not succinylated WGA or Con A, caused inhibition of the oxidative burst in neutrophils. The specificity of neutrophil depression resulting from binding of sialic acid-specific ligands was further tested using increasing concentrations of bovine submaxillary mucin, a source of soluble sialic acid-containing conjugates. Lectins incubated with mucin caused less neutrophil depression compared with lectins used alone; there was an indirect correlation between the concentration of mucin and the amount of neutrophil depression (Table 5.3). These data strongly suggest that just attachment of HA to one or more types of sialic acid-containing receptors on neutrophils, rather than fusion of viral envelope with the host cell plasma membrane, is sufficient to cause neutrophil dysfunction due to virus. The identity of the specific receptor(s) that influenza virus interacts with to cause neutrophil dysfunction remains to be determined.

Studies are underway to determine which steps along the activation pathway are altered by influenza virus. We have noted that influenza A virus inhibited the fusion of primary and secondary granules with plasma membrane components (Fig. 5.2; 65, 72). While inhibition of lysosome–phagosome fusion had been noted before in cells exposed to *Toxoplasma gondii* and *Mycobacteria tuberculosis* (92, 93), this finding was unique in that lysosomes fused with endosomes containing virus, but when neutrophils were exposed to subsequent stimuli (e.g. *S. aureus* or FMLP) fusion of lysosomes with phagosomes and other plasma membrane components did not occur. Inhibition of lysosome–phagosome fusion directly corre-

Table 5.3   Competitive inhibition of neutrophil depression by lectins after preincubation with mucin[a]

Condition	Mucin (μg)	% Depression of chemiluminescence	
		Experiment 1	Experiment 2
Limax flavus + mucin	0	41	59
	50	27	60
	100	4	36
Mucin alone	100	—	8
Limulus polyphemus + mucin	0	25	21
	50	7	0
	100	11	0
Mucin alone	100	0	0

[a] Bovine submaxillary mucin, at the indicated concentrations, was preincubated with 10 μg of either *Limax flavus* or *Limulus polyphemus* lectins. Neutrophils were incubated with the lectin–mucin mixtures for 20 min before the addition of PMA. All the incubations were at 25 °C. Per cent depression of chemiluminescence is the peak response of neutrophils preincubated with lectin and/or mucin divided by the peak response of control cells × 100. Experiments 1 and 2 represent responses of neutrophils from two different donors. Table copied from reference 69 with permission.

lated with depression of end-stage cellular functions. This is not surprising, since the secretory process has been shown to be involved in chemotactic (94) and oxidative (95) responses. The virus has also been shown to inhibit both fluid- and receptor-mediated endocytosis in neutrophils (96).

The effect of influenza virus on many of the activation steps which occur prior to lysosome–phagosome fusion has also been studied. The phosphorylation and dephosphorylation of intracellular proteins in neutrophils appears to have a major regulatory role in activation of neutrophil responses to a variety of stimulating agents which activate the cell through different pathways (e.g. FMLP and PMA). Since influenza virus inhibits end-stage functions in neutrophil exposed to a number of different stimuli, including FMLP and PMA, the effect of the virus on protein phosphorylation was examined. Influenza virus was noted to markedly inhibit the phosphorylation or dephosphorylation of multiple membrane and cytosolic proteins (Figs 5.3 and 5.4; 73). One such protein that demonstrated decreased phosphorylation in virus-treated cells stimulated with either FMLP or PMA was a 47 kDa phosphoprotein which has been shown to be involved in the oxidative burst; this protein is absent from the PMN of most patients with the autosomal recessive/cytochrome-*b*-positive form of chronic granulomatous disease and there are other forms of this disease where the 47 kDa protein is present, but is not phosphorylated to the

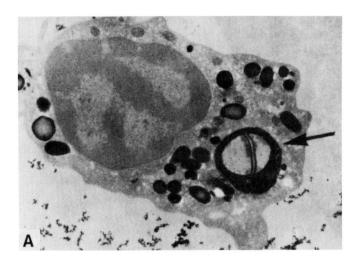

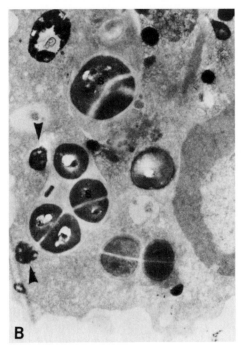

Fig. 5.2 The deposition of myeloperoxidase (MPO) in neutrophils exposed to (A) *S. aureus* alone for 30 min or (B) influenza virus for 30 min followed by *S. aureus*. MPO is demonstrated in these electron micrograph sections using diaminobenzidine. (A) MPO is found in both azurophil granules and phagosomes containing the bacteria and (B) MPO is found in endosomes containing the virus, whereas very little MPO is seen in phagosomes containing the bacteria. Similar electron micrographs are contained in reference 72.

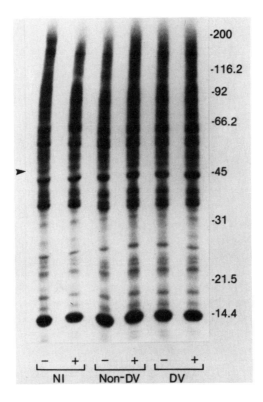

Fig. 5.3 Phosphorylation of neutrophil cytosolic proteins in cells exposed to influenza virus without (−) or with (+) subsequent stimulation with FMLP. Neutrophils were pre-labelled with ^{32}P, treated with buffer (NI), a non-depressing harvest of influenza virus (non-DV) or a depressing harvest of influenza virus (DV) for 30 min and then stimulated with 10^{-6} M FMLP or solvent for 30 s. The cells were then fractionated. A representative autoradiogram demonstrates decreased phosphorylation and dephosphorylation of multiple proteins (densitometry data from this autoradiogram are shown in Fig. 5.4). Similar results were obtained when phosphorylation of membrane-associated proteins was examined and when PMA, rather than FMLP, was used as the cell stimulant. M_r markers, to the right are in kDa. Arrowhead shows the position of the 47 kDa phosphoprotein. This figure was copied with permission from reference 73, © by Williams and Wilkins (1988).

normal extent (97). Virus-induced alterations in the phosphorylation of this regulatory protein could be an important step in the proposed pathway by which virus causes PMN dysfunction [see Fig. 5.5 (this pathway is discussed later on in this section of the chapter)].

Since influenza virus could interfere with phosphorylation by altering the activity of protein kinases (or phosphatases in the case of dephosphorylation), the effect of the virus on early events in the signal transduction

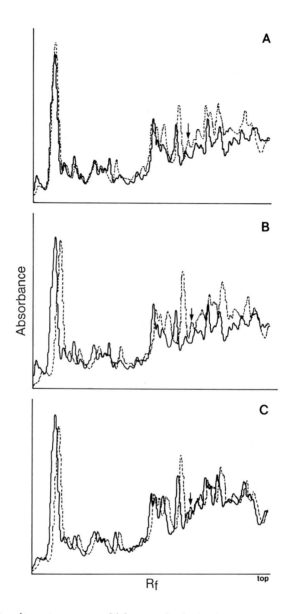

Fig. 5.4. Densitometry scans which quantitatively demonstrate the decreased phosphorylation seen in Fig. 5.3 when neutrophils are exposed to virus followed by FMLP. Densitometry scans of all lanes of Fig. 5.3 are superimposed to illustrate the effect of FMLP stimulation on phosphorylation of cytosolic proteins. (A) Cytosols from buffer-treated PMN without (——) and with (---) FMLP stimulation; (B) cytosols from non-DV-treated PMN without (——) and with (---) FMLP; (C) cytosols from DV-treated PMN without (——) and with (---) FMLP. Arrows show the position of the 47 kDa protein. This figure was copied with permission from reference 73, © by Williams and Wilkins (1988).

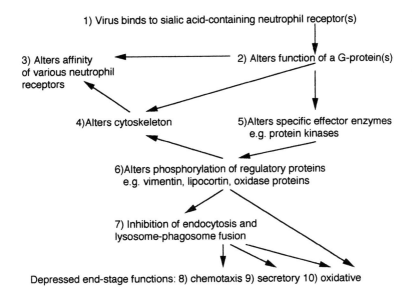

1) Virus binds to sialic acid-containing neutrophil receptor(s)

3) Alters affinity of various neutrophil receptors

2) Alters function of a G-protein(s)

4) Alters cytoskeleton

5) Alters specific effector enzymes e.g. protein kinases

6) Alters phosphorylation of regulatory proteins e.g. vimentin, lipocortin, oxidase proteins

7) Inhibition of endocytosis and lysosome-phagosome fusion

Depressed end-stage functions: 8) chemotaxis 9) secretory 10) oxidative

Fig. 5.5 Potential pathway by which virus-induced alterations in G proteins lead to depressed chemotactic and metabolic activities in neutrophils exposed to receptor-mediated stimuli (e.g. FMLP). Several lines of evidence indicate that the virus is affecting neutrophils at the point of G protein regulation (step 2). The alterations in phosphorylation of multiple cellular proteins (step 6) suggest that the virus is affecting a very early step in cell activation. Both influenza virus and HA decrease GTPase activity in neutrophils stimulated with FMLP. Additionally, influenza virus alters FMLP receptor affinity yet does not decrease the total number of FMLP receptors on the cell plasma membrane (step 3); see text for additional discussion of these points. Finally, G proteins appear to regulate other steps which the virus is known to affect including F-actin polymerization and cytoskeleton activation (step 4), phosphorylation of cellular proteins (step 6), endocytosis and fusion of lysosomes with plasma membrane components (step 7), chemotaxis (step 8), degranulation (step 9) and the respiratory burst (step 10).

pathway contributing to the activity of these enzymes was examined. The virus did not alter the number of FMLP receptors, transmembrane potential, or cAMP levels in neutrophils upon exposure of cells to FMLP (73). The effect of virus on intracellular calcium levels remains unclear. Both Hartshorn *et al.* (74) and our group (73) have noted increased intracellular $[Ca^{2+}]$ in neutrophil exposed to virus alone. However, upon addition of FMLP they noted decreased intracellular $[Ca^{2+}]$, while we found the intracellular $[Ca^{2+}]$ to be increased. The virus inhibits the cell's response to PMA, a stimulant of neutrophil activation not associated with a rise in intracellular $[Ca^{2+}]$ (98, 99). Additionally, decreased intracellular $[Ca^{2+}]$ does not appear to inhibit FMLP-induced chemotactic activity (100), a function which the virus does inhibit. Therefore, whatever the actual effect of the virus is on intracellular $[Ca^{2+}]$, it is unlikely to be the primary mechanism by which the virus alters neutrophil function.

The alteration in phosphorylation of multiple membrane and cytosol proteins in neutrophils suggested that virus disrupts an early step in the activation pathway of neutrophils. We therefore decided to study the effect of influenza virus and its purified viral HA on G protein function in neutrophils for the following reasons: (i) a number of trimeric G proteins (G proteins that contain α, β, and γ subunits) have been identified in various cell types including neutrophils, and they function to link receptors on the plasma membrane of neutrophils to effector enzymes which then start the activation cascade (101); (ii) influenza virus causes depressed cell function to stimuli (e.g. FMLP, opsonized zymosan) which are known to activate the cell through trimeric G protein-dependent pathways (102, 103). The virus also alters the neutrophil response to PMA which is not known to be associated with a trimeric G protein. While at least a portion of the activation pathway for PMA is different to that for FMLP, the virus could alter a G protein(s) which functions at a point where the two pathways might convrege or affect a G protein(s) that is unique to the PMA pathway. For example, evidence is accumulating that monomeric (low mol. wt) G proteins in neutrophils function at points along the activation pathway distal to where trimeric G protein-controlled ligand–plasma membrane receptor interaction occurs (e.g. 104); the virus could be affecting a monomeric G protein(s); (iii) influenza virus alters FMLP receptor affinity yet does not decrease the total number of FMLP receptors on the cell plasma membrane. This finding is consistent with what would be expected if the virus interferes with normal G protein function (103, 105); and (iv) the effect of pertussis toxin (PT) and influenza virus on neutrophil end-stage functions are very similar. Neutrophils have at least two pertussis toxin-sensitive G proteins (106) which appear to participate in the regulation of cellular chemotaxis (107), respiratory burst activity (108), exocytic secretion (109), endocytosis (110), and membrane fusion (110), but not the process of particle phagocytosis (111). A more detailed discussion of how G proteins function can be found in Chapter 3. Our studies on the effect of PT and influenza virus on neutrophils demonstrate a competitive interaction of these two inhibitors. This observation suggests, but does not prove, that influenza virus is interacting with the neutrophil at an activation point that is also affected by a PT-sensitive G protein(s).

Both influenza virus and HA were found to alter G protein function significantly, as measured using a GTPase assay. The GTPase assay, as described by Feltner *et al.* (112), was used because it provides a simple, convenient, and direct assessment of G protein function (113). Additionally, since there are multiple G proteins in neutrophils it was desirable to measure the total activity of al G proteins in the cell, since we did not know which of these proteins the virus was affecting. In the original experiments neutrophils were treated with influenza virus (100 µg/10^8 cells) or buffer for 20 min. Isolated plasma membranes were then prepared by fractionation through discontinuous sucrose gradients. Basal GTPase activity was significantly decreased in membranes prepared from virus-treated cells at all time points measured (0, 2, 4, 10 min) except baseline. At 4 and 10 min approximately 50 per cent of the basal GTPase activity was blocked. When FMLP was added to the plasma membranes of virus-treated cells, the GTPase activity was also significantly decreased (55 per cent) at 4 and 10 min compared with the corresponding control. Similar results were noted when plasma membrane fractions were exposed to influenza virus and when HA was used instead of influenza virus. While these data suggest that virus is altering one or more G proteins in neutrophils, this assay is not capable of determining the specific G protein(s) which the virus affects or the factors that are causing the alteration.

Preliminary studies have been done to examine the mechanism by which the virus causes decreased GTPase activity. The virus could interfere with one of the functional domains of a G protein(s) and thereby alter its function. As noted above, PT and virus cause similar end-stage dysfunction in neutrophils stimulated with FMLP. PT inhibits neutrophil function by inducing ADP-ribosylation of a cysteine residue near the C terminus of the α subunit of PT-sensitive G proteins (114); see Section 3.2 for further discussion of the effect of PT on neutrophils. The virus could induce a similar result by affecting ADP-ribosyltransferases found in neutrophils (115). Preliminary evidence suggests that one or more of the G proteins altered by the virus is PT-sensitive, but, to date, the data do not implicate ribosylation of the α subunit as the mechanism by which the virus affects G proteins. Phosphorylation of certain G protein subunits appears to occur and it has been postulated that this process participates in the regulation of G proteins (113, 116). This is especially interesting, since our data show that influenza virus alters phosphorylation of multiple membrane and cytosol proteins in neutrophils. Multiple other factors regulate the function of trimeric G proteins. The rate of release of GDP may be the rate-limiting step in G protein activation (113) and intracellular $[Mg^{2+}]$ appears to be important in regulating this step; in other words, low $[Mg^{2+}]$ facilitates guanine nucleotide exchange, while high $[Mg^{2+}]$ prevents dissociation of bound nucleotide (117). The intracellular concentrations of GDP and GTP (118, 119), the rate of binding of GTP to the α subunit (113), and intrinsic GTPase activity (113) are also important in regulation of the G proteins. Studies are underway to examine whether influenza virus is exerting its effect at any of these points.

As noted above, a group of low molecular weight (20–28 kDa) monomeric G proteins also exists. These proteins, which have been identified by molecular cloning, include the ras, rac, rho and rap gene products. The functions of these monomeric G proteins are just beginning to be delineated and they appear to be involved in control of a diverse set of cellular functions including proliferation, cytoskeletal organization, vesicle endocytosis, and secretion. Investigators have shown that rac and rap1 are present in neutrophils (120, 121). At least in the case of rap1, $[Mg^{2+}]$ appears to regulate the conformation of the nucleotide-binding site. Guanosine triphosphatase (GTPase) activity is enhanced by a GTPase-activating protein (GAP) and appears not to be affected by phosphorylation. Preliminary data suggest that rap1 and rac may be involved in oxidative and secretory functions, respectively (120–122). Studies are needed to determine the effect of influenza virus on monomeric G proteins.

It is likely that influenza virus is affecting more than one G protein since the virus depresses the neutrophil response to a number of stimuli which activate the cell by different pathways (e.g. FMLP and PMA). Virus-induced alterations in just one of the factors noted above (e.g. intracellular guanine nucleotide levels) could affect many, if not all, of the G proteins in the cell. Alternatively, Gilman (123) has proposed a subunit exchange hypothesis which predicts that activation of one G protein-dependent pathway causes inhibition of effector molecules that are controlled by other G proteins. Indeed, evidence exists showing that the β/γ subunit from one type of G protein, once it has dissociated from the α subunit, can inhibit the function of effector enzymes which interact with other types of G proteins (124). One model which is consistent with available data, and explains how virus-induced alterations in the function of a G protein(s) could lead to end-stage neutrophil dysfunction is shown in Fig. 5.5.

While the exact mechanism by which influenza A virus disrupts neutrophil function remains to be further defined, the above findings indicate that this virus is interfering with an early step in the signal transduction pathway of neutrophils. We therefore decided to examine the ability of agents which prime neutrophils (i.e. increase the neutrophil response to various cell stimuli, but do not by themselves cause metabolic responses in the cell) for their capacity to overcome virus-induced neutrophil dysfunction. These agents could potentially overcome the effect of the virus on neutrophils through direct mechanisms (i.e. amplifying a signal transduction pathway previously muted by the virus) or indirect mechanisms (i.e. augmenting other activation pathways not altered by the virus). Several priming agents [e.g. granulocyte-macrophage colony-stimulating factor (GM-CSF), guanosine triphosphate (GTP), 1-oleoyl-2-acetylglycerol (OAG)] were capable of partially or totally overcoming influenza virus-induced neutrophil dysfunction in cells stimulated with either FMLP or PMA, as measured using the luminol-enhanced chemiluminescence assay (75). There was a strong direct correlation between the amount of priming caused by an agent and its capacity to overcome virus-induced neutrophil dysfunction (Fig. 5.6). Similar results were noted in other studies where granulocyte colony-stimulating factor (G-CSF) was used as the priming

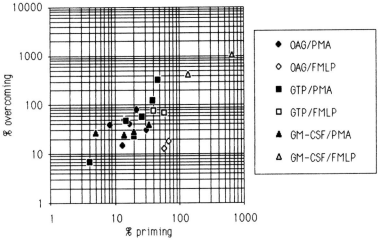

Fig. 5.6 The relationship between a compound's (e.g. GM-CSF, GTP, or OAG) ability to prime neutrophils and its capacity to overcome influenza virus-induced depression of the cell's chemiluminescence response to influenza virus. Neutrophils were exposed to virus for 30 min, followed by each priming agent, and then PMA or FMLP. Each point on this figure represents data from an individual experiment. There was a strong correlation between a compound's ability to prime neu-trophils and its capacity to overcome the virus-induced neutrophil dysfunction ($r = 0.85$, $P < 0.001$). This figure was copied from reference 75 with permission.

agent. The mechanism by which influenza A virus is altering neutrophil function could not be determined from these data, since not all of the priming agents which were effective in overcoming virus-induced neutrophil dysfunction appear to exert their effect through the same signal transduction pathway [e.g. GM-CSF primes neutrophils through a G protein-sensitive pathway (125), while OAG primes neutrophils, at least in part, through activation of protein kinase C (126)]. However, the fact that GM-CSF and G-CSF are capable of overcoming influenza A virus-induced neutrophil dysfunction provides a unique opportunity to explore further the role of virus-induced neutrophil dysfunction in the pathogenesis of bacterial superinfections. Studies are now underway in which the ability of GM-CSF, as well as other cytokines which are more specific for the neutrophil (G-CSF) and monocyte (M-CSF), are tested in an animal model for their ability to overcome influenza A virus-induced neutrophil dysfunction and prevent the associated bacterial superinfections.

3.2   Bacteria and mycobacteria

The study of bacterial and mycobacterial infections is not complete without surveillance of the many mechanisms by which these microbes resist host immunity. While some microbes are passive in nature and persist by merely evading host immunity (e.g. normal respiratory flora), others actively inhibit host immunity and thus have the potential to predispose the host to invasive infection with other pathogens. Table 5.4 lists bacteria and fungi which are known to inhibit some aspect of neutrophil function. In spite of considerable *in vitro* studies on these pathogens and the mechanisms of their virulence, there is very little clinical correlation demonstrating that impaired neutrophil function induced by these organisms leads to susceptibility to other infections. In this respect, bacterial and mycobacterial infections are quite different from viral infections such as HIV-1 and influenza virus where there is a clear-cut relationship between viral inhibition of cellular function and secondary bacterial and fungal infection. This difference may be explained by two factors. First, except for fulminant cases, bacterial and mycobacterial infection tends to be focal. In most cases neutrophil-inhibiting factors are secreted in the microenvironment only, and thus immune dysfunction may escape clinical detection. Viral infections which are known to induce immune dysfunction tend to do so on a more widespread basis (i.e. effect one or more types of immune cells both at local sites of infection and systemically). Second, even when bacterial infection becomes disseminated, the period of immune suppression is usually of insufficient duration for secondary infections to develop. Chronic bacterial infections such as those in cystic fibrosis, chronic sinusitis etc. are exceptions and potentially could induce long-term immune suppression in the microenvironment. These particular diseases are in fact associated with mixed infections but there are little direct data to prove that the immunosupressive effect of the initial organism promotes the development of superinfections with other organisms.

There are multiple mechanisms by which bacteria inhibit neutrophil function and are potentially culpable for inducing secondary infections. Examples include (i) the elaboration of a variety of toxins [e.g. pertussis toxins (128), adenylate cyclase inhibitor (128, 129), staphylococcal and streptococcal toxins (144–6, 148, 149)]; (ii) production of inhibitors of opsonization [staphylococcal protein A and pseudomonas mucoexopolysaccharide (141, 156): see Chapter 4 for extensive discussion of this topic]; (iii) inhibitors of chemotaxins [Capnocytophagia, group A and B streptococcus (130, 157, 158)]; and (iv) bacteria may indirectly diminish neutrophil function by primarily interacting with other immune cells. It has been shown, for instance, that human monocytes and lymphocytes when exposed to the peptidoglycan fraction of staphylococci produced an inhibitor of neutrophil chemotaxis (159). Further, the effects of bacteria on neutrophil function may be indirect. The sepsis syndrome is an example of how bacterial induced processes may indirectly lead to diminution of neutrophil responses (160). The release of humoral factors such as lipopolysaccharide, tumour necrosis factor, GM-CSF, and interleukin-1 are thought to modulate this process (161, 162). These diverse mechanisms lead to different functional effects on neutrophils. The study of individual effects of bacteria on PMN, particularly the study of toxins, has helped distinguish and provide clues to precise mechanisms of inhibition. In this section we will focus on the effect of PT on neutrophils. Excellent reviews can be found which offer special details on the effects of toxins and other microbial products on neutrophils (146, 163).

Bordetella pertussis, the bacteria which produces whooping cough, is an excellent example of an organism that demonstrates a variety of neutrophil-inhibiting effects. While pertussis infection is now less common because of widespread vaccination programmes, outbreaks still occur and are associated with overwhelming disease and death (164). Dual infections with *B. pertussis* and other agents (viral and bacterial) have been described (165) suggesting that immunosuppressive effects of *B. pertussis* may be clinically relevant. *B. pertussis* has been shown to survive in PMN, through interference with lysosome–phagosome fusion (128). The elaboration of at least three different factors helps lead to abnormal neutrophil function and prolonged survival of the organism. These factors include PT, *B. pertussis* adenylate cyclase and lipopolysaccharide. The enormous explosion of knowledge about PT has allowed precise knowledge of several neutrophil-activation pathways and has demonstrated the widespread effects this toxin may have on neutrophil function.

PT has a number of properties which are recognized to be clinically relevant including increased sensitization of cells to the effects of histamine and bradykinin and the induction of leukocytosis (151). In addition, animal studies have shown that the chemotactic activity of neutrophils from animals treated with PT is inhibited (166). These phenomena are clearly related to the effects of the toxin on the signal transduction pathways of target cells.

PT is made up of two major components: (i) the B component, a pentamer which has a membrane-binding function and (ii) the A component responsible for ADP-ribosyltransferase and NAD glycohydrolase activities. Membrane binding appears to occur on sialic acid residues explaining in part its lectin-like qualities (167, 168). The site of ADP-ribosylation in neutrophils is a cysteine amino acid on the C terminus of the α subunit of the trimeric G_i protein (see Chapter 3 for detailed discussion of the function of trimeric and monomeric G proteins). Other G proteins without the cysteine modification site on the C-terminal end of the α protein do not appear to be PT-sensitive (169). These include the smaller 'ras'-related proteins (20–26 kDa) responsible for cell growth and metabolism (169, 170).

Clear descriptions of the intracellular actions of PT have recently emerged (see 151, 169 and 171 for excellent reviews). It is now clear that PT interferes with the transformation of ATP to cAMP by adenylate cyclase (172, 173) and blocks inhibitory responses by guanine nucleotides

Table 5.4 Bacterial, fungal, and mycobacterial agents associated with *in vitro* neutrophil dysfunction: specific end-stage functions and signal transduction steps that are altered

Agent	End-stage functions impaired[a]	Transduction steps altered	Agent attaches/ enters PMN	References
Bacteria				
Bacteroides spp	CT	Membrane depolarization		127
Bordetella pertussis				
Pertussis toxin	OX, CT, BACT, SEC	G protein	Yes	128
Adenylate cyclase	OX, CT, BACT, SEC	Phagosome–lysosome fusion	Yes	128, 129
Capnocytophaga	CT	?		130
C. perfringens theta toxins	OX, CT	?Membrane permeabilization		131
E. coli				
Haemolysin	Viability	Membrane poration		132
Heat-sensitive enterotoxin	CT	Increased cAMP		133
Haemophilus pleuropneumoniae	Viability			134
Neisseria gonococcus	BACT	MPO inhibition		135
Pasturella haemolytica				
Leukotoxin	OX	Membrane permeabilization		136, 137

Pseudomonas				
Pyocyanine	?Oxidase	Yes	OX	138
Cytotoxin	Membrane pores		Viability	139
Elastase	Anti-complement protease	No	CT	140
Staphylococcus				
Protein A	Binds Fc of free IgG		PHAG	141
Mucopeptide	Anti-kinins		CT	142, 143
Alpha toxin	ADP-ribosylation, poration		?All	144, 145
'Leukotoxin'	ADP-ribosylation		?All	144
'Leukocidin'	Membrane depolarization, ionic leak	Yes	All	146
S. pneumoniae	Elastase inhibitor	Yes	SEC	147
S. pyogenes				
O toxin	Membrane poration	Yes	SEC	148
S toxin	Transmembrane ionic leak	Yes	SEC	149
Vibrio cholera	Decreased receptor binding		CT	150
	ADP-ribosylation of G_s			151
Fungi and mycobacteria				
Candida albicans	Hyphal inhibitory product (CHIP)		OM, SEC	152, 153
Aspergillus	?		CT, BACT	154
M. tuberculosis	Cord factor		CT	155

[a] Abbreviations: adherence (ADH), bactericidal (BACT), chemotaxis (CT), oxidative (OX), phagocytosis (PHAG), secretory (SEC).

on the adenylate cyclase in non-myeloid cells (151). Inhibitory receptors are shown to be disengaged from the adenylate cyclase by PT (151). The specific mechanism for this effect may lie in the ability of PT to decrease GTPase activity of the α subunit, leaving the α subunit in a tonically 'on' position and thereby disrupting the G_i/receptor relationship The ribosylation of a $G_{i\alpha}$-like membrane protein has been shown in guinea-pig neutrophils (174, 175) and in human cells ribosylation of a 41 kDa α subunit of a G protein was correlated with inhibitory effects of PT (176). Interestingly, only a small amount of this protein was modified. Functional abnormalities in PT-treated neutrophils include reduction in FMLP, IL-1, and other agonist stimulated secretory, chemotactic, and oxidative responses (177, 178). Neither Ca ionophore nor PMA oxidative responses were reduced by PT (179), and the level of cAMP did not differ in PT-treated neutrophils compared with controls following FMLP stimulation. Both decreased (150) and no change (176) in the number of FMLP receptors have been found after PT treatment of neutrophils. The effect of PT on the distribution of low and high affinity receptors is also controversial. A number of other effects on second messengers such as phosphoinositol pathway products and calcium (179, 180) have been noted in PT treated cells and are thought to occur as a direct consequence of $G_{i\alpha}$ dysfunction. A second G protein (G_O) has been isolated and is also thought to be a substrate for PT. Its specific role in adenylate cyclase activity and other cell functions is still emerging. Further the role PT has in influencing the function of GAP proteins is still being defined, although it is not thought to have a direct effect.

Knowledge about this toxin continues to increase. The most significant revelation has been the important tie to G protein dysfunction which is emerging as a common theme in a number of processes by which microbes and drugs inhibit cell function.

3.3   Fungi

Fungi are known to secrete certain substances which inhibit PMN function although these have not been as well studied for fungi as for bacteria. An inhibitor of neutrophil function known as CHIP (candida hyphal inhibitory product) has been isolated and demonstrated to inhibit both the respiratory burst and receptor-mediated degranulation (152, 153). *Aspergillus* spores have been shown to inhibit PMN function (154) presumably through aflatoxins or gliotoxins. Other work has focused on the cryptococcal capsule (181, 182) and its ability to block phagocytosis but clear-cut inhibition of neutrophil function following heterologous stimuli has not been shown. In fungi which are not typically pathogenic for humans, there have been a number of families of fungi which inhibit neutrophil aggregation (183). The persistent nature of many fungal infections would make them ideal agents to produce secondary clinical infections since the normal host is vulnerable to phagocytic dysfunction especially if it occurs over long periods of time. Since many fungal infections develop in the neutropenic patient or the patient with dysfunctional neutrophils, fungal organisms may promote growth of other pathogens or perpetuate their own growth through secreting factors which inhibit neutrophil function. At this time, no evidence exists to support these speculations, although they remain an importat research focus.

4   Pharmacological compounds which induce neutrophil disorders

Pharmacological compounds induce neutrophil disorders by either reducing neutrophil numbers or function (Table 5.5). In some cases this is a desired goal, in others it is an undesired consequence of therapy. Alterations in the normal proliferation of PMN in the marrow result in neutropenia, either as a general phenomena associated with cytopenias of other cell lines or as a selective process only affecting myeloid lines. This may occur by direct toxic effects of chemotherapy or radiation. Not only anti-myeloplastic drugs but more benign drugs such as anti-inflammatory and antibiotic preparations are well recognized to induce neutropenia. In addition to direct toxic effects, drugs may induce autoimmune antibodies against neutrophil precursors through hapten-like behaviour or by directly influencing suppressor cells so that suppression of anti-neutrophil antibodies is reduced (184). The mechanisms are unknown in most cases, and withdrawal of the offending drug results in normalization of neutrophil counts within 1–2 weeks. Drugs well known to cause neutropenia include the penicillins, cephalosporins, sulphonamides, anti-inflammatory drugs, and phenothiazines but a wide number of pharmaceutical compounds are noted to interfere with normal neutrophil numbers (reviewed in 185, 186).

The role of drugs in inhibiting PMN function has been widely studied both for the intentional inhibition sought with drugs like salicylates, corticosteroids, and colchicine but also for the unintentional side effects caused by antibiotics.

The uncontrolled cellular response of neutrophils leading to the devastating consequences of arthritis, ARDS, and leukocytoclastic vasculitis are well described in Chapter 7. The necessity for drugs which could inhibit inflammation have yielded drugs which modulate inflammation by multiple mechanisms.

Salicylates and related compounds were initially thought to impair neutrophil function by altering arachidonic acid pathways and minimizing the liberation of pro-inflammatory prostaglandins. It is now believed that additional pathways of inflammation are inhibited by salicylates and non-

Table 5.5   Examples of pharmacologically induced neutrophil disorders

Neutropenia	
Direct toxic effects	Chemotherapy–cytoxan, methotrexate
	Antimicrobials–penicillins,
	cephalosporins, sulfas
	Phenothiazides, NSAIDs, and others
Autoimmune	Antimicrobials–semisynthetic
	penicillins
Neutrophil dysfunction	
G protein dysfunction	NSAID
Cyclooxygenase/lipoxygenase	
inhibition	NSAID, corticosteroids
Impaired receptor upregulation	Corticosteroids
Microtubular dysfunction	Colchicine
Microfilament dysfunction	Cytochalasins
Impaired adherence	CD11b/CD18 inhibitors, corticosteroids
Altered calcium metabolism	Tetracyclines
Reduced oxidative burst	Trimethoprim, sulfas
Unknown	Rifampin

steroidal anti-inflammatory drugs (NSAID). These anti-inflammatory effects only occur at higher doses of these drugs and not at the doses sufficient to inhibit prostaglandin synthesis. It is proposed that these anti-inflammatory effects occur through the capacity of the NSAIDs to insert directly into the lipid bilayer of the cell membrane and disrupt signal transduction (187). Thus events such as superoxide generation (188), aggregation (189), and related post-transduction events are uncoupled. Studies have been performed which show that the effect of PT is inhibited by NSAIDs (190), suggesting that both inhibitors share a common pathway of inhibition. This continues the theme of the role of G proteins in a number of different situations in which neutrophil dysfunction occurs.

Corticosteroids are a second group of drugs classically proposed as having direct effects which reduce neutrophil function. It has been argued (191) that corticosteroids, acting through a cytoplasmic steroid receptor, directly induce nuclear generation of new proteins (such as macrocortin) which would directly inhibit cellular enzymes (such as phospholipase A_2). This would lead to a depression in the generation of important cellular messages (LTB_4 and PGE_2) responsible for normal inflammatory responses (such as chemotaxis). While initial studies suggested that steroids impaired neutrophil function, more recent reports (192, 193) have cast doubt on the role of corticosteroids in directly suppressing neutrophil function. Earlier studies in which steroids impaired neutrophil function utilized supraphysiological doses of drug, often used non-human sources for neutrophils and employed short incubations of a drug that requires several hours (for the process of nuclear signalling, expression of message, and translation of modulatory proteins) to induce its effects. Newer studies have shown a much smaller range of effects of corticosteroids on neutrophil functions. Schleimer *et al.* have shown no effects of physiologic doses of dexamethasone on degranulation, chemotaxis, or LTB_4 production (193). Further, they noted no differences in adherence of stimulated neutrophils to endothelial cells. However, there was a significant difference in dexamethasone-treated neutrophil adherence in unstimulated cells. Other studies have shown that neutrophils cultured for 24 h or more have decreased expression of INFγ-induced FcγRI and CR_3 following exposure to dexamethasone (195). Thus, our understanding of the mechanisms by which steroids inhibit tissue accumulation of neutrophils remains incomplete and controversial. Further studies are needed which are relevant to the microenvironment of circulating and tissue-localized neutrophils and which take into account the possible inhibition of chemotactic factor production by other immune cells.

The mechanisms by which another drug, colchicine, inhibits neutrophil function is more clear cut. This drug and its analogues act directly on the microtubular network to depress neutrophil motile activity. Other functions of neutrophils such as LTB_4 production are decreased by colchicine but appear to be depressed through direct inhibition of the microtubular network (196). This drug is most often used to treat gout, but wider use of this drug has been suggested in diseases where neutrophilic inflammation is present, such as leukocytoclastic vasculitis.

The pharmaceutical industry is actively trying to develop other potential weapons against neutrophilic inflammation by using compounds which block the activity of cell adhesion molecules of the CD18 or MAC1 family. By blocking or modulating the cell-surface adhesion molecules with monoclonal antibodies or smaller peptides, a number of neutrophil-driven processes such as asthma, reperfusion injury, and autoimmune disorders may be attenuated (197). This is discussed in detail in Chapter 8.

The undesired inhibition of neutrophil function by antimicrobial agents has been studied for some time and initial *in vitro* studies found that many antibiotics induced neutrophil dysfunction. However, as has been repeatedly argued (194, 198–199) many of these results were noted in experiments wherein clinically irrelevant levels of drugs were used. The present consensus is that a relatively small number of antimicrobials can reproducibly induce neutrophil dysfunction. Rifampin by unknown mechanisms, and tetracyclines by interference with calcium metabolism are thought to inhibit neutrophil chemotaxis, while sulphonamides and trimethoprim are thought to interfere with intracellular killing by interference with the hydrogen peroxide-generating system (199). Inconsistencies in studies on aminoglycosides prevent clear conclusions to be drawn for this class of drug (194, 199). Most importantly, it is not clear that the findings of decreased neutrophil function with any of these antimicrobial agents have any clinical significance, since the modest impairment in neutrophil function is overshadowed by the clinical benefit from the antimicrobial effect of the antibiotic. As noted in Chapter 6, nearly total inhibition of oxidative–metabolic neutrophil function may be required for a patient to develop infections. In studies where antibiotics depress neutrophil functions, only partial (and generally minimal) dysfunction is noted.

5   Summary

Acquired disorders of neutrophil number and function that occur as a result of periodic host interactions with micro-organisms and pharmaceutical compounds are prevalent. The last decade has yielded important information regarding the mechanisms by which micro-organisms and drugs induce neutrophil disorders. With the pathophysiology of these processes now being unravelled, an opportunity to reverse and/or control the neutrophil response to disease is now possible. Chapter 8 will discuss at length the potential avenues that may soon be available for management of neutrophil defects, both congenital and acquired.

References

1 Pizzo, P.A. (1981). Infectious complications in the child with cancer. Pathophysiology of the compromised host and the initial evaluation and mangement of the febrile cancer patient. *J. Pediatr.*, **98**, 341–54.

2 Yang, K. D. and Hill, H.R. (1991). Neutrophil function disorders: pathophysiology, prevention and therapy. *J. Pediatr.*, **119**, 343–54.

3 Henderson, F. W., Collier, A. M., Sanyal, M. A., Watkins, J. M., Fairclough, D. L., Clyde, W. A., Jr, and Denny, F. W. (1982). A longitudinal study of respiratory viruses and bacteria in the etiology of acute otitis media with effusion. *N. Engl. J. Med.*, **306**, 1377–83.

4 Ramsey, B. W., Marcuse, E. K., Foy, H. M., Cooney, M. K., Allan, I., Brewer, D., and Smith, A. L. (1986). Use of bacterial antigen detection in the diagnosis of pediatric lower respiratory tract infections. *Pediatrics*, **78**, 1–9.

5 Paisley, J. W., Lauer, B. A., McIntosh, K., Glode, M. P., Schachter, J., and Rumack, C. (1984). Pathogens associated with acute lower respiratory tract infection in young children. *Pediatr. Infect. Dis.*, **3**, 14–9.

6 Krasinski, K., Nelson, J. D., Butler, S., *et al.* (1987). Possible association of mycoplasma and viral respiratory infections with bacterial meningitis. *Am. J. Epidemiol.*, **125**, 499–508.

7 Hietala, J., Uhari, M., Tuokko, H., and Leinonen, M. (1989). Mixed

bacterial and viral infections are common in children. *Pediatr. Infect. Dis. J.*, **8**, 683–91.

 8 Korppi, M., Leinunen, M., Makela, P. H., and Launiala, K. (1991). Mixed infections are common in children with respiratory adenovirus infection. *Acta Paediatr. Scand.*, **80**, 413–17.

 9 Chatterjee, S. N., Fiala, M., Weiner, J., Stewart, J. A., Stacey, B., and Warner, N. (1978). Primary cytomegalovirus and opportunistic infections: incidence in renal transplant recipients. *J. Am. Med. Assoc.*, **240**, 2446–9.

10 Hamilton, J. R., Overall, J. C., Jr, and Glasgow, L. A. (1976). Synergistic effect on mortality in mice with murine cytomegalovirus and *Pseudomonas aeruginosa, Staphylococcus aureus,* or *Candida albicans* infections. *Infect. Immun.*, **14**, 982–9.

11 Bale, J. F., Jr, Kern, E. R., Overall, J. C., Jr, and Baringer, J. R. (1983) Impaired migratory and chemotactic activity of neutrophils during murine cytomegalovirus infection. *J. Infect. Dis.*, **148**, 518–25.

12 Dearth, J. C. and Rhodes, K. H. (1980). Infectious mononucleosis complicated by severe mycoplasma pneumonia infection. *Am. J. Dis. Child.*, **134**, 744–6.

13 DuBois, D. R. and Bachner, R. L. (1979). Infectious mononucleosis associated with beta hemolytic streptococcal infection. *Clin. Pediatr.*, **18**, 511–12.

14 Levitt, L. P., Bond, J. O., Hall, I. E. Jr, Dame, G. M., Buff, E. E., Marston, C., and Prather, E. C. (1970). Meningococcal and ECHO-9 meningitis. Report of an outbreak. *Neurology*, **20**, 45–51.

15 Sferra, T. J. and Pacini, D. L. (1988). Simultaneous recovery of bacterial and viral pathogens from cerebrospinal fluid. *Pediatr. Inf. Dis.*, **7**, 552–6.

16 Maggiore, G., De Giacomo, C., Marconi, M., Sacchi, F., and Scotta, M. S. (1983). Defective neutrophil motility in children with chronic liver disease. *Am. J. Dis. Child.*, **137**, 768–70.

17 Boisjoly, H. M., Pavan-Langston, D., Kenyon, K. R., and Baker, A. S. (1983). Superinfections in herpes simplex keratitis. *Am. J. Opthalmol.*, **96**, 354–61.

18 Preblud, S. R., Orenstein, W. A., and Bart, K. J. (1984). Varicella: clinical manifestations, epidemiology and health impact in children. *Pediatr. Infect. Dis.*, **3**, 505–9.

19 Russler, S. K., Tapper, M. A., Knox, K. K., Lipeins, A., and Carrigan, D. R. (1991). Pneumonitis associated with coinfection by human herpes virus 6 and legionella in an immunocompetent adult. *Am. J. Pathol.*, **138**, 1405–11.

20 Report of a National Heart, Lung, and Blood Institute workshop. (1984). Pulmonary complications of the acquired immunodeficiency syndrome. Special report. *N. Engl. J. Med.*, **310**, 1682–8.

21 Bernstein, L. J., Krieger, B. N., Novick, B., Sicklick, M. J., and Rubinstein, A. (1985). Bacterial infection in the acquired immunodeficiency syndrome of children. *Pediatr. Infect. Dis.,* **4,** 472–5.

22 Valone, F. H., Payan, D. G., Abrams, D. I., and Goetzl, E. J. (1984). Defective polymorphonuclear leukocyte chemotaxis in homosexual men with persistent lymph node syndrome. *J. Infect. Dis.,* **150,** 267–71.

23 Kaplan, S. L., Taber, L. H., Frank, A. L., and Feigin, R. D. (1981). Nasopharyngeal viral isolates in children with *Haemophilus influenzae* type B meningitis. *J. Pediatr.,* **99,** 591–3.

24 Young, L. S., LaForce, M., Head, J. J., Fealey, B. S., and Bennet, J. V. (1972). A simultaneous outbreak of meningococcal and influenza infections. *N. Engl. J. Med.,* **287,** 5–9.

25 Fischer, J. J. and Walker, D. H. (1979). Invasive pulmonary aspergillosis associated with influenza. *J. Am. Med. Assoc.,* **241,** 1493–4.

26 Pearson, H. E., Eppinger, E. C., Dingle, J. H., and Enders, J. F. (1941). A study of influenza in Boston during the winter of 1940–1941. *N. Engl. J. Med.,* **225,** 763–70.

27 Cartwright, K. A., Jones, D. M., Smith, A. J., Stuart, J. M., Kaczmarski, E. B., and Palmer, S. R. (1991). Influenza A and meningococcal disease. *Lancet,* **338,** 554–7.

28 Abramson, J. S., Giebink, G. S., Mills, E. L., and Quie, P. G. (1981). Polymorphonuclear leukocyte dysfunction during influenza virus infection in chinchillas. *J. Infect. Dis.,* **143,** 836–45.

29 Abramson, J. S., Giebink, G. S., and Quie, P. G. (1982). Influenza A virus induced polymorphonuclear leukocyte dysfunction in the pathogenesis of experimental pneumococcal otitis media. *Infect. Immun.,* **36,** 289–96.

30 Gardner, I. D. (1980). Effect of influenza virus infection on susceptibility to bacteria in mice. *J. Infect. Dis.,* **142,** 704–7.

31 Klein, J. O. and Teele, D. W. (1976). Isolation of viruses and mycoplasmas from middle ear effusions: a review. *Ann. Otol. Rhinol. Laryngol.,* **85 (Suppl 25),** 140–4.

32 Michaels, R. H., Myerowitz, R. L., and Klaw, R. (1977). Potentiation of experimental meningitis due to *Haemophilus influenzae* by influenza A virus. *J. Infect. Dis.,* **135,** 641–5.

33 Jakab, G. J., Warr, G. A., and Knight, M. E. (1979). Pulmonary and systemic defenses against challenge with *Staphylococcus aureus* in mice with pneumonia due to influenza A virus. *J. Infect. Dis.,* **140,** 105–8.

34 Giebink, G. S., Berzins, I. K., Marker, S. C., and Schiffman, G. (1980). Experimental otitis media following nasal inoculation of *Streptococcus pneumoniae* and influenza A virus in chinchillas. *Infect. Immun.,* **30,** 445–50.

35 Klein, B. S., Dollete, F. R., and Yolken, R. H. (1982). The role of respiratory syncytial virus and other viral pathogens in acute otitis media. *J. Pediatr.*, **101**, 16–20.

36 Glezen, W. P. (1982). Serious morbidity and mortality associated with influenza epidemics. *Epidemiol. Rev.*, **4**, 25–44.

37 Centers for Disease Control. (1986). Toxic shock syndrome associated with influenza–Minnesota. *MMWR*, **35**, 143.

38 Dagan, R., Hall, C. B., and Menegus, M. A. (1985). Atypical bacterial infections explained by a concomitant virus infection. *Pediatrics*, **76**, 411–14.

39 Giebink, G. S. and Wright, P. F. (1983). Different virulence of influenza A virus strains and susceptibility to pneumococcal otitis media in chinchillas. *Infect. Immun.*, **41**, 913–20.

40 Silverberg, B. A., Jakab, G. J., Thomason, R. G., Warr, G. A., and Boo, K. S. (1979). Ultrastructural alterations in phagocytic functions of alveolar macrophages after parainfluenza virus infection. *J. Reticuloendothel. Soc.*, **25**, 405–16.

41 Jakab, G. J. and Green, G. M. (1976). Defect in intracellular killing of *Staphylococcus aureus* within alveolar macrophages in Sendai virus-infected murine lungs. *J. Clin. Invest.*, **57**, 1533–9.

42 Edwards, K. M., Dundon, M. C., and Altemeier, W. A. (1983). Bacterial tracheitis as a complication of viral croup. *Pediatr. Infect. Dis.*, **2**, 390–1.

43 Korppi, M., Leinonen, M., Koskela, M., Makela, H., and Launiala, K. (1989). Bacterial coinfection in children hospitalized with respiratory syncytial virus infections. *Pediatr. Infect. Dis. J.*, **8**, 687–92.

44 Arola, M., Ziegler, T., Ruuskanen, O., Mertsola, J., Nanto-Sulonen, K., and Halonen, P. (1988). Rhinovirus in acute otitis media. *J. Pediatr.*, **113**, 693–5.

45 Lecce, J. G., Balsbaugh, R. A., Clare, D. A., and King, M. G. (1982). Rotavirus and hemolytic enteropathogenic *Escherichia coli* in weanling diarrhea of pigs. *J. Clin. Microbiol.*, **16**, 715–23.

46 Olson, R. W. and Hodges, G. R. (1975). Measles pneumonia:bacterial suprainfection as a complicating factor. *J. Am. Med. Assoc.*, **232**, 363–5.

47 Hussey, G. and Simpson, J. (1990). Nosocomial bacteremias in measles. *Pediatr. Infect. Dis. J.*, **9**, 715–17.

48 Fishbacher, M. and Green, S. T. (1987). Varicella and life-threatening streptococcal infection. *Scand. J. Infect. Dis.*, **19**, 519.

49 Bale, J. F., O'Neil, M. E., and Greiner, T. (1985). The interaction of murine cytomegalovirus with murine neutrophils: effect on migratory and phagocytic activities. *J. Leukocyte Biol.*, **38**, 723–34.

50 Tolone, C., Toraldo, R., Catalanotti, P., Ianniello, R., D'Avanzo, M., Galdiero, F., and Iafusco, F. (1989). Decreased adherence of

polymorphonuclear neutrophils in children with viral infections. *Acta Paediatr. Scand.*, **78**, 907–10.

51 Dankner, W. M., McCutchan, J. A., Richman, D. D., Hirata, K., and Spector, S. A. (1990). Localization of human cytomegalovirus in peripheral blood leukocytes by in situ hybridization. *J. Infect. Dis.*, **161**, 31–6.

52 Solberg, C. O., Kalager, T., Hill, H. R., and Glette, J. (1982). Polymorphonuclear leukocyte function in bacterial and viral infections. *Scand. J. Infect. Dis.*, **14**, 11–18.

53 Bultmann, B. D., Haferkamp, O., Eggers, H. J., and Gruler, H. (1984). Echo 9 virus-induced order–disorder transition of chemotactic response of human polymorphonuclear leukocytes: Phenomenology and molecular biology. *Blood Cells*, **10**, 79–106.

54 Vierucci, A., DeMartino, M., Graziani, E., Rossi, M. E., London, W. T., and Blumberg, B. S. (1983). A mechanism for liver cell injury in viral hepatitis: effects of hepatitis B virus on neutrophil function in vitro and in children with chronic active hepatitis. *Pediatr. Res.*, **17**, 814–20.

55 Vierucci, A., DeMartino, M., London, W. T., and Blumberg, B. S. (1977). Neutrophil function in children who are carriers of hepatitis-B surface antigen. *Lancet*, **i**, 157–60.

56 Saunders, S. J., Dowdle, E. B., Fiskerstrand, C., Bassendine, M., and Walls, R. (1978). Serum factors affecting neutrophil function during acute viral hepatitis. *Gut*, **19**, 930–4.

57 Hoar, D. I., Bowen, T., Matheson, D., and Poon, M. C. (1985). Hepatitis B virus DNA is enriched in polymorphonuclear leukocytes. *Blood*, **66**, 1251–3.

58 Ellis, M., Gupta, S., Galant, S., Hakim, S., VandeVen, C., Toy, C., and Cairo, M. (1988). Impaired neutrophil function in patients with AIDS or AIDS-related complex: A comprehensive evaluation. *J. Infect. Dis.*, **158**, 1268–76.

59 Murphy, P. M., Lane, H. C., Fauci, A. S., and Gallin. (1988). Impairment of neutrophil bactericidal capacity in patients with AIDS. *J. Infect. Dis.*, **158**, 627–9.

60 Roilides, E., Mertins, S., Eddy, J., Walsh, T. J., Pizzo, P. A., and Rubin, M. (1990). Impairment of neutrophil chemotactic and bactericidal function in children infected with human immunodeficiency virus type 1 and partial reversal after in vitro exposure to granulocyte-macrophage colony-stimulating factor. *J. Pediatr.*, **117**, 531–40.

61 Spear, G. T., Ou, C. Y., Kessler, H. A., Moore, J. L., Schochetman, G., and Landay, A. L. (1990). Analysis of lymphocytes, monocytes, and neutrophils from human immunodeficiency virus (HIV)-infected persons for HIV DNA. *J. Infect. Dis.*, **162**, 1239–44.

62 Rabson, A. R., Whiting, D. A., Anderson, R., Glover, A., and

Koornhof, H. J. (1977). Depressed neutrophil motility in patients with recurrent herpes simplex virus infections: in vitro restoration with levamisole. *J. Infect. Dis.*, **135**, 113–16.

63 Faden, H., Sutyla, P., and Ogra, P. L. (1979). Effect of viruses on luminol-dependent chemiluminescence of human neutrophils. *Infect. Immun.*, **24**, 673–8.

64 Van Strip, J. A. G., Vankessel, K. P. M., Vander Tol, M. E., and Verhoef, J. (1989). Complement mediated phagocytosis of herpes simplex virus by granulocytes: Binding or ingestion. *J. Clin. Invest.*, **84**, 107–12.

65 Abramson, J. S., Parce, J. W., Lewis, J. C., Lyles, D. S., Mills, E. L., Nelson, R. D., and Bass, D. A. (1984). Characterization of the effect of influenza virus on polymorphonuclear leukocyte membrane responses. *Blood*, **64**, 131–8.

66 Abramson, J. S., Wiegand, G. L., and Lyles, D. S. (1985). Neuraminidase activity is not the cause of influenza virus-induced neutrophil dysfunction. *J. Clin. Microbiol.*, **22**, 129–31.

67 Abramson, J. S., Mills, E. L., Giebink, G. S., and Quie, P. G. (1982). Depression of monocyte and polymorphonuclear leukocyte oxidative metabolism and bactericidal capacity by influenza A virus. *Infect. Immun.*, **35**, 350–5.

68 Abramson, J. S., Lyles, D. S., Heller, K. A., and Bass, D. A. (1982). Influenza A virus-induced polymorphonuclear leukocyte dysfunction. *Infect. Immun.*, **37**, 794–9.

69 Cassidy, L. F., Lyles, D. S., and Abramson, J. S. (1989). Depression of polymorphonuclear leukocyte functions by purified influenza virus hemagglutinin and sialic acid-binding lectins. *J. Immunol.*, **142**, 4401–6.

70 Hartshorn, K. L., Karnad, A. B., and Tauber, A. I. (1990). Influenza A virus and the neutrophil: a model of natural immunity. *J. Leukocyte Biol.*, **47**, 176–86.

71 Henricks, P. A. J., van der Tol, M. E., van Kessel, K. P. M., and Verhoef, J. (1984). Effect of influenza virus on human polymorphonuclear leukocytes: virus-induced dysfunction is not mediated by oxygen metabolism. In *Modulation of phagocytic cell function: involvement of receptors, oxygen species and arachidonic acid metabolites* (ed. P. A. J. Henricks), pp. 37–54. Drukkerij Elinkwijk, B.V., Utrecht.

72 Abramson, J. S., Lewis, J. C., Lyles, D. S., Heller, K. A., Mills, E. L., and Bass, D. A. (1982). Inhibition of neutrophil lysosome–phagosome fusion associated with influenza virus infection in vitro: role in depressed bactericidal activity. *J. Clin. Invest.*, **69**, 1393–7.

73 Caldwell, S. E., Cassidy, L. F., and Abramson, J. S. (1988). Alterations in cell protein phosphorylation in human neutrophils exposed to

influenza A virus: A possible mechanism for depressed cellular end-stage function. *J. Immunol.*, **140**, 3560–7.

74 Hartshorn, K. L., Collamer, M., Auerbach, M., Myers, J. B., Pavlotsky, N., and Tauber, A. I. (1988). Effects of influenza A virus on human neutrophil calcium metabolism. *J. Immunol.*, **141**, 1295–301.

75 Abramson, J. S., Wagner, M. P., Ralston, E. P., Wei, Y., and Wheeler, J. G. (1991). The ability of polymorphonuclear leukocyte priming agents to overcome influenza A virus-induced cell dysfunction. *J. Leukocyte Biol.*, **50**, 160–6.

76 Ruutu, P., Vaheri, A., and Kosunen, T. U. (1977). Depression of human neutrophil motility by influenza virus in vitro. *Scand. J. Immunol.*, **6**, 897–906.

77 Wheeler, J. G., Winkler, L. S., Seeds, M., Bass, D. A., and Abramson, J. S. (1990). Influenza A virus alters structural and biochemical functions of the neutrophil cytoskeleton. *J. Leukocyte Biol.*, **47**, 332–43.

78 Merchant, D. J. and Morgan, H. R. (1950). Inhibition of the phagocytic action of leucocytes by mumps and influenza viruses. *Proc. Soc. Exp. Biol. Med.*, **74**, 651–3.

79 Davies, D. H., McCarthy, A. R., and Keen, K. L. (1986). The effect of parainfluenza virus type 3 and *Pasteurella haemolytica* on oxygen-dependent bactericidal mechanisms of bovine pulmonary phagocytic cells. *Vet. Microbiol.*, **12**, 147–59.

80 Jakab, G. J., Warr, G. A., and Sannes, P. L. (1980). Alveolar macrophage ingestion and phagosome–lysosome fusion defect associated with virus pneumonia. *Infect. Immun.*, **27**, 960–8.

81 Craft, A. W., Reid, M. M., and Low, W. T. (1976). Effect of virus infections on polymorph function in children. *Br. Med. J.*, **1**, 1570.

82 Baynes, R. D., Bezwoda, W. R., and Mansoor, N. (1988). Neutrophil lactoferrin content in viral infections. *Am. J. Clin. Pathol.*, **89**, 225–8.

83 Anderson, R., Rabson, A. R., Sher, R., and Koornhof, H. J. (1976). Defective neutrophil motility in children with measles. *J. Pediatr.*, **89**, 27–32.

84 Szanton, E. and Sarov, I. (1985). Interaction between polymorphonuclear leukocytes and varicella–zoster virus-infected cells. *Intervirology*, **24**, 119–34.

85 Abramson, J. S. and Mills, E. L. (1988). Depression of neutrophil function induced by viruses and its role in secondary microbial infections. *Rev. Infect. Dis.*, **10**, 326–41.

86 Douglas, R. G. (1990). Prophylaxis and treatment of influenza. *N. Engl. J. Med.*, **32**, 443–50.

87 (1989). Influenza vaccination levels in selected states—behavioural risk factor surveillance system, 1987. *MMWR*, **38**, 124–36.

88 Lipscomb, M. F., Yeakel-Houlihan, D., Lyons, C. R., Gleason, R. R.,

and Stein-Streilein, J. (1983). Persistence of influenza as an immunogen in pulmonary antigen-presenting cells. *Infect. Immun.*, **42**, 965–72.

89 Mills, E. L., Debets-Ossenkopp, Y., Verbrugh, H. A., and Verhoef, J. (1981). Initiation of the respiratory burst of human neutrophils by influenza virus. *Infect. Immun.*, **32**, 1200–5.

90 Ewetz, L., Palmblad, J., and Thore, A. (1981). The relationship between luminol chemiluminescence and killing of *Staphylococcus aureus* by neutrophil granulocytes. *Blut*, **43**, 373–81.

91 Horan, T. D., English, D., and McPherson, T. A. (1982). Association of neutrophil chemiluminescence with microbicidal activity. *Clin. Immunol. Immunopathol.*, **22**, 259–69.

92 Armstrong, J. A. and Hart, P. D. (1971). Response of cultured macrophages to *Mycobacteria tuberculosis*, with observations on fusion of lysosomes with phagosomes. *J. Exp. Med.*, **134**, 713–40.

93 Jones, T. C. and Hirsch, J. G. (1972). The interaction between *Toxoplasma gondii* and mammalian cells. II. The absence of lysosomal fusion with phagocytic vacuoles containing living parasites. *J. Exp. Med.*, **136**, 1173–94.

94 Fletcher, M. P. and Gallin, J. I. (1983). Human neutrophils contain an intracellular pool of putative receptors for the chemoattractant N-formyl-methionyl-leucyl-phenylalanine. *Blood*, **62**, 792–9.

95 Edwards, S. W. and Swan, T. F. (1986). Regulation of superoxide generation by myeloperoxidase during the respiratory burst of human neutrophils. *Biochem. J.*, **237**, 601–4.

96 Abramson, J. S., Wheeler, J. G., Parce, J. W., Rowe, M. J., Lyles, D. S., Seeds, M., and Bass, D. A. (1986). Suppression of endocytosis in neutrophils by influenza A virus in vitro. *J. Infect. Dis.*, **154**, 456–63.

97 Heyworth, P. G. and Segal, A. W. (1986). Further evidence for the involvement of a phosphoprotein in the respiratory burst oxidase of human neutrophils. *Biochem. J.*, **239**, 723–31.

98 Tauber, A. I. (1987). Protein kinase C and the activation of the human neutrophil NADPH-oxidase. *Blood*, **69**, 711–20.

99 Shaafi, R. I., White, J. R., Molski, T. F. P., Schefcyk, K., Volip, M., Naccache, P. H., and Feinstein, M. B. (1983). Phorbol-12-myristate 13-acetate activates rabbit neutrophils without an apparent rise in the level of intracellular free calcium. *Biophys. Biochem. Res. Commun.*, **114**, 638–45.

100 Zigmond, S. H., Slonczewski, J. L., Wilde, M. W., and Carson, M. (1988). Polymorphonuclear leukocyte locomotion is insensitive to lowered cytoplasmic calcium levels. *Cell Motil. Cytoskel.*, **9**, 184–9.

101 Freissmuth, M., Casey, P. J., and Gilman, A. G. (1989). G proteins control diverse pathways of transmembrane signaling. *FASEB J.*, **3**, 2125–31.

102 Kanaho, Y., Kermode, J. C., and Becker, E. L. (1990). Comparison of stimulation by chemotactic formyl peptide analogs between GTPase activity in neutrophil plasma membranes and granule enzyme release from intact neutrophils. *J. Leukocyte Biol.*, **47**, 420–8.

103 Feltner, D. E. and Marasco, W. A. (1989). Regulation of formyl peptide receptor binding to rabbit neutrophil plasma membranes: use of monovalent cations, guanine nucleotides and bacterial toxins to discriminate among different states of the receptor. *J. Immunol.*, **142**, 3963–70.

104 Dexter, D., Rubins, J. B., Manning, E. C., Khachatrian, L., and Dickey, B. F. (1990). Compartmentalization of low molecular mass GTP-binding proteins among neutrophil secretory granules. *J. Immunol.*, **145**, 1845–50.

105 Koo, C., Lefkowitz, R. J., and Snyderman, R. (1983). Guanine nucleotides modulate the binding affinity of the oligopeptide chemoattractant receptor on human polymorphonuclear leukocytes. *J. Clin. Invest.*, **72**, 748–53.

106 Corey, S. J. and Rosoff, P. M. (1989). Granulocyte-macrophage colony stimulating factor primes neutrophils by activating a pertussis toxin-sensitive G-protein not associated with phosphatidyl inositol turnover. *J. Biol. Chem.*, **264**, 14165–72.

107 Verghese, M. W., Charles, L., Jakoi, L., Dilllon, S. B., and Snyderman, R. (1987). Role of guanine nucleotide regulatory protein in the activation of phospholipase C by different chemoattractants. *J. Immunol.*, **138**, 4374–80.

108 Siefert, R., Rosenthal, W., and Schultz, G. (1986). Purine and pyrimidine nucleotides potentiate activation of NADPH oxidase and degranulation via chemotactic peptides and induce degranulation of human neutrophils via G proteins. *FEBS Lett.*, **205**, 161–5.

109 Barrowman, M. M., Cockroft, S, and Comperts, B. D. (1986). Two roles for guanine nucleotides in the stimulus–secretion sequence of neutrophils. *Nature*, **319**, 504–7.

110 Mayorga, L. S., Diaz, R., and Stahl, P. S. (1989). Regulatory role for GTP-binding proteins in endocytosis. *Science*, **244**, 1475–7.

111 Lad, P. M., Olson, C. V., and Grewal, I. S. (1986). A step sensitive to pertussis toxin and phorbol ester in human neutrophils regulates chemotaxis and capping but not phagocytosis. *FEBS Lett.*, **200**, 91–6.

112 Feltner, D., Smith, R. H., and Marasco, W. A. (1986). Characterization of the plasma membrane bound GTPase from rabbit neutrophils. *J. Immunol.*, **137**, 1916–20.

113 Milligan, G. (1988). Techniques used in the identification and analysis of function of pertussis toxin-sensitive guanine nucleotide binding proteins. *Biochem. J.*, **255**, 1–13.

114 McKenzie, F. R., Mullaney, I., Unson, O. G., Spiegel, A. M., and

Milligan, G. (1988). The use of anti-peptide antisera to probe interactions between receptors and guanine nucleotide binding proteins. *Biochem. Soc. Trans.*, **16**, 434–7.

115 Obara, S., Mishima, K., Yamada, K., Taniguchi, M., and Shimoyama, M. (1989). DNA-regulated arginine-specific mono (ADP-ribosyl)ation and de-ADP-ribosylation of endogenous acceptor proteins in human neutrophils. *Biochem. Biophys. Res. Commun.*, **163**, 452–7.

116 Gilman, A. G. (1987). G proteins: transducers of receptor-generated signals. *Annu. Rev. Biochem.*, **56**, 615–49.

117 Hall, A. and Self, A. J. (1986). The effect of Mg^{2+} on the guanine nucleotide exchange rate of p21 N-ras. *J. Biol. Chem.*, **261**, 10963–5.

118 Cockcroft, S. and Stutchfield, J. (1989). The receptors for ATP and fMetLeuPhe are independently coupled to phospholipases C and A2 via G-protein(s). Relationship between phospholipase Ca and A2 activation and exocytosis in HL60 cells and human neutrophils. *Biochem. J.*, **263**, 715–23.

119 English, D., Rizzo, Mt., Tricot, S., and Hoffman, R. (1989). Involvement of guanine nucleotides in superoxide release by fluoride-treated neutrophils. Implications for a role of a guanine nucleotide regulatory protein. *J. Immunol.*, **143**, 1685–91.

120 Bokoch, G. M. and Quilliam, L. A. (1990). Guanine nucleotide binding properties of rap1 purified from human neutrophils. *Biochem. J.*, **267**, 407–11.

121 Didsbury, J., Weber, R. F., Bokoch, G. M., Evans, T., and Snyderman, R. (1989). Rac, a novel ras-related family of proteins that are botulism substrates. *J. Biol. Chem.*, **264**, 16378–82.

122 Quinn, M. T., Parkos, C. A., Walker, L., Orkin, S. H., Dinauer, M. C., and Jesaitis, A. J. (1989). Association of a ras-related protein with cytochrome B of human neutrophils. *Nature*, **342**, 198–200.

123 Gilman, A. G. (1989). G proteins and regulation of adenyl cyclase. *J. Am. Med. Assoc.*, **262**, 1819–25.

124 Katada, T., Kusakabe, K., and Oinuma, M., *et al.* (1987). A novel mechanism for the inhibition of adenylate cyclase via inhibitory GTP-binding proteins. *J. Biol. Chem.*, **262**, 11897–900.

125 Steinbeck, M. J. and Roth, J. A. (1987). Neutrophil activation by recombinant cytokines. *Rev. Infect. Dis.*, **11**, 549–68.

126 Bass, D. A., Gerard, C., Olbrantz, P., Wilson, J., McCall, C. E., and McPhail, L. C. (1987). Priming of the respiratory burst of neutrophils by diacylglycerol. *J. Biol. Chem.*, **262**, 6643–9.

127 Novak, M. J. and Cohen, H. J. (1991). Depolarization of polymorphonuclear leukocytes by *Porphyromonas (Bacteroides) gingivalis* 381 in the absence of respiratory burst activation. *Infect. Immun.*, **59**, 3134–42.

128 Steed, L. L., Setareh, M., and Friedman, R. H. (1991). Intracellular survival of virulent *Bordetella pertussis* in human polymorphonuclear leukocytes. *J. Leukocyte Biol.*, **50**, 321–31.

129 Friedman, R. L., Fiederlein, R. L., Glasser, L., and Galgiani, J. N. (1987). *Bordetella pertussis* adenylate cyclase. Effects of affinity-purified adenylate cyclase on human polymorphonuclear leukocyte functions. *Infect. Immun.*, **55**, 135–40.

130 Shurin, S. B., Socransky, S. S., Sweeny, E., *et al.* (1979). Neutrophil disorder induced by capnocytophaga, a dental microorganism. *N. Engl. J. Med.*, **301**, 849–54.

131 Stevens, D. L., Mitten, J., and Henry, C. (1987). Effects of alpha and θ toxins from *Clostridium perfringens* on human polymorphonuclear leukocytes. *J. Infect. Dis.*, **156**, 324–33.

132 Bhakdi, S. and Martin, E. (1991). Superoxide generation by human neutrophils induced by low doses of *Escherichia coli* hemolysin. *Infect. Immun.*, **59**, 2955–62.

133 Bergman, M. J., Guerrant, R. L., Murad, F., Richardson, S. H., Weaver, D., and Mandell, G. L. (1978). The interaction of polymorphonuclear neutrophils with *Escherichia coli. J. Clin. Invest.*, **61**, 227.

134 Rosendale, S., Devenish, J., MacInnes, J. I., Lumsden, J. H., Watson, S., and Xun, H. (1988). Evaluation of heat-sensitive, neutrophil-toxic, and hemolytic activity of *Haemophilus (Actinobacillus) pleuropneumoniae. Am. J. Vet. Res.*, **49**, 1053–8.

135 Quie, P. G. (1983). Perturbation of the normal mechanisms of intra-leukocytic killing of bacteria. *J. Infect. Dis.*, **148**, 189–93.

136 Czuprynski, C. J. and Noel, E. J. (1990). Influence of *Pasteurella haemolytica* A1 crude leukotoxin on bovine neutrophil chemiluminescence. *Infect. Immun.*, **58**, 1485–7.

137 Hendricks, P. A. J., Binkhorst, G. J., Drijver, A. A., Van Der Vliet, H., and Nijkamp, F. P. (1990). The effect of *Pasteurella haemolytica* cytotoxin on bovine polymorphonuclear leukocytes can be attenuated by β-adrenoceptor antagonists. *Veterin. Microbiol.*, **22**, 259–66.

138 Sorensen, R. U. and Klinger, J. D. (1987). Biological effects of *Pseudomonas aeruginosa* phenazine pigments. *Antibiot. Chemother.*, **39**, 113–24.

139 Bishop, M. B., Baltch, A. L., Hill, L. A., Smith, R. P., Lutz, F., and Pollack, M. (1987). The effect of *Pseudomonas aeruginosa* cytotoxin and toxin A on human polymorphonuclear leukocytes. *J. Med. Microbiol.*, **24**, 315–24.

140 Schultz, D. R. and Miller, K. D. (1974). Elastase of *Pseudomonas aeruginosa*: Inactivation of complement components and complement derived chemotactic and phagocytic factors. *Infect. Immun.*, **10**, 128.

141 Peterson, P. K., Verhoef, J., Sabbath, L. D., and Quie, P. G. (1977).

Effect of protein A on staphylococcal opsonization. *Infect. Immun.,* **15,** 760.

142 Weksler, B. B. and Hill, M. J. (1968). Inhibition of leukocyte migration by a staphylococcal factor. *J. Bacteriol.,* **98,** 1030.

143 Easmon, C. S. F., Hamilton, J., and Glynn, A. A. (1973). Mode of action of a staphylococcal anti-inflammatory factor. *Br. J. Exp. Pathol.,* **54,** 638.

144 Kato, I. and Noda, M. (1989). ADP-ribosylation of cell membrane proteins by staphylococcal alpha-toxin and leukocidin in rabbit erythrocytes and polymorphonuclear leukocytes. *FEBS Lett.,* **255,** 59–62.

145 Bhakdi, S. and Tranum-Jensen, J. (1991). Alpha-toxin of *S. aureus. Microbiol. Rev.,* **55,** 733–51.

146 Densen, P. and Mandell, G. (1980). Phagocyte strategy vs. microbial tactics. *Rev. Infect. Dis.,* **2,** 817–38.

147 Dal Nogare, A. R., Vial, W. C., and Toews, G. B. (1988). Bacterial species-dependent inhibition of human granulocyte elastase. *Am. Rev. Respir. Dis.,* **137,** 907–11.

148 Bernheimer, A. W. (1954). Streptolysins and their inhibitors. In *Streptococcal Infection* (ed. M. McCarty), pp. 19–38. Columbia University Press, New York.

149 Sullivan, G. W., Sullivan, J. A., and Mandell, G. L. (1978). Leukotoxic streptococci and neutrophil degranulation. *Clin. Res.,* **26,** 407A.

150 Hensler, T., Koller, M., and Konig, W. (1991). Regulation of leukotriene B4 generation from human polymorphonuclear granulocytes after stimulation with formyl-methionyl-leucyl phenylalanine: effects of pertussis and cholera toxins. *Infect. Immun.,* **59,** 3046–52.

151 Moss, J. and Vaughan, M. (1988). ADP-Ribosylation of guanyl nucleotide-binding regulatory proteins by bacterial toxins. *Adv. Enzymol. Rel. Areas Mol. Biol.,* **61,** 303–79.

152 Smail, E. H., Melnick, D. A., Ruggeri, R., and Diamond, R. D. (1988). A novel natural inhiitor from *Candida albicans* hyphae causing dissociation of the neutrophil respiratory burst response to chemotactic peptides from other post-activation events. *J. Immunol.,* **140,** 3893–9.

153 Smail, E. H., Kolotila, M. P., Ruggeri, R., and Diamond, R. D. (1989). Natural inhibitor from *Candida albicans* blocks release of azurophil and specific granule contents by chemotactic peptide-simulated human neutrophils. *Infect. Immun.,* **57,** 689–92.

154 Robertson, M. D., Seaton, A., Raeburn, J. A., and Milne, L. J. (1987). Inhibition of phagocyte migration and spreading by spore diffusates of *Aspergillus fumigatus. J. Med. Vet. Mycol.,* **25,** 389–96.

155 Allgower, M. and Bloch, H. (1949). The effect of tubercle bacilli on the migration of phagocytes in vitro. *Am. Rev. Tuber.,* **59,** 562.

156 Garner, C. V., DesJardins, D., and Pier, G. B. (1990). Immunogenic properties of *Pseudomonas aeruginosa* mucoid exopolysaccharide. *Infect. Immun.,* **58,** 1835–42.

157 Wexler, D. E. and Cleary, P. P. (1985). Purification and characteristics of the streptococcal chemotactic factor inactivator. *Infect. Immun.,* **50,** 757–764.

158 Bignold, L. P., Rogers, S. D., Siaw, T. M., and Bahnisch, J. (1991). Inhibition of chemotaxis of neutrophil leukocytes to interleukin-8 by endotoxins of various bacteria. *Infect. Immun.,* **59,** 4255–8.

159 Donabedian, H. (1985). Human mononuclear cells exposed to staphylococci rapidly produce an inhibitor of neutrophil chemotaxis. *J. Infect. Dis.,* **152,** 24–32.

160 Link, A. S., Bass, D. A., and McCall, C. E. (1979). Altered neutrophil migration during bacterial infection associated with a serum modulator of cellular motility. *J. Infect. Dis.,* **76,** 5896–900.

161 Fasano, M. B., Cousart, S., and McCall, C. E. (1991). Increased expression of the interleukin 1 receptor on blood neutrophils of humans with the sepsis syndrome. *J. Clin. Invest.,* **88,** 1452–9.

162 Tennenberg, S. and Solomkin, J. S. (1988). The relationship between fMet-Leu-Phe receptor mobilization and oxidative activity. *Arch. Surg.,* **123,** 171–5.

163 Krause, K.-H. and Lew, D. P. (1988). Bacterial toxins and neutrophil activation. *Sem. Hematol.,* **25,** 112–22.

164 Feigin, R. D. and Cherry, J. D. (1987). Pertussis. In *Text book of pediatric infectious diseases* (ed. R. D. Feigen and J. D. Cherry), pp. 1227–38. W. B. Saunders, Philadelphia.

165 Nelson, W. L., Hopkins, R. S., Roe, M., and Glode, M. (1986). Simultaneous infection with *Bordetella pertussis* and respiratory syncytial virus in hospitalized children. *Pediatr. Infect. Dis.,* **5,** 540–4.

166 Nourshargh, S. and Williams, T. J. (1990). Evidence that a receptor-operated event on the neutrophil mediates neutrophil accumulation in vivo. *J. Immunol.,* **145,** 2633–8.

167 Witvliet, M. H., Burns, D. L., Brennan, M. J., Poolman, J. T., and Manclark, C. R. (1989). Binding of pertussis toxin to eucaryotic cells and glycoproteins. *Infect. Immun.,* **57,** 3324–30.

168 Tyrell, G. J., Peppler, M. S., Bonnah, R. A., Clark, C. G., Chong, P., and Armstrong, G. D. (1989). Lectinlike properties of pertussis toxin. *Infect. Immun.,* **57,** 1854–7.

169 Simon, M. I., Strathmann, M. P., and Gautam, N. (1991). Diversity of G proteins in signal transduction. *Science,* **252,** 802–8.

170 Bokoch, G. M. and Parkos, C. A. (1988). Identification of novel GTP-binding proteins in the human neutrophil. *FEBS Lett.,* **227,** 66–70.

171 Milligan, G. (1988). Techniques used in the identification and analysis of function of pertussis toxin-sensitive guanine nucleotide binding proteins. *Biochem. J.*, **255**, 1–13.

172 Gilman, A. G. (1984). Guanine nucleotide binding regulatory proteins and dual control of adenylate cyclase. *J. Clin. Invest.*, **73**, 1–4.

173 Katada, T. and Ui, M. (1981). Islet-activating protein; a modifier of receptor-mediated regulation of rat islet adenylate cyclase. *J. Biol. Chem.*, **256**, 8310–17.

174 Bokoch, G. M. and Gilman, A. G. (1984). Inhibition of receptor-mediated release of arachidonic acid by pertussis toxin. *Cell*, **39**, 301–8.

175 Okajima, F., Katada, T., and Ui, M. (1985). Coupling of the guanine nucleotide regulatory protein to chemotactic peptide receptors in neutrophil membranes and its uncoupling by islet-activating protein, pertussis toxin. *J. Biol. Chem.*, **260**, 6761–8.

176 Okajima, F. and Ui, M. (1984). ADP-ribosylation of the specific membrane protein by islet-activating protein, pertussis toxin, association of inhibition of a chemotactic peptide-induced arachidonate release in neutrophils. *J. Biol. Chem.*, **259**, 13863–71.

177 Lad, P. M., Olson, C. V., and Smiley, P. A. (1985). Association of the n-formyl-met-leu-phe receptor in human neutrophils of a GTP binding protein sensitive to pertussis toxin. *Proc. Natl Acad. Sci. USA*, **82**, 869–73.

178 Chedid, M., Shirakawa, F., Naylor, P., and Mizel, S. B. (1989). Involvement of a pertussis toxin sensitive GTP-binding protein in the activation of adenylate cyclase. *J. Immunol.*, **142**, 4301–6.

179 Becker, E. L., Kermode, J. C., Naccache, P. H., Yassin, R., Munoz, J. J., Marsh, M. L., *et al.* (1986). Pertussin toxin as a probe of neutrophil activation. *Fed. Proc.*, **45**, 2151–5.

180 Lad, P. M., Olson, C. V., and Grewal, I. S. (1986). Role of a pertussis toxin substrate in the control of lectin-induced cap formation in human neutrophils. *J. Biochem.*, **238**, 29–36.

181 Diamond, R. D. (1988). Fungal surfaces: effects of interactions with phagocytic cells. *Rev. Infect. Dis.*, **10 suppl 2**, S428–31.

182 Kozel, T. R., Pfrommer, G. S., Guerlain, A. S., Hisghison, B. A., and Highison, G. J. (1988). Strain variation in phagocytosis of *Cryptococcus neoformans*: dissociation in susceptibility of phagocytosis from activation and binding of opsonic fragments of C3. *Infect. Immun.*, **56**, 2794–800.

183 Pinto, A., Cirono, G., Meli, R., Senatore, F., and Capasso, F. (1988). Inhibitory effects of fungi on aggregation of rabbit platelets and rat polymorphonuclear leucocytes in vitro. *J. Ethnopharmacol.*, **22**, 91–9.

184 Weitzman, S. A. and Stossel, T. P. (1978). Drug-induced immunological neutropenia. *Lancet,* **i,** 1068–72.

185 Lubran, M. M. (1989). Hematologic side effects of drugs. *Ann. Clin. Lab. Sci.,* **19,** 114–21.

186 Nefel, K., Hauser, S., and Muller, M. (1985). Inhibition of granulopoiesis in vivo and in vitro by beta-lactam antibiotics. *J. Infect. Dis.,* **152,** 90–8.

187 Abramson, S. and Weisman, G. (1989). The mechanisms of action of nonsteroidal antiinflammatory drugs. *Arthritis Rheum.,* **32,** 1–9.

188 Biemond, P., Swaak, A. G., Penders, J. A., Beindroff, C. M., and Koster, J. F. (1986). Superoxide production by polymorphonuclear leucocytes in rheumatoid arthritis and osteoarthritis: in vivo inhibition by the antirheumatic drug prioxicam due to interference with the activation of the NADPH-oxidase. *Ann. Rheum. Dis.,* **45,** 249–55.

189 Abramson, S., Korchak, H. M., Ludewig, R., Edelson, H., Haines, K., Leven, R., *et al.* (1985). Modes of action of aspirin-like drugs. *Proc. Natl Acad. Sci. USA,* **82,** 7227–31.

190 Abramson, S., Haines, K., Leszczynska, J., Reibman, J., and Weissmann, G. (1988). Nonsteroidal antiinflammatory drugs inhibit neutrophil (PMN) functions via effects at the G protein of the plasma membrane (abstract). *Clin. Res.,* **36,** 548A.

191 Townley, R. G. and Suliaman, F. (1987). The mechanism of corticosteroids in treating asthma. *Ann Allergy,* **58,** 1–8.

192 Mukwaya, G. (1988). Immunosuppressive effects and infections associated with corticosteroid therapy. *Pediatr. Infect. Dis.,* **7,** 499–504.

193 Schleimer, R. P., Freeland, H. S., Peters, S. P., Brown, K. E., and Derse, C. P. (1989). An assessment of the effects of glucocorticoids on degranulation, chemotaxis, binding to vascular endothelium and formation of leukotriene B4 by purified human neutrophils. *J. Pharm. Exp. Therapeut.,* **250,** 598–605.

194 Labro, M. T. and El Benna, J. (1991). Effects of anti-infectious agents on polymorphonuclear neutrophils. *Eur. J. Clin. Microbiol. Infect. Dis.,* **10,** 124–31.

195 Petroi, K. C., Shen, L., and Guyre, P. M. (1988). Modulation of human polymorphonuclear leukocyte IgG Fc receptors and Fc receptor-mediated functions by IFN-gamma and glucocorticoids. *J. Immunol.,* **140,** 3467–72.

196 Ouyant, Y., Wang, W., Shuta, S., and Changy, Y. (1989). Mechanism of action of colchicine. VI: Effect of colchincine on generation of leukotriene B4 by human polymorphonuclear leukocytes. *Clin. Exp. Rheumatol.,* **7,** 397–402.

197 Osborn, L. (1990). Leukocyte adhesion to endothelium in inflammation. *Cell,* **62,** 3–6.
198 Mandell, L. A. (1982). Effects of antimicrobial and antineoplastic drugs on the phagocytic and microbicidal function of the polymorphonuclear leukocyte. *Rev. Infect. Dis.,* **4,** 683–97.
199 van den Broek, P. J. (1989). Antimicrobial drugs, microorganisms, and phagocytes. *Rev. Infect. Dis.,* **11,** 213–45.

6 Congenital neutrophil deficiencies

E. L. MILLS and F. J. D. NOYA

1 Clinical case: congenital neutropenia

A 9-year-old girl born of non-consanguineous parents presented at 11 days of age with a staphylococcal cellulitis of the heel and inguinal adenitis. At that time, her initial peripheral blood count revealed a white cell count of 15.4×10^9 cells/l, with no PMN, and bone marrow aspiration revealed maturation of PMN precursors only to the myelocyte stage. During the next 5 years, the patient required 19 hospitalizations for respiratory tract infections and bacteraemias as well as for periorbital cellulitis, ethmoid sinusitis, and *Pseudomonas* osteomyelitis. At the age of 4, she had *Pseudomonas* pneumonia that required lobectomy, and at the age of 5 she had a severe cellulitis of the abdominal wall. Her other medical problems included osteopenia, chronic mouth ulcerations, and severe failure to thrive. Laboratory studies showed the following: consistent peripheral blood absolute PMN counts of zero, with total white cell counts usually of 4.7×10^9 cells/l (monocytes 0.15–0.4 and eosinophils 0.05–0.1); a hypercellular bone marrow with a maturational arrest in the PMN lineage at the promyelocyte/myelocyte level; normal erythroid, lymphoid, and megakaryocytic lineages; a normal chromosomal analysis; and the absence of anti-neutrophil antibodies.

In 1988, at the age of 5, she began treatment with RhG-CSF, as part of a clinical trial. She gradually responded to initial i.v. administration of the drug with absolute PMN counts of more than 1×10^9 cells/l, and then subsequently, to initial daily s.c. injections of RhG-CSF, with absolute PMN counts of more than 3×10^9 cells/l. On long-term maintenance therapy, her absolute PMN counts remained at $0.35–1.2 \times 10^9$ cells/l. Her clinical response to therapy had been a dramatic improvement in quality of life, with an absence of recurrent, serious infections, and regular attendance at school. However, in late 1989 she began requiring progressive increases in her dose of RhG-CSF to maintain her absolute PMN count at $0.4–0.8 \times 10^9$ cells/l; no anti-neutrophil antibodies were present. By mid 1991, her absolute PMN count was consistently less than 0.5×10^9 cells/l and was unresponsive to increasing doses of RhG-CSF, and she began having low-grade fevers. A liver abscess was diagnosed and responded to surgical drainage and antibiotics; at the time of diagnosis her absolute

PMN count was less than 0.1×10^9 cells/l. With resolution of the liver abscess, she is again able to maintain absolute PMN counts of more than 0.5×10^9 cells/l and has remained infection free.

2   Introduction

Neutrophils, the most abundant of the phagocytic cells in circulating blood, are the first to arrive at sites of infection where they avidly ingest and efficiently kill a variety of microbial pathogens. PMN are critical to host defence against tissue-invading bacteria and fungi. Individuals who lack PMN have long been recognized to be at risk for recurrent and life-threatening infections. In the past 25 years, a growing number of disease entities marked by frequent infections despite normal numbers of PMN, have been recognized as having underlying PMN dysfunction (1–3). *In vitro* studies of PMN from these patients have led to a wealth of information concerning the PMN functional activities of adherence, migration, phagocytosis, secretion, the respiratory burst, and intracellular killing. Pathologic defects in one or other of these cellular functions have been correlated with characteristic clinical syndromes. These congenital PMN disorders which are listed in Table 6.1, have served as models for understanding the essential contribution of PMN to host defence, and to the process of inflammation. New technology in the past decade has been successfully applied to reveal one or more molecular lesions responsible for the disturbed cellular function in some of these disorders.

The clinical manifestations of individuals who lack PMN are similar in many ways to those who possess defective PMN. In both groups, the skin and mucous membranes, areas of the body often colonized with microbes, provide a portal of entry for bacteria and fungi to establish infections. Among the most common pathogens to both groups are *Staphylococcus aureus, Pseudomonas* species, enteric organisms, and *Candida* and *Aspergillus* species. The two groups, however, differ strikingly in their ability to contain localized infection (4, 5). In neutropenic patients, such as the case noted above, organisms frequently escape from localized soft tissue infections to become blood-borne and bacteraemia progresses to life-threatening septicemia. In contrast, infections in patients with defective PMN function tend to remain localized within the superficial tissues, or the lymph nodes and the liver, and uncommonly become generalized (6, 7).

The time lapse between bacterial invasion and the mobilization of phagocytic cells to the site of invasion is critical to the prevention or at least the containment of the infectious process; animal studies have shown that this crucial time-window is between 2 and 4 h (8). Hence, patients who lack PMN or those with disorders of PMN migration, are unable to provide the

Table 6.1 Major congenital neutrophil disorders

Disease	Inheritance[a]	Cellular defect	Clinical features
Chronic granulomatous disease	XR AR AD	Bactericidal defect for catalase-positive microbes; inability to generate superoxide and reduce nitroblue tetrazolium (NBT)	Severe infections of skin, lungs, liver and bone with catalase-positive micro-organisms (e.g. staphylococci, enteric Gram-negative bacteria, *Candida* and *Aspergillus* species. Abscesses in any organ; granuloma may obstruct gastrointestinal or genitourinary tract.
Myeloperoxidase deficiency	AR	Absent myeloperoxidase	No symptoms unless has another defect (e.g. diabetes mellitus), then risk for fungal infections
Leukocyte adhesion deficiency	AR	Deficient adherence, aggregation, chemotaxis, and ingestion	Delayed separation of umbilical cord; neutrophilia; bacterial infections without pus; periodontitis
Chédiak–Higashi syndrome	AR	Giant granules; decreased chemotaxis, degranulation and microbicidal activity; increased O_2 consumption and H_2O_2 production; decreased cathepsin G and elastase	Neutropenia. Recurrent bacterial infections especially with *S. aureus*; periodontal disease; partial oculocutaneous albinism; progressive peripheral neuropathy; during adolescence may develop an accelerated, fatal lymphoma-like phase
Specific granule deficiency	AR	Abnormal or absent specific granules; decreased degranulation, chemotaxis, and bactericidal activity; absent gelatinase granules and defensins	Exceedingly rare disorder. Recurrent infections of skin, mucous membranes, and lungs. Neutrophils have bilobed nuclei, lack granules on Wright stain

[a] Autosomal recessive (AR), X-linked recessive (XR), autosomal dominant (AD).

timely infiltration of PMN at sites of minute breaks in the skin, mucous membranes, and gastrointestinal tract. Patients with profound impairment of phagocytic cell mobilization such as those with leukocyte adhesion deficiency, are unable to form pus at sites of infection, and the infected tissue is typically necrotic or gangrenous and devoid of PMN (6). Infected sites show little evidence of an inflammatory response, but the infectious process may be deceptively aggressive and lead to destruction of cutaneous, subcutaneous, and periodontal tissue. Patients with disorders of mild or intermittent impairment of PMN migration such as those with the hyper-IgE (Job's) syndrome, tend to form abscesses containing large numbers of PMN and mononuclear leukocytes, cells which have presumably arrived too late at the infected site to prevent infection (9). In contrast, individuals with disorders of PMN and monocyte microbicidal activity such as those with chronic granulomatous disease characteristically develop widespread abscesses which are frequently deep-seated (10). The abscesses may contain granulomas with or without purulent material. Skin and soft tissue infections are typically pustular and the signs and symptoms of inflammation are preserved.

3   Congenital neutropenia

Congenital neutropenia is a heterogeneous group of disorders characterized by decreased production or release of mature PMN from the bone marrow, resulting in persistently or intermittently low counts of circulating PMN. There is no clear definition of congenital neutropenia. In practice, we consider congenital neutropenia as that detected during infancy or early childhood and is not secondary to infection, drugs, toxins, neoplasia, antineutrophil antibodies, autoimmune disorders, or other acquired conditions. The known disorders associated with congenital neutropenia are listed in Table 6.2. Neutropenia may be the only abnormality or it may be associated with other hereditary disorders or phenotypical syndromes. In children, neutropenia is defined as an absolute PMN count in peripheral blood of less than 1.8×10^9 cells/l during the first week of life, less than 1.0×10^9 cells/l in infants between 2 weeks and 1 year of life, and less than 1.5×10^9 cells/l thereafter (11, 12). Black individuals may have lower PMN counts than age-matched whites (12). The lower normal limits for PMN counts in blacks are considered to be from 0.2×10^9 to 0.6×10^9 cells/l lower than those cited above (12).

The spectrum of disease observed in patients with congenital neutropenia is very broad and varies from life-threatening infections (Kostmann's syndrome) to an asymptomatic course (chronic benign neutropenia) where the neutropenia is often an incidental finding. The degree of neutropenia is also variable and may be characterized as mild ($1.0–1.5 \times 10^9$ cells/l),

Table 6.2 Disorders associated with congenital neutropenia

1. Severe congenital neutropenia (Kostmann's syndrome)
2. Chronic benign neutropenia
3. Reticular dysgenesis
4. Cyclic neutropenia
5. Severe chronic neutropenias
    (a) Myelokathesis
    (b) Neutropenia associated with immunoglobulinopathies
        X-linked agammaglobulinaemia
        Hyper-IgM immunodeficiency syndrome
        Hyperimmunoglobulinaemia A with arthropathy
    (c) Neutropenia associated with phenotypic abnormalities
        Cartilage-hair hypoplasia
        Schwachman–Diamond syndrome
        Dyskeratosis congenita
        Chédiak–Higashi syndrome
        Fanconi's syndrome
        Osteopetrosis
    (d) Neutropenia associated with metabolic disorders
        Hyperglycinaemia
        Isovaleric acidaemia
        Methylmalonic acidaemia
        Propionic acidaemia
        Gaucher's disease
        Type Ib glycogenosis

moderate ($0.5–1.0 \times 10^9$ cells/l), or severe ($<0.5 \times 10^9$ cells/l) (12). Only patients with severe neutropenia have increased susceptibility to life-threatening infections, especially if it lasts more than a few days. Some patients with chronic severe neutropenia remain remarkably free of serious infections. While the resistance to infection in these patients has never been explained, it is likely that other host defence mechanisms, such as the mononuclear phagocytic, humoral, and cellular immune systems compensate for the lack of PMN.

The most frequent infections that occur in patients with significant neutropenia are those due to bacteria which form part of their own normal endogenous flora, such as *S. aureus, Escherichia coli,* and other enterobacteria, and *Pseudomonas aeruginosa* (4). Mixed bacterial infections are not uncommon, particularly those originating in the oral cavity or anal canal. Significantly, neutropenia does not increase the susceptibility to infections with viruses, parasites, or intracellular bacteria such as *Listeria monocytogenes.* Likewise, the neutropenic state by itself does not favour invasion of the central nervous system. The most common types of infection seen in these patients are skin and soft tissue infections such as cellulitis and furuncles, pneumonia, lung or liver abscesses, and septicaemia (12). Also common are ulcerative stomatitis, gingivitis, perirectal, or vulvar inflammation, urinary tract infections, and otitis media. These infections tend to recur, or to become chronic, and they respond poorly to antimicrobial therapy. Fever is almost always present in early infection. Of the cardinal signs of inflammation at infected sites, pain and erythema are preserved, but warmth, oedema, and exudation or suppuration are usually less evident in neutropenic patients than they are in normal hosts (13). As in the case presented at the beginning of this chapter, abscess formation can be poor. This patient's liver abscess was ill defined and had no discrete areas of liquefaction, all of which made surgical drainage difficult.

3.1   Severe congenital neutropenia (Kostmann's syndrome)

Also known as infantile genetic agranulocytosis, severe congenital neutropenia (SCN) is a syndrome first described by Rolf Kostmann in Sweden in 1956 (14, 15) in infants dying from recurrent infections resulting from severe neutropenia. The features of this syndrome are outlined in Table 6.3. This uncommon disorder of autosomal recessive mode of inheritance, is characterized by persistent severe absolute neutropenia (0.5×10^9 cells/l or less) and maturation arrest of PMN myelopoiesis at the promyelocyte or myelocyte stage in the bone marrow. There is an absence of post-mitotic cells of PMN lineage (metamyelocytes, banded and segmented PMNs). The promyelocytes are frequently morphologically abnormal with vacuolization and atypical nuclei. Affected patients may also have monocytosis, eosinophilia, hypergammaglobulinaemia, and thrombocytosis. One can

Table 6.3   Features of severe congenital neutropenia

1. Rare disorder, autosomal recessive inheritance
2. Persistent absolute neutropenia $<0.5 \times 10^9$ cells/l
3. Bone marrow: maturational arrest of PMN lineage at promyelocyte stage
4. Severe bacterial infections beginning in early infancy
5. Chronic gingivitis, stomatitis, perirectal inflammation
6. High mortality due to infections
7. Response to treatment with haematopoietic growth factors:
   RhGM-CSF: Monocytosis, eosinophilia, no increase in PMN count
   RhG-CSF: Increase in PMN count to $>1.0 \times 10^9$ cells/l
            Interindividual variation in dose requirement
            Cycling of PMN count frequently observed
            Prevents the majority of infections, chronic infections resolve

only speculate about the contribution these 'compensatory' responses offer to host defence in neutropenic patients.

Infants with SCN are symptomatic in early infancy with frequent and severe bacterial infections, often leading to a fatal outcome despite appropriate antimicrobial therapy. Typically, these patients present during the first few months of life with fever, irritability, omphalitis, and subcutaneous abscesses. Subsequently they may experience pneumonia, otitis media, gingivitis, perineal, and urinary tract infections. The recurrence or chronicity of these localized infections and the progression to septicaemia, visceral abscesses, or severe enteritis accounts for the high morbidity and mortality in infants and young children with this disease. Fifty per cent die from infection before 7 months of age, and only 10 per cent survive long term (16). A few patients with SCN have developed leukaemia (12). Several treatment modalities have been used unsuccessfully in an attempt to stimulate PMN production, such as plasma transfusions, leukocyte transfusions, glucocorticosteroids, androgenic steroids, vitamin B6, and lithium. Before the advent of recombinant haematopoietic growth factors, only bone marrow transplantation had resulted in correction of the defect (17). At present, treatment trials with RhG-CSF promises to alter such a dismal prognosis (18–21) (see Chapter 8, Section 5). The patient described above in fact participated in one of these clinical trials (18). Before RhG-CSF therapy, she had been hospitalized 19 times during her 5 years of life. Once treatment with RhG-CSF induced and maintained an adequate PMN count, she was free of major infections and did not require hospitalization for 2.5 years until the development of the liver abscess. Interestingly, over the 9 months preceding this event, her PMN count had decreased to less than 0.1×10^9 cells/l. It is very likely that the development of the liver abscess is causally related to low PMN counts. Presently, we do not understand why she became less responsive to RhG-CSF.

The nature of the defect in SCN is unknown. Most likely, this syndrome comprises a heterogeneous group of defects all resulting in maturational arrest of the PMN lineage at the promyelocyte level, hence, the absence of mature PMNs. The familial occurrence and autosomal recessive pattern of transmission of SCN indicate a genetic defect (14, 15). Serum inhibitors or anti-neutrophil antibodies have not been found in affected patients. Correction of this disorder by bone marrow transplantation (17) suggests a stem cell defect. On the other hand, there is evidence suggestive of a stromal origin of the defect, that is, in the accessory cell system in the bone marrow that supports the growth and differentiation of the haematopoietic precursors (see below).

Bone marrow cells from patients with SCN are capable of *in vitro* generation of normal numbers of colony-forming units-granulocyte/macrophage (CFU-GM); although, these colonies can be devoid of PMN and contain only macrophages and eosinophils (18). Nevertheless, stimulation with crude conditioned media of undefined colony-stimulating activity, such as phytohaemagglutinin-stimulated conditioned media, induces PMN maturation in such colonies (22). Such findings suggest that bone marrow cells of SCN patients have the capacity for normal proliferation and differentiation to mature myeloid cells. Indeed, *in vitro* stimulation with RhG-CSF of bone marrow cells from patients with SCN, alone (23, 24), or together with IL-3 (25), resulted in formation of colonies with normal PMN maturation. In patients responding to RhG-CSF with significant increases in blood PMN counts, bone marrow examination showed varying degrees of maturation, although the developmental arrest was not completely eliminated in any patients (18, 19). That is, the proportion of promyelocytes in bone marrow remained elevated, whereas the proportions of myelocytes, metamyelocytes, and mature PMN remained low (18).

Cell differentiation in long-term bone marrow cultures is dependent on the formation of an adherent layer of accessory cells which provides nurturing (or 'stromal') influences to the haematopoietic colonies. In contrast, colony development in short-term cultures is dependent on exogenous sources of colony-stimulating activity and evidently is not subject to stromal influences because a stromal adherent layer does not develop in these cultures. Coulombel *et al.* (22) have hypothesized that the defect in late granulocyte differentiation is of stromal origin, rather than of stem cell derivation, because long-term bone marrow cultures from patients with SCN have reproduced the *in vivo* differentiation defect, whereas short-term cultures of the same patients have yielded colonies with normal differentiation (22).

All the above *in vivo* and *in vitro* observations have led many to speculate that the defect responsible for SCN is either an inadequate production of G-CSF by the bone marrow microenvironment, or a defective response of myelopoietic precursors to G-CSF (Table 6.4). The results of clinical studies have supported the hypothesis of deficient production since:

Table 6.4   Postulated mechanisms for maturational defect in severe congenital neutropenia

---

1. Impaired production of biologically active G-CSF
    (a) Absent or non-functional gene
    (b) Inability to secrete G-CSF
    (c) Production of biologically inactive molecule
2. Defective response of PMN precursors to G-CSF
    (a) Decreased expression of G-CSF receptors
    (b) Decreased binding affinity of receptors for G-CSF
    (c) Impaired intracellular signal transduction
3. Defective co-factor needed for G-CSF-induced PMN maturation

---

(i) patients with SCN treated with RhG-CSF demonstrated a dose-dependent increase in blood PMN counts (18–21); (ii) bone marrow myelopoietic progenitor cells of patients with SCN were capable of differentiating into mature PMN *in vitro* (22, 23, 25); and (iii) low serum G-CSF concentrations were found in patients with SCN (18, 21, 26). Nevertheless, the theory of deficient production now seems unlikely with the information obtained using more sensitive techniques to measure G-CSF to concentrations as low as 5 pg/ml. One group of investigators has shown that patients with SCN are capable of synthesizing and secreting biologically active G-CSF (27). They demonstrated that patient-derived peripheral blood mononuclear cells, stimulated *in vitro* with lipopolysaccharide, produced G-CSF proliferative activity (measured by the induction of proliferation in a leukaemia cell line); the G-CSF activity was specifically inhibited by anti-G-CSF antiserum. Furthermore, they demonstrated that G-CSF protein and G-CSF mRNA, as analysed by Western and Northern blot analysis, respectively, were indistinguishable from those of normal controls. Moreover, they showed that serum of patients with SCN contained higher concentrations of G-CSF (150–910 pg/ml) compared with healthy individuals (<5–100 pg/ml), when measured by Western blotting and by the leukaemia cell line proliferation assay (28). Finally, during treatment with RhG-CSF, serum G-CSF levels in these patients fell significantly, compared to before treatment, to levels within the range of healthy individuals.

Possible molecular mechanisms for decreased precursor responsiveness to G-CSF are outlined in Table 6.4. If the mechanism responsible for the PMN maturation defect in SCN is not a defective production of G-CSF, a logical alternative explanation is a defective response of PMN precursors to G-CSF. Although there is no direct evidence for any of these hypotheses, decreased responsiveness to G-CSF in these patients is suggested by: (i) the requirement for pharmacological doses of RhG-CSF as high as 3–120 µg/kg/day to achieve blood PMN counts of 1.0×10^9 cells/l; and (ii) by the variability observed between patients in dose requirement and in pattern of response. By comparison, dosages equal to or greater than 10 µg/kg/day induce PMN counts above 5.0×10^9 cells/l in neutropenic cancer patients (29). We cannot exclude the possibility that abnormalities in other factors, different from G-CSF but indispensable for G-CSF to induce terminal PMN differentiation, are involved in the pathogenesis of SCN.

3.2   Chronic benign neutropenia

Under this umbrella is a heterogeneous group of disorders characterized, as the name implies, by a benign course with no or only mild infections of skin and mucous membranes (30). PMN counts vary from 0.2 to 2.0×10^9 cells/l. The PMN count remains relatively stable over the course of years;

spontaneous remissions have been reported in children, usually between 2 and 4 years of age (31). No genetic pattern is discernible in most children with this condition, except for some familial cases where transmission has been described as autosomal dominant (12). A genetically transmitted benign neutropenia exists among Yemenite Jews (12). Bone marrow morphology and *in vitro* studies have yielded variable results among patients, and in the same patient over time. Because of the benign course of this condition, no treatment is indicated.

3.3   Reticular dysgenesis

Reticular dysgenesis is an autosomal recessive disorder due to a selective failure of stem cells committed to differentiate along myeloid and lymphoid lineages, whereas erythroid and platelet development are normal (32). As a consequence of the profound failure of leukocyte production, affected patients lack PMN and both B and T lymphocytes, and are agammaglobulinaemic. The thymus is underdeveloped and there is absence of lymphoid elements in the lymph nodes, tonsils, spleen, and gut. These patients die of severe infections during the first few months of life. At present, the only hope of survival for affected infants is bone marrow transplantation (33).

3.4   Cyclic neutropenia

Cyclic neutropenia is a rare disorder characterized by regular cyclic fluctuations (usually every 21 days) in the number of blood PMN, with periods of absolute neutropenia ($<0.2 \times 10^9$ cells/l) lasting 3–10 days (referred to as the nadir of the cycle), alternating with periods of normal PMN counts (Table 6.5 and ref. 34). Seventy per cent of patients have 21 day cycles, but the range of cycles observed have varied from 14 to 36 days. In individual patients the cycle length is usually constant. Other cell counts may also oscillate in cycles of the same length, although not necessarily in phase with the PMN. For example, monocytosis and eosinophilia may coincide with the nadir of the PMN cycle, whereas, fluctuation of platelets and reticulocytes may occur in phase with that of PMN. Evaluation of the bone marrow reveals cyclic oscillations of haematopoietic progenitors, most notably of elements of PMN lineage. A paucity of mature PMN is observed during the nadir, whereas normal maturation is found during periods of normal PMN counts (35). Bone marrow myeloid progenitors (CFU-GM) which have also been found to cycle, are present in higher concentrations than normal, and the highest levels coincide with the nadirs of neutropenia (36). The cellular composition of these CFU-GM was similar to those of normal controls.

Table 6.5 Features of cyclic neutropenia

---

1. Congenital form (70% of cases)
    (a) Childhood onset
    (b) Familial occurrence, autosomal dominant inheritance
2. Acquired form (30% of cases)
    (a) Adult onset
    (b) May have clonal proliferation of large granular lymphocytes
    (c) Some respond to corticosteroids
3. Absolute neutropenia occurs in cycles, usually every 3 weeks
4. Monocytes and eosinophils cycle asynchronously with PMN
5. Recurrent symptoms coincide with nadir of neutropenia: fever, malaise,
    mouth ulcers, pharyngitis, lymphadenopathy
6. Skin infections and sometimes more serious bacterial infection may occur
7. Bone marrow myelopoietic progenitors and serum G-CSF levels increase
    during neutropenic phase
8. Treatment with RhG-CSF reduces degree and duration of neutropenia but
    may not abolish cycling

The features of cyclic neutropenia are summarized in Table 6.5. Characteristically, the majority of patients become symptomatic during the periods of neutropenia. Fever, malaise, mucosal ulcers, sore throat, and lymph node enlargement recur regularly with each cycle. Skin infections, or sometimes, more severe infections may occur during the neutropenic phase. The symptoms resolve as the PMN count returns to normal. Although many patients live full lives, with some having a gradual amelioration of symptoms and less noticeable cycles, up to 10 per cent of patients die of infectious complications (12). Usually the disorder is familial, with onset during childhood. Genetic transmission is autosomal dominant with variable expression in 25 per cent of families (12). An adult onset form has been described (34), which has been shown to respond to low dose corticosteroid therapy, and has been associated with clonal proliferation of large granular lymphocytes (37).

Grey collie dogs have cyclic haematopoiesis very similar to the human disorder with the exception that the cycle is 14 days long (38). The disease is transferable by bone marrow transplantation in both humans and dogs, and curable by bone marrow transplantation in dogs (39). In humans, curative bone marrow transplantation has not been attempted, but a leukaemic child receiving bone marrow from a sibling with cyclic neutropenia developed this disorder. These observations suggest a stem cell disorder in which periodic failure of cell production results in neutropenia. The cause of cyclic neutropenia is uncertain. One thought is that the defect is one of dysregulation of haematopoiesis due to disordered feedback, with more noticeable consequences on PMN myelopoiesis. The mechanisms underlying the abnormalities in feedback have not been well defined. Defective production of G-CSF does not appear to have a role because serum G-CSF levels are usually elevated, particularly during the neutropenic period of the cycle (40–42). Compared to marrow myelopoietic progenitors from normal individuals, those from patients with cyclic neutropenia have been found to be less responsive *in vitro* to G-CSF and GM-CSF (36, 43). The decreased responsiveness to these growth factors appears to be restricted to cells of PMN lineage since macrophage colony generation is not affected.

Although the pathogenesis of cyclic neutropenia is not well defined, it is known that therapy with haematopoietic growth factors can significantly ameliorate both the intermittent neutropenia of this disorder and its clinical consequences. In humans with cyclic neutropenia, several investigators have demonstrated a salutary effect of therapy with RhG-CSF (35, 40, 41, 44, 45). In brief, treatment resulted in increased PMN counts throughout the cycle, decrease in duration of neutropenia, shortening of the cycle, and marked clinical improvement. Cycling persisted, particularly in patients with the childhood-onset or congenital form of the disorder. Therapy with RhGM-CSF at conventional doses induced marked eosinophilia but no change in PMN counts in a patient who subsequently responded to RhG-CSF (44) (see Chapter 8 for further discussion).

3.5   Other forms of congenital neutropenia

Myelokathesis is a rare form of congenital neutropenia characterized by persistent neutropenia, recurrent infections, and peculiar morphology of the PMN in the bone marrow (46). Examination of the bone marrow reveals a large reservoir of segmented PMN containing pyknotic nuclei and very thin chromatin filaments connecting the nuclear lobes. Kinetic studies have shown increased intramedullary destruction of PMN, which is probably the underlying mechanism of neutropenia in this disorder. One patient with myelokathesis responded to treatment with RhGM-CSF with normalization of the PMN count and clinical improvement (47). Other forms of congenital neutropenia are those associated with immunoglobulinopathies, with phenotypic abnormalities, or with inherited metabolic disorders, as outlined in Table 6.2. The readers are referred to other sources for descriptions of these disorders (12, 48, 49).

4   Chronic granulomatous disease

Chronic granulomatous disease (CGD) is a group of inherited disorders which affects the oxygen-dependent microbicidal activity of PMN and other phagocytic cells (monocytes, macrophages, and eosinophils) and leads to severe, recurrent bacterial and fungal infections (5, 50). The microbicidal activity of PMN resides primarily with nicotinamide adenine dinucleotide phosphate (NADPH) oxidase, which when activated generates superoxide (O_2^-) anion and other highly reactive forms of reduced oxygen (51, 52) (see Chapter 3 for details regarding the normal function of the PMN oxidative systems). PMN of patients with CGD have a defective NADPH oxidase system which fails to generate O_2^- and renders the cells profoundly ineffective in killing intracellular organisms. Since the oxidase consists of several components, the phenotype of CGD can result from different genetic defects affecting one or another of the individual constitutive proteins (53). The classic form of this disease is an X-linked recessive disorder, but a clinically indistinguishable variant affecting both males and females, exhibits an autosomal recessive mode of inheritance (54). The intense search over several decades for the biochemical and more recently, the molecular basis of CGD, has contributed enormously to identifying the enigmatic nature of the components and the processes used by normal PMN to generate antimicrobial oxidants. Although CGD is a rare disease, estimated to occur in 1 in 1 000 000 persons, it is a prototype for abnormalities of phagocyte oxidative metabolism and its biochemical basis is the most completely understood of the PMN disorders (5, 50, 53).

4.1 Clinical manifestations

In its classic form, CGD becomes apparent early in childhood with more than 75 per cent of affected individuals developing symptoms in the first year of life, and almost 90 per cent being identified before their second birthday (7). The disease, however, may occasionally present in adolescence or adulthood with the oldest reported individual presenting in the sixth decade of life (55). Individuals who present after childhood, may have had recurrent though non-fatal infections since infancy, a minimal history of infection, or rarely, been perfectly well prior to the development of severe or unusual infections later in life (5, 55, 56).

The major manifestations of the disease are similar for all patients, independent of age at onset or mode of transmission (10). Abscess formation is the hallmark of CGD and has been reported to occur in every organ in the body. Infections predominate in the skin, lung, and mucous membranes, areas of the body which interface with the environment and are easily colonized by micro-organisms. Common infectious manifestations are recurrent pneumonia and lung abscesses, skin and soft tissue infections, lymphadenopathy and suppurative lymphadenitis, visceral abscesses, and osteomyelitis usually involving the small bones of the hands and feet (10, 50, 57). Septicaemia and meningitis are less common. In general, infections of the lung and the liver follow a protracted course with a slow response to antibiotics. Cutaneous infections are associated with persistent drainage, prolonged healing and residual scarring. Mucous membrane complications include ulcerative stomatitis, persistent rhinitis, and conjunctivitis. Diarrhoea is a relatively common manifestation of CGD and enteritis and colitis, although infrequent, occur and may be indistinguishable from Crohn's disease. Infections of the genitourinary tract and the central nervous system are relatively uncommon, although renal, perinephric, and brain abscesses have been documented.

Physical findings commonly include dermatitis, adenopathy and hepatosplenomegaly (10). Routine laboratory studies show anaemia of chronic disease and hypergammaglobulinemia. The patient with CGD has a delayed response to infection but eventually develops fever, an appropriate localized inflammatory response, leukocytosis, and an elevated erythrocyte sedimentation rate. Typically, in the absence of early warning signs of osteomyelitis, the disease may be moderately advanced at the time of diagnosis with extensive bony destruction evident radiographically. Similarly, intra-abdominal abscesses, particularly liver abscesses, may progress almost silently until the patient presents with a spiking fever pattern but few other signs and symptoms, and a large abscess cavity visualized by imaging studies (10, 57). Incomplete resolution of the inflammatory response may contribute to the formation of granulomas, lesions characterized by collections of phagocytes and giant cells sometimes loaded with pigmented lipid material. Granulomas can develop in virtually any organ system and occasionally, when strategically situated they cause oesophageal, antral, or genitourinary tract obstruction.

Although an infectious pathogen is not isolated in many of the febrile episodes of CGD, the causative agents recovered are distinctive of this disorder: the overwhelming majority are catalase-positive organisms such as *S. aureus*, enteric Gram-negative rods and *Aspergillus* species, with a paucity of catalse-negative organisms such as *Streptococcus pneumoniae* and *Haemophilus influenzae* (58). This strikingly peculiar set of pathogens could be predicted from the nature of the biochemical lesion of CGD. Once ingested into the phagocytic vacuole, catalase-producing bacteria enter a safe haven: microbial H_2O_2, generated by all bacteria as a waste product, is neutralized by microbial catalase and cellular antioxidant systems. Thus, neither the cell nor the ingested micro-organism generate toxic oxygen radicals. As a result, 80–100 per cent of ingested catalase-positive organisms may remain viable in the phagolysosome after a 2 h incubation (59). In contrast, catalase-negative pathogens such as pneumococci produce large amounts of unneutralized H_2O_2 within the phagocytic vacuole, which in turn drives intracellular oxygen-dependent microbicidal reactions, and promotes microbial 'suicide' (60). As a result of delayed intracellular killing and degradation, catalase-positive organisms persist within phagolysomal vacuoles and form a nidus for chronic inflammation and granuloma formation.

With the exception of the respiratory burst and intracellular killing, the other functional activities of PMN and monocytes are normal in the vast majority of patients studied. These functions include adherence, chemotaxis, phagocytosis, lysosomal content, and degranulation (2).

4.2   Laboratory studies used to diagnose CGD

The diagnosis of CGD is based on the demonstration of an absent, or near absent, respiratory burst in stimulated phagocytic cells. Of the many methods available to measure respiratory burst activity, the assays most frequently used to diagnose CGD are those which measure nitroblue tetrazolium (NBT) dye reduction, chemiluminescence response and O_2^- anion production. Confirmatory evidence of CGD is a demonstrated inability of phagocytic cells to kill ingested catalase-positive bacteria (59).

The NBT dye reduction assay is a widely available screening test for CGD (61). In this semiquantitative assay, PMN are activated and the O_2^- generated by the respiratory burst reduces the yellow nitroblue tetrazolium dye to blue formazan that precipitates on the activated cell as a deep blue pigment: the ability of individual cells to reduce NBT is assessed microscopically. Since CGD cells generate little or no O_2^- they remain unstained, (or in rare variants, weakly positive), and the NBT test is negative (53). The qualitative NBT slide test, particularly the modified version employing PMA is a simple, sensitive, and specific screening test which will, when properly performed, identify virtually all patients with CGD. It should be noted, however, that detection of the weak activity present in the variant CGD PMN requires that the unstimulated PMN have low background activity, and that the positive control PMN be optimally activated with a potent stimulus (such as PMA) to attain strong positivity (53, 62, 63). The NBT slide test provides unique information in classifying variant forms of CGD, as well as in detecting the carrier state in X-linked CGD families (53, 64). Nevertheless, identification of the carrier state in X-linked CGD may be difficult with the NBT test (or luminol-enhanced chemiluminescence described below) under two circumstances': (i) low degree of inactivation of the abnormal X-chromosome; and (ii) CGD which arises from a spontaneous mutation in a parental germline (54). The NBT test has also been used for prenatal diagnosis to test blood obtained at fetoscopy (65). The results of a negative NBT test in a suspected case of CGD should be confirmed with the cytochrome *c* assay for O_2^- production.

The chemiluminescence assay is a highly sensitive but non-specific indicator of the respiratory burst and is a useful screening test for CGD (2, 66, 67). The respiratory burst of stimulated PMN is associated with the generation of unstable oxygen radicals which react with oxidizable substrates constitutive to the (particulate or soluble) stimuli to form unstable intermediates: these intermediates return to their ground state by emission of light energy measurable as chemiluminescence (68). Light emission is conveniently measured in a scintillation counter. Photomultiplier tubes easily detect the low levels of light emission generated by stimulated PMN, but native chemiluminescence can be multiplied 1000-fold by the addition to the phagocytic mixtures of oxidizable substrates such as luminol (5-amino-2,3-dihydro-1,4-phthalazinedione) (69). This exogenous organic molecule serves as a substrate for reduction–oxidation reactions in the MPO–H_2O_2–halide system to generate electronically excited products; relaxation of these products to ground state produces chemiluminescence. CGD cells generate essentially no chemiluminescence, and this assay is used, with or without amplification, as a rapid, sensitive method to identify CGD patients. Similar to the NBT test, diagnosis of variant CGD may be difficult even using the more sensitive luminol-amplified chemilumin-escence assay (62). The luminol-enhanced assay is useful for detecting heterozygous carriers but is subject to the same limitations as those de-scribed above for the NBT test (64, 67).

Specific assessment of the integrity of the NADPH oxidase can be made with the quantitative analysis of O_2^- formation by measurement of O_2^- dismutase-inhibitable cytochrome c reduction. Superoxide production analysed in response to soluble (e.g. PMA) or to particulate stimuli (e.g. opsonized zymosan) is typically undetectable in most patients with CGD (70, 71). In variant forms of CGD with diminished levels of cytochrome b_{558}, low levels of O_2^- of 0.5–10 per cent of control, have been present (72). To distinguish CGD including variant forms from other PMN dis-orders with partial deficiency of the respiratory burst, it is necessary to measure O_2^- production in response to a soluble stimulus in a continuous assay, and response to a particulate stimulus in an end-point assay (71).

The laboratory studies for classification of CGD will be briefly noted here and have been described in detail by Curnutte (53, 71). Using intact cells, cytochrome b can be measured by spectral analysis on Triton X-100 extracts of intact PMN by means of a dithionite reduced minus oxidized absorbance spectrum. The presence or absence of the 91 and 22 kDa subunits of the cytochrome can be confirmed by Western blot analysis and the presence of mRNAs for the cytochrome b subunits can be analysed with Northern blots. In all CGD patients reported to date, defects in PMN oxidase activity could be localized to either the membrane or the cytosol fractions (53). The subcellular location of the genetic lesion can be deter-mined by using a cell-free oxidase system reconstituted from subcellular fractions of unactivated PMN. In this assay, PMN cell membrane and cytosol are combined in the presence of certain activating agents and co-factors, and O_2^- production is measured in the presence of NADPH. Variant forms of CGD can be detected when one subcellular fraction is prepared from CGD PMN and the other fraction from normal PMN. Two sets of studies should be performed on PMN disrupted into subcellular fractions. In the first set, the cells are activated prior to disruption and the level of NADPH oxidase determined. Only in the rare CGD variant will NADPH oxidase activity be detectable and in those cells the Michaelis constant (K_m) for NADPH oxidase can be determined. In the second set of studies, the cells are not activated prior to disruption. The cytosol, membrane, and granule fractions are obtained and analysed in the cell-free activation system to determine the subcellular location of the genetic lesion.

4.3 Molecular basis of CGD and mode of inheritance

The initial case reports of boys with severe, recurrent, local infections and hypergammaglobulinaemia appeared in 1954 but the familial nature of the disease was not documented until 1965 when a series of 18 boys in 10 families with the disease were described (73–75). It was discovered shortly thereafter that the PMN of patients with CGD were markedly abnormal in their ability to kill intracellular micro-organisms, a defect attributed to a virtual absence of stimulatable oxidative metabolism (59, 76). When mothers of these patients were found to have intermediate levels of these cellular functions, the mode of inheritance was established as X-linked recessive. However with documentation of families in which several girls or siblings of both sexes were affected, an autosomal recessive pattern of inheritance for CGD was also recognized (7, 54).

The discovery that CGD PMN did not undergo a burst in oxygen consumption during bacterial ingestion (76), singled out the 'respiratory burst' as the key to the cellular defect of this disorder. The inability of the CGD phagocytes to produce oxidizing radical species specifically focused attention on the NADPH oxidase, the enzyme system responsible for O_2^- formation during the respiratory burst (51). Multiple reports have now confirmed that defects in the NADPH oxidase cause CGD, and that abnormalities in its constituent proteins alter enzyme activity (53). The biochemical and clinical phenotype of CGD can arise from any number of genetic defects affecting a single essential component of the NADPH oxidase.

The demonstration by spectral analysis that a membrane-bound low-potential b cytochrome, designated cytochrome b_{558} and unique to phagocytic cells, was absent in most patients with X-linked CGD but was present in patients with autosomal CGD, implied two genetically distinct forms (77–79). Nevertheless, the subsequent identification of patients with X-linked inheritance patterns and measurable levels of this cytochrome, as well as other patients with autosomal inheritance patterns and no detectable levels of cytochrome b_{558} strongly suggested more than two genetic forms (80–82). With the development of cell-free NADPH oxidase systems, our comprehension of the multi-component oxidase escalated and so did the potential number of genetic lesions in the enzyme (53, 83). The various defective or absent oxidase proteins which result from the many genetic lesions which form the molecular basis of the CGD syndrome are listed in Table 6.6 and are discussed in detail in Chapter 3, Section 1.

Genetic defects leading to CGD have now been defined in each of the four identified constituents of the NADPH oxidase: the α and β chains of the membrane cytochrome b_{558}, and the cytosolic proteins p47 and p67 (53, 71). The genetic variants of CGD may be organized (Table 6.6) according to the subcellular location of the defective oxidase components in the resting cell (53, 71). The membrane fraction of the oxidase contains at a minimum, the subunits of the cytochrome b_{558}, a large 91 kDa glyco-protein β subunit termed gp91-*phox* (glycoprotein subunit, 91 kDa mass, of the phagocyte oxidase) and a 22 kDa protein α subunit (p22-*phox*) (83–88). A 22 kDa *ras*-like G protein, termed *rap*, is intimately associated with the cytochrome and may also be an obligatory component of the oxidase (89). Those oxidase components that reside in the cytosol in the resting cell include the p47-*phox* and p67-*phox* referred to above, the NADPH-binding protein, and potentially an unidentified fourth component (90). Addition of an activating agent to a cell-free system, or stimulation of an intact cell, causes assembly of all these components into a catalytically functioning oxidase on the plasma membrane.

In almost two-thirds of individuals with CGD, the cellular defect can be localized to a membrane component of the oxidase in a cell-free activation system (71, 91–94) (Table 6.6). All of these individuals appear to have abnormalities in either the gp91-*phox* or p22-*phox* subunit of the cytochrome b_{558}, to have less than 1 per cent activatable oxidase in the cell-free system, and to have the presence of variable amounts of cytochrome b on spectral analysis. At least half of all cases of CGD are due to defects in gp91-*phox* and inheritance is in an X-linked fashion (53, 71). In classic X-linked CGD, the most common form of the disorder accounting for 50 per cent of all cases of the disease, cytochrome b_{558} is completely missing as demon-strated by spectroscopy or by immunoblot analysis using antibodies directed at either subunit. Only about 5 per cent of cases of CGD are due to defects in p22-*phox* and inheritance of these defects is autosomal re-cessive (94, 96).

The gene encoding gp91-*phox* has been identified within the Xp21 locus in the short arm of the X chromosome, the cDNA has been cloned and the protein purified (84–86, 97). mRNA for gp91-*phox* is found only in cells of phagocytic lineage (84). As indicated in Table 6.6, the lesion in the gene encoding gp91-*phox* can lead to the absence of the protein product, the presence of a non-functional protein, a partial deficiency of gp91-*phox*, or the assembly of an abnormal oxidase (K_m mutant) with no detectable haem spectrum. In the great majority of cases of X-linked CGD, the defect in the gene encoding gp91-*phox* leads to the absence of the protein product

Table 6.6 Diagnostic features of chronic granulomatous disease

Type of CGD	Intact cell superoxide production (% normal)	Cytochrome b spectrum (% normal)	Cell-free system activity (% normal)		Prevalence (% of CGD cases)
			Membrane	Cytosol	
X-linked inheritance					
Membrane cytochrome b 91 kDa subunits					
Absent	<1	0	0	100	52
Non-functional	<1	100	0	100	3
Partial deficiency	1–10[a]	8–15	<1	100	2
K_m defect	1–10[a]	0	0	100	<
Autosomal recessive inheritance					
Membrane cytochrome b 22 kDa subunit					
Absent	<1	0–4	0	100	5
Non-functional	<1	100	0	100	<1
Cytosol component 46 kDa protein					
Absent	<1	100	100	≤2	33
Cytosol component 67 kDa protein					
Absent	<1	100	100	≤2	5
Cytosol component unclassified					
K_m variant	1–4*	100	100	<2	<1

[a] Nitroblue tetrazolium (NBT) reduction is zero in all types of CGD except those types indicated in which >60% of NBT score may be weakly positive.

(96, 98). But partial or complete gene deletions are rare, and the majority of patients have a grossly intact gp91-*phox* gene on Southern blot analysis (99). Many of these patients lack the gp91-*phox* mRNA transcript (100), other patients have the gp91-*phox* mRNA but produce little or no detectable protein (101). In a small number of mRNA-positive patients, point mutations have been identified near the gp91-*phox* C terminus with normal levels of a functionally defective cytochrome (55, 102). In contrast, missense mutations identified in other gp91-*phox* domains have been associated with low levels or absence of the cytochrome (103). Lesions in gp91-*phox* that lead to the total absence of the protein or to an abnormal protein, completely eliminate O_2^- production in the intact PMN. On the other hand, in variant forms of gp91-*phox* CGD in which the genetic lesion leads to a partial deficiency of gp91-*phox*, the corresponding levels of cytochrome b_{558} are diminished to between 8 and 15 per cent of normal (71, 72), and the quantity of O_2^- produced and of NBT reduced, is proportional to the level of measurable cytochrome. Genetic lesions in gp91-*phox* that lead to the assembly of an abnormal oxidase with an altered K_m for NADPH and very low (or non-detectable) levels of cytochrome b_{558}, may still have sufficient amounts of the cytochrome for electron transport (104–108). PMN of these patients produce minimal quantities of O_2^- and have weakly positive NBT scores.

Cytochrome b_{558} is intrinsic to the membrane and its two subunits are tightly associated together and co-purify on chromatography. The full expression of either subunit of the cytochrome appears to require the presence of the companion subunit. The majority of cases of X-linked CGD have a grossly intact gp91-*phox* gene but the protein product is absent. In both the X-linked and the autosomal forms of CGD missing the cytochrome, both cytochrome subunits are absent by immunoblotting (83, 96, 98). In summary, an absence of gp91-*phox* results in no detectable p22-*phox* and, therefore, no detectable levels of cytochrome b_{558}. Similarly, when p22-*phox* is absent, the gp91-*phox* subunit is not detectable.

Defects in p22-*phox* account for approximately 5 per cent of the described cases of CGD (94, 96). Genetic defects are inherited in an autosomal recessive fashion and p22-*phox* is encoded on chromosome 16. While gp91-*phox* is found only in PMN and monocytes, stable mRNA for p22-*phox* but not translated protein, is found in all cell types (87). Hence, normal levels of p22-*phox* protein appear to require steady-state levels of gp91-*phox* protein. In only four individuals examined to date have the molecular mechanisms leading to p22-*phox* CGD been identified. One patient was homozygous for a large deletion in the p22-*phox* gene while the other three had grossly normal mRNA on Northern blot analysis (94, 109). Of the mRNA-positive patients, two had point mutations with no gp91-*phox* or p22-*phox* protein detected despite abundant message for both. The third mRNA-positive patient had a point mutation in the p22-*phox* that caused the substitution of a glutamine for a proline at residue 156 (109); the cytochrome b_{558} protein was present in normal amounts but appeared to be non-functional.

In approximately 40 per cent of individuals with CGD, the cytosolic fraction of the PMN is found to be defective when analysed by a cell-free system (53, 95). All cases described have had an autosomal recessive inheritance pattern and normal levels of membrane cytochrome b_{558} by spectral analysis. NBT reduction by intact PMN and O_2^- production are usually absent, although low but measurable levels ($\leqslant 1$ per cent of normal) have been reported in a few cases (71). Analysis in a cell-free assay system has shown that the activity of the membrane fractions of the cells is completely normal but the cytosol fractions from the same cells have a marked decrease in activity (typically $\leqslant 2$ per cent of normal) (110). Some genetic carriers of cytosol-deficient CGD have been detected by analysis in a cell-free system (110). Of the cytosol-deficient CGD patients reported to date, all were found to have defects in either p47-*phox* or p67-*phox* (95). Deficiency of p47 is far more common than that of p67 and accounts for about one-third of all patients with CGD (95). All five patients reported with p47-*phox*-deficient CGD and examined by Northern blotting appeared to have adequate amounts of a normal sized mRNA transcript despite the absence of any detectable p47-*phox* protein (111). Recombinant p47-*phox* fusion proteins as well as purified cytosol fractions containing p47-*phox* are able to restore cell-free oxidase activity to cytosols from deficient patients (90, 111–115). A few patients with cytosol-deficient CGD, and 5 per cent of all patients with CGD, lack detectable levels of p67-*phox* as shown by immunoblotting (95). Similar to p47-*phox*-deficient CGD, the nature of the genetic lesion in these patients is unknown and Northern blot analysis demonstrates the presence of apparently normal amounts of mRNA despite an absence of detectable protein by immunoblotting (116). Likewise, recombinant p67-*phox* fusion proteins and purified cytosol fractions containing p67-*phox* are able to restore activity to cytosol from deficient patients (90, 116). The clinical course of patients with autosomal recessive forms of CGD is typically milder and begins later in childhood (53, 117). Interestingly, factors other than the magnitude of the O_2^- production must influence the severity of the clinical course, since patients with X-linked, partially deficient cytochrome b_{558} generate O_2^- at rates of up to 10 per cent of normal but have severe clinical disease.

Until recently, management of CGD had been aimed at prevention of infection and early recognition and aggressive treatment of infections and their complications. Allogeneic bone marrow transplantation has been successfully used in a small number of patients with CGD (118–120). An exciting new approach to therapy is the use of INFγ to prevent infection in these patients. Recombinant human INFγ was recently shown in a randomized double-blind, placebo-controlled study to be an effective and well-tolerated treatment that reduces the frequency of serious infections in CGD patients (121). The use of INFγ is discussed in detail in Chapter 8, section 6.

5   Hereditary myeloperoxidase deficiency

Neutrophil myeloperoxidase (MPO) deficiency has only recently been recognized as the most common of the congenital PMN disorders, occurring with a prevalence of approximately 1 in 2000 of the general population (122, 123). The fact that otherwise healthy individuals with complete MPO deficiency are not at increased risk for infection precluded recognition of this disorder in the past. However, the introduction of automated flow cytochemistry systems for routine determination of white cell differentials (a method that uses peroxidase staining of leukocytes) has facilitated the screening of large populations and has led to an appreciation of the true prevalence of the disorder (124, 125). Of all the individuals recognized with MPO deficiency, only six have been reported to have serious infections (125, 126). Four of these six patients had visceral or disseminated candidiasis, and three of the four had diabetes mellitus. These clinical findings correlate with *in vitro* studies of MPO-deficient phagocytic cells. Stimulated MPO-deficient PMN exhibit a supranormal respiratory burst and normal but delayed bactericidal activity, indicating that these cells use a MPO-independent system to kill bacteria that is slower than the MPO–H_2O_2–halide system but one that is ultimately effective (123). In contrast, MPO-deficient PMN do not kill *Candida* species *in vitro*. Thus, an alternative PMN candidacidal system that functions in the absence of MPO, appears to protect the vast majority of individuals with MPO deficiency from fungal infections. Only the presence of an additional insult to host defences, such as that of diabetes mellitus, increases the risk for infection in MPO-deficient patients.

The genetic lesion underlying hereditary MPO deficiency has not been established. Kindred studies of MPO-deficient individuals suggest that this is an autosomal recessive disorder, although the heterogeneous expression of the defect is consistent with polygenic control of MPO gene expression (123). Normal MPO is the product of a single gene on chromosome 17. There is evidence that both pre-translational (127) and post-translational (128) defects may underlie the genetic defect. Western blots of PMN from completely MPO-deficient subjects demonstrated no immunochemical evidence of mature MPO, in contrast to partially MPO-deficient individuals who had approximately 50 per cent of the mature MPO subunits found in normal persons (129). MPO-deficient PMN contained proMPO suggesting that the defect was post-translational. Completely MPO-deficient PMN have also been found to have normal amounts of normal sized mRNA for MPO, and to have no gross defect or rearrangement of the MPO gene on Southern blots of genomic DNA (128). Evidence for a pre-translational defect was recently reported in a completely MPO-deficient patient who lacked immunochemical evidence for any MPO-related proteins and only trace mRNA for MPO in bone marrow cells (127). For the purposes of clinically defining MPO deficiency, the presence of MPO in PMN can be evaluated by several assays. The easiest method is by automated flow cytochemical analysis, but the most widely available method for estimating the amount of MPO is by histochemical staining of peripheral blood smears.

6   Leukocyte adhesion deficiency

6.1   Clinical manifestations

Leukocyte adhesion deficiency (LAD) is a disorder of autosomal recessive heredity characterized by recurrent, life-threatening bacterial infections, impaired pus formation and wound healing, and a wide array of functional abnormalities of cells of myeloid and lymphoid lineage. The features of this disorder are summarized in Table 6.7. As the name suggests, the functional

Table 6.7   Features of leukocyte adhesion deficiency

---

1. Autosomal recessive heredity
2. Two phenotypes have been identified
    (a) Severe, commonly present with omphalitis and delayed umbilical cord severance
        Susceptible to life-threatening infections, usually die during infancy
        Undetectable CD11/CD18 on leukocyte surfaces
    (b) Moderate, less severe infections, usually survive into adulthood
        Chronic severe gingivitis and periodontitis
        Surface expression of CD11/CD18 is 3–10% of normal
3. Patients have recurrent, necrotic infections of skin, soft tissues, and mucous membranes; infections may progress locally or systemically despite antimicrobial therapy
4. Pus formation and wound healing are poor, PMN fail to migrate to infected tissues
5. Marked peripheral blood neutrophilia, 5- to 20-fold higher than normal
6. Profound impairment of many leukocyte functions *in vitro*, particularly those dependent on adhesion
7. Absent or very reduced expression of CD11/CD18 glycoproteins on leukocytes
8. Genetic defect localized in β subunit gene, several classes of mutations have been recognized

---

abnormalities of LAD are those that depend on adhesion to other cells or to substrate. One of the most striking features of this disorder is the inability of phagocytes to accumulate at extravascular inflammatory sites in the face of marked peripheral blood leukocytosis, indicating the failure of phagocytes to adhere and traverse the endothelium in response to chemotaxis. The molecular basis of LAD has been extensively characterized thanks to the pioneering work of several investigators. It is now well recognized that LAD is due to absent or deficient expression on the cell surface of a group of glycoproteins related to each other functionally and structurally (130–132). These molecules are the leukocyte integrins or leukocyte adhesion molecules, present only on cells of myeloid and lymphoid lineage, which normally function to mediate cellular adherence reactions in inflammation and host defence.

The characteristics and nomenclature of the three glycoproteins collectively referred to as leukocyte integrins or leukocyte adhesion molecules are summarized in Table 2.1; Chapter 2, Section 3.2 contains a detailed discussion of the biophysical nature of these molecules. These glycoproteins are homologous to other integrins, such as the fibronectin receptor, and are important mediators of leukocyte adhesion. CD11a/CD18, also known as the lymphocyte function-associated antigen 1 (LFA-1) is present in all leukocytes and is primarily involved in adhesion of leukocytes to other cells. CD11b/CD18, also termed MAC-1 or Mo-1, is a receptor for the complement fragment iC3b (complement receptor 3, CR_3) and mediates the binding and phagocytosis of particles opsonized with iC3b. CD11c/CD18 or p150,95 can also bind iC3b, but the biological significance of this activity is not well understood. All three receptors mediate cell adhesion to other cells or to a variety of substrates, including adhesion to surfaces, adhesion to endothelial or to epithelial cells, adhesion to target cells by killer cells (antigen-specific cytotoxic T cells, NK cells, and in antibody-dependent killing by K cells and PMN), and homotypic aggregation of PMN and lymphocytes. The use of monoclonal antibodies to the leukocyte integrins to inhibit adhesion, results in inhibition of a variety of functions related to host defence and inflammation, such as surface migration of phagocytes, accumulation of PMN at sites of inflammation, phagocytosis of foreign particles, PMN secretory activity resulting from attachment to a surface, some helper T cell functions, and attachment and killing of target cells.

Since 1974 several investigators have reported patients with a severe immunodeficiency state related to impaired leukocyte adherence and absent expression of certain cell surface glycoproteins (130–132). Absent or very reduced expression of the CD11/CD18 glycoproteins on the cell surface of leukocytes has been confirmed in more than 30 patients, and their clinical and functional abnormalities constitute what has been defined as LAD. Another 26 patients, including many of the patients first reported but now deceased, are presumed to have had LAD but CD11/CD18 deficiency was not documented.

Patients with LAD have recurrent necrotic and indolent infections of soft tissues primarily involving the skin, mucous membranes, and intestinal tract (130, 131). Superficial infections may become invasive, locally or systemically. Skin lesions start as small, erythematous, non-purulent nodules that may progress to large ulcers that fail to heal, or do so very slowly leaving dysplastic scars. Surgical wounds also heal poorly. One patient had progression to gas gangrene requiring amputation. Omphalitis with delayed umbilical cord severance is a characteristic feature of LAD; its presence is strongly suggestive of this disorder. In many instances, the umbilical cord had to be removed surgically. Septicaemia or extension of the infection into the abdominal cavity may occur as complications of omphalitis (133). Severe gingivitis and periodontitis are a constant feature in patients that survive infancy. The oral disease becomes chronic and progressive, leading to gingival proliferation and severe loss of alveolar bone and teeth. Facial or deep neck cellulitis may occur as a complication. Recurrent otitis and sinusitis are common. Progression of otitis to mastoiditis and facial nerve palsy has been reported. Perirectal abscess or cellulitis occurs frequently and may progress to peritonitis and septicaemia. Recurrent pneumonia is the most common deep-seated infection. Other infections that have been observed are appendicitis, necrotizing enterocolitis, intestinal ulceration, bacterial tracheitis, candida oesophagitis, and erosive gastritis.

A wide spectrum of Gram-positive and -negative bacteria are isolated from both superficial and deep infections. The most common pathogens are staphylococci, enteric Gram-negative bacilli, and *Pseudomonas* species, not unlike the neutropenic disorders. Yeast infections of the skin or mucosal surfaces are not infrequent. Infections with *Aspergillus* species have also been observed (132). LAD patients do not appear to be more susceptible to viral infections, at least not to the degree they are for bacterial and fungal infections (6). Several patients have had self-limited courses of varicella, herpes simplex, cytomegalovirus, or viral respiratory infections. No untoward effects of live viral vaccines have been observed among LAD patients who have received them.

Two clinical phenotypes have been identified, and designated severe deficiency and moderate deficiency (6). The severity of clinical infectious complications appears to be directly related to the degree of glycoprotein deficiency. Severely deficient patients have essentially undetectable expression of CD11/CD18 (<1 per cent of normal) on their leukocytes. Patients with moderate deficiency, on the other hand, display 3–10 per cent of the normal surface expression of CD11/CD18. Affected individuals within a kindred are either all severely deficient or all moderately deficient.

Severely deficient patients usually succumb to overwhelming infections during the first few years of life. Most of these patients present with omphalitis and delayed severance of the umbilical cord. Moderately deficient patients also suffer from recurring infections, however, they have a much better prognosis and usually survive to adulthood. Although skin infections may recede during childhood in some patients, and only recur occasionally thereafter, severe gingivitis is a universal problem in patients with moderate deficiency. Nevertheless, patients with moderate deficiency who survive to adulthood may still die from complications of severe infections.

6.2   Laboratory diagnosis

At present, the diagnosis of LAD can be easily confirmed by flow cytometric analysis of peripheral blood PMN, using monoclonal antibodies specific for one of the CD11 or CD18 subunits. Tests of PMN function will reveal profound defects in adhesion-dependent functions such as adherence to substrates and spreading, chemotaxis, aggregation, CR_3-dependent binding and phagocytosis of iC3b-coated particles, as well as the respiratory burst triggered by such particles (130, 133). Conversely, adhesion-independent functions are normal, such as intracellular microbicidal activity, and the respiratory burst and degranulation mediated by soluble stimuli (such as phorbol esters). Examination of infected tissues reveals a profound impairment of leukocyte mobilization into extravascular inflammatory sites. Infected tissues contain inflammatory infiltrates totally devoid of PMN in the face of a marked peripheral blood neutrophilia (6). Neutrophilia, 5- to 20-fold higher than normal, is a constant feature and hallmark of LAD. This inability of PMN to emigrate out of the blood vessels has been confirmed using Rebuck skin windows. This test is no longer recommended in the evaluation of suspected LAD because *in vitro* tests are superior; further, there exists the possibility of infectious complications or poor healing at the skin test site. Serum immunoglobulin levels, antibody responses, and delayed hypersensitivity reactions have been normal in those patients studied except for one who had impaired antibody responses to vaccination (130).

6.3   Molecular basis

Although an early report suggested X-linked inheritance, analysis of most other cases indicate autosomal recessive transmission. The lines of evidence consistent with autosomal recessive heredity are: (i) equal numbers of male and female patients; (ii) a high frequency of consanguineous marriages; and (iii) half-normal levels of CD11/CD18 expression (heterozygous carriers) in parents and many unaffected siblings (130). Other than the few kindreds described, the incidence of LAD shows no geographic or ethnic clusters. LAD patients of diverse ethnic origins have been identified over North America, Europe, and Japan (130).

It is now clear that LAD is due to heterogeneous defects in the β subunit (CD18) (134–139). These defects result in (i) absence, (ii) insufficient quantity, or (iii) abnormal structure of the β subunit precursor, the consequence of which is failure of association of the β precursor with the α precursor in the endoplasmic reticulum. Such association is a prerequisite for further processing of the heterodimer to a mature glycoprotein in the Golgi apparatus for transportation to the cell surface or the intracellular granules. The first clues to the molecular basis of LAD came from biosynthetic 'pulse and chase' studies of metabolically labelled cells, which showed that cell lines derived from LAD patients synthesized apparently normal LFA-1 α subunit precursor, but the precursor did not undergo subsequent carbohydrate processing, and it did not associate with β subunit to form α/β heterodimers; consequently, neither subunit was expressed on the cell surface (140, 141). In these early studies, the β subunit was undetectable in patient cell lines. These findings suggested that impaired biosynthesis of the β subunit was the fundamental molecular lesion of LAD. However, because the monoclonal antibodies used to immunoprecipitate the β subunit did not seem to recognize the β subunit precursor in normal cell lines, it was impossible to establish whether the β subunit precursor was present or not in the defective cells. The α subunit is apparently degraded in the absence of the β subunit.

Further evidence that the primary defect is in the β subunit was provided by studies which demonstrated that human LFA-1 α subunit could associate with murine β subunits and be expressed at the cell surface of hybrids formed by fusion of human and murine cells (142). Surface expression of the α subunit but not the β subunit of patients cells was rescued by the formation of interspecies α/β complexes, whereas in hybrids of normal human cells both α and β subunits of human origin could associate with their murine counterpart and be expressed at the cell surface. These findings indicated that the α subunit from LAD cells is competent for surface expression in the presence of an appropriate β (mouse) subunit, therefore, the genetic defect in LAD affects the β subunit. This and a subsequent study (143) mapped the α subunit gene to chromosome 16 and the β subunit gene to chromosome 21. In fact, the genes for the three CD11 α subunits form a cluster in the short arm of chromosome 16.

The development of sophisticated molecular probes has permitted further characterization of the molecular defects underlying LAD. Two groups of investigators working independently cloned the β subunit cDNA and developed rabbit monospecific antisera that immunoprecipitates β subunit precursors. Using these tools they were able to study β subunit mRNA expression and genomic organization with the first probe and to study the biosynthesis of the β subunit precursor with the second probe (134, 135). Dana *et al.* studied four patients and found that their B cells had a single normal sized β subunit mRNA and that these cells synthesized a normal sized β subunit precursor (134). These investigators concluded that the defect in these four unrelated patients was due to a defective β gene resulting in abnormal post-translational processing of the synthesized precursor. Kishimoto *et al.* studied 10 patients and found five distinct β subunit phenotypes (see Table 6.8) in which either the precursor and the mRNA were not detected, both were present in very low amounts, or mRNA levels were normal with β precursor of normal, aberrantly large, or aberrantly small size (135). In all patients the β subunit gene was detected and no gross deletions were found. It appears that the mutations responsible for the patterns observed, affect either the amount of β subunit precursor synthesized or, after its synthesis, affect the ability of the β subunit to associate with the α subunit in the endoplasmic reticulum.

Patients with the first β subunit phenotype produce no detectable β subunit mRNA or protein precursor and, as expected, have severe deficiency. In contrast, the patient with the second pattern, characterized by very low levels of β subunit precursor and its mRNA, has moderate deficiency. It seems that the low levels of β subunit produced are sufficient to allow the expression of approximately 10 per cent of the normal amount of mature αβ complexes on leukocyte surfaces. The genetic defect in patients with these two β subunit phenotypes may affect either RNA transcription, processing, or stability. Four patients of one kindred with moderate deficiency expressed the third phenotype, defined by a β subunit which is aberrantly small. Further investigations in these patients, using powerful polymerase chain reaction techniques (136), have shown a single base pair substitution in an intron splice site within the β subunit gene. This substitution results in the deletion of a 30 amino acid segment in a highly conserved region of the extracellular domain of the β subunit polypeptide. A small amount of normally spliced message was also detected, which

Table 6.8   Correlation between β subunit and clinical phenotypes in leukocyte adhesion deficiency

β subunit phenotype		Clinical phenotype
β subunit precursor	β subunit mRNA	
Not detectable	Not detectable	Severe
Trace	Low level	Moderate
Aberrantly small	Normal level	Moderate
Aberrantly large	Normal level	Severe
Normal size	Normal level	Severe or moderate

explains the low levels of LFA-1 expressed on the cell surface, hence, the moderate phenotype. In the fourth phenotype, the aberrantly large β subunit precursor is thought to be due to the presence of an extra glycosylation site. Such defective glycosylation may effect conformational changes of the β subunit precursor impeding its association with the α subunit. Patients with this mutation have severe deficiency. Patients expressing the fifth β subunit phenotype may have moderate or severe deficiency. This suggests that there are several distinct mutations within this group resulting in defective processing and association of the α and β subunit precursors. The patients studied by Dana *et al.* (134) belong to this group. Other investigators have identified patients with β subunit abnormalities consistent with the first, second, and fifth phenotypes (137).

Through recombinant DNA techniques, the genetic defects of some patients with the fifth phenotype have been clearly defined. Two mutant alleles were found in one patient with moderate deficiency (138), each representing a point mutation in the β subunit gene resulting in single amino acid substitutions in two highly conserved regions of the extracellular domain of the β subunit. Similarly, two other patients have been found to have one point mutation each resulting in single amino acid substitutions in distinct but adjacent sites of one of the highly conserved regions of the β subunit (139), the same region that contains the deletion responsible for the third phenotype (136). These findings suggest that these highly conserved regions of the β subunit are critical for association with the α subunit.

At present, the only effective therapy for LAD is bone marrow transplantation. Other potential strategies such as gene therapy are discussed in Chapter 8.

7 Chédiak–Higashi syndrome

7.1 Clinical diagnosis

Chédiak–Higashi syndrome is an autosomal recessive disorder characterized by: (i) partial oculocutaneous albinism, (ii) the presence of giant lysosomal granules in all granular cells, (iii) frequent pyogenic infections, (iv) neutropenia, (v) mild bleeding diathesis, (vi) neurologic abnormalities, and (vii) an accelerated lymphoma-like phase before 10 years of age (12, 144, 145). The distribution of this syndrome is world-wide, with cases described in North America, Latin America, Europe, and Asia (144). Remarkably, no cases have been reported in black individuals.

The infections commonly observed in patients with Chédiak–Higashi syndrome involve the skin and soft tissues, respiratory tract, and mucous membranes (12). Less frequent are sepsis, gingivitis, and infections of the gastrointestinal or the urinary tract. Febrile episodes occur frequently; an infection can be demonstrated in about 60 per cent of these. Infections in these patients are caused by Gram-positive and -negative bacteria as well as fungi, however, S. aureus accounts for 70 per cent of all infections (145). The increased susceptibility to infection is due to defective phagocytic function, which may be compounded by neutropenia.

The physical appearance of patients with this disorder is characteristic due to an abnormality of pigmentary dispersion (partial oculocutaneous albinism) (145). The hair colour varies from blond to dark brown, but it always exhibits a distinctive silvery tint. Abnormal dispersion of ocular pigment is manifested by an increased red reflex, photophobia, and rotatory nystagmus in bright light. Skin colour tends to be lighter than in parents and siblings, and there is increased susceptibility for sunburn. Patients with long-standing disease may have neurologic abnormalities, including peripheral neuropathy, ataxia, and seizures. Most patients exhibit a mild bleeding diathesis manifested by occasional petechiae and prolonged bleeding time, and this is usually not a problem until the accelerated phase of the disease (described below) develops. Neutropenia, thrombocytopenia, and haemolytic anaemia are uniformly seen during the accelerated phase, but they may be found before it develops, particularly neutropenia. Neutropenia is thought to be due to increased intramedullary destruction of PMN (145). Serum immunoglobulins are usually elevated, particularly IgG and IgA (144). A few patients have had hypogammaglobulinemia.

The accelerated phase occurs during the first decade of life in about 85 per cent of those who survive other complications of this disorder (12, 144–146). The outcome is almost invariably fatal. The accelerated phase is characterized by widespread tissue infiltrates of lymphoid and histiocytic cells, which do not appear malignant on histopathologic examination. This phase is manifested by fever, hepatosplenomegaly, lymphadenopathy, pancytopenia due to hypersplenism and bone marrow infiltration, and severe bleeding diathesis. The pathogenesis of the accelerated phase remains undefined.

7.2   Laboratory diagnosis

The hallmark of this disorder is the presence of large intracellular inclusions of lysosomal origin in granule-containing cells, most notably leukocytes (147). These giant granules are seen in granulocytes, monocytes, and lymphocytes on Wright's stained smears of blood or bone marrow. In PMN these granules contain MPO and other markers of primary granules, as well as markers of secondary granules. The abnormal granules are formed during myelopoiesis by aggregation and fusion mainly of primary azurophilic granules, but also of secondary granules. Monocytes, lymphocytes, and platelets also contain giant granules. Other cell types affected by this disorder are Schwann cells, melanocytes, and granular cells found in the renal tubular epithelium, gastric mucosa, pancreas, and thyroid. The tendency of granules to fuse is thought to be due to an abnormality of cellular membranes, both plasma membrane and organelle membranes (148). Membrane-related abnormalities that have been described include increased membrane fluidity, elevated cAMP levels, disordered assembly of microtubules (12).

7.3 Molecular basis

The molecular basis of the cellular abnormalities in Chédiak–Higashi syndrome is still a mystery. Some of the consequences of these abnormalities are defective phagocyte function, abnormal platelet function, altered pigmentation, and neuropathy. Phagocytes show impaired chemotaxis and decreased and delayed intracellular killing of bacteria, despite a normal phagocytic capacity and normal to elevated oxidative burst (149). The chemotactic defect is thought to be due, at least in part, to mechanical interference by the giant granules, whereas the bactericidal defect may be related to ineffective delivery of lysosomal contents to the phagocytic vacuole. NK cell activity and antibody-dependent cytotoxic activity are also defective (12). Impaired pigmentary dispersion is due to abnormal aggregation of melanin granules within melanocytes (144).

Bone marrow transplantation resulted in clinical and immunological recovery in three patients (146) and a small number of other patients have now been similarly treated. Treatment with ascorbic acid has resulted in clinical amelioration and improvement of PMN function in some patients but not in others (144). Corticosteroids and cytotoxic therapies have not proved to be of benefit (12, 144). Definition of the molecular pathogenesis will be needed to develop effective therapy for this serious disorder.

8 PMN-specific granule deficiency

Specific granule deficiency (SGD) is a rare congenital disorder of PMN characterized by susceptibility to recurrent and severe infections of the skin, mucous membranes, and lungs (12, 144, 146). Most commonly, these infections are due to *S. aureus*, enteric Gram-negative bacilli, *P. aeruginosa* and *C. albicans*. As the name of this disorder suggests, the PMN of these patients appear to lack specific granules on Wright's stained smear, but have demonstrable azurophilic granules on peroxidase staining (150). In addition, nuclear morphologic abnormalities are present such as bilobulation, multilobulation, and nuclear blebs, clefts, and pockets. Spitznagel *et al.* described the first case in 1972 (151), and a few other cases have been reported subsequently (150). Although one patient had an acquired deficiency associated with a myeloproliferative syndrome (151), the others appear to have an inherited disorder, probably in an autosomal recessive pattern (150). Despite the recurrent infections, most of these patients survive when their infections are treated promptly and aggressively (12).

Cytochemical studies of SGD PMN have suggested the absence of specific granules. Instead, what are found on ultrastructural studies are small, elongated granules that appeared late in maturation and that lack the normal constituents of specific granules such as lactoferrin, cytochrome *b* and vitamin B_{12} binding protein (150). Abnormalities of azurophil granules have been found as well. Azurophil granule fractions sediment abnormally (150), lack defensins (152), and the subpopulation of peroxidase-positive granules (the one associated with defensins) are smaller in size (153). A tertiary granule protein, gelatinase, is also deficient (150). The molecular defect or defects underlying these abnormalities have not been clearly defined. Lomax *et al.* have shown that the deficiency of lactoferrin synthesis in SGD PMN is secondary to an abnormality of RNA production (154); lactoferrin RNA transcripts were of normal size but were markedly reduced in amount. This abnormality is specific to myeloid cells since lactoferrin is secreted normally into tears, nasal secretions, and saliva in SGD patients (154, 155).

The impact of these granule abnormalities on PMN function is reflected in the increased susceptibility to infections among SGD patients. Many PMN functional abnormalities have been reported, of which the most consistent have been impaired chemotaxis and deficient bactericidal activity (150). The defect in microbicidal activity may be due in part to the deficiency of defensins mentioned above. Upon PMN activation, specific granules fuse with the plasma membrane and its contents are secreted to the extracellular environment (degranulation). The release of granule contents is important in promoting and modulating inflammation because granules contain activators of complement, monocyte chemoattractants, lactoferrin (which may play a role in hydroxyl radical generation, facilitate adhesiveness, and inhibit myelopoiesis), and certain other enzymes. Two other important consequences of degranulation are: (i) the addition of new membrane to the cell surface, which may be important to processes such as chemotaxis, diapedesis, and phagocytosis; (ii) the translocation of membrane-associated molecules from intracellular pools (granules) to the cell surface. Examples of such molecules are CR_3 (CD11b/CD18), cytochrome *b*, and the receptor for the chemoattractant FMLP (152). It is thought that failure to 'upregulate' these molecules to the cell surface during cell activation is, at least in part, responsible for many of the functional defects of SGD PMN.

9 Acknowledgement

This work was supported in part by a National Health Research and Development Program grant.

References

1 Malech, H. L. and Gallin, J. I. (1987). Neutrophils in human diseases. *N. Engl. J. Med.,* **317**, 687–94.

2 Anderson, D. C. (1987). Infectious complications resulting from phagocytic cell dysfunction. In *Textbook of pediatric infectious diseases* (ed. R. D. Feigin and J. D. Cherry), 2nd edition. W. B. Saunders, Philadelphia.

3 Lehrer, R. I., Ganz, T., Selsted, M. E., Babior, B. M., and Curnutte, J. T. (1988). Neutrophils and host defense. *Ann. Intern. Med.,* **109**, 127–42.

4 Howard, M. W., Strauss, R. G., and Johnston, R. B., Jr (1977). Infections in patients with neutropenia. *Am. J. Dis. Child.,* **131**, 788–90.

5 Tauber, A. I., Borregaard, N., Simons, E., and Wright, J. (1983). Chronic granulomatous disease: a syndrome of phagocyte oxidase deficiencies. *Medicine,* **62**, 286–309.

6 Anderson, D. C., Schmalstieg, F. C., Finegold, M. J., Hughes, B. J., Rothlein, R., Miller, L. J. *et al.* (1985). The severe and moderate phenotypes of heritable Mac-1, LFA-1 deficiency: Their quantitative definition and relation to leucocyte dysfunction and clinical features. *J. Infect. Dis.,* **152**, 668–89.

7 Johnston, R. B., Jr and Newman, S. L. (1977). Chronic granulomatous disease. *Pediatr. Clin. North Am.,* **24**, 365–76.

8 Miles, A. A., Miles, E. M., and Burke, J. (1957). The value and duration of defense reactions of the skin to the primary lodgement of bacteria. *Br. J. Exp. Pathol.,* **38**, 79–93.

9 Donabedian, H. and Gallin, J. I. (1983). The hyperimmunoglobulin E recurrent-infection syndrome. *Medicine,* **62**, 195–208.

10 Donowitz, G. R. and Mandell, G. L. (1983). Clinical presentation and unusual infections in chronic granulomatous disease. In *Advances in host defense mechanisms* (ed. J. I. Gallin and A. S. Fauci), pp. 5–75. Raven Press, New York.

11 Hajjar, F. M. (1990). Neutrophils in the newborn: normal characteristics and quantitative disorders. *Semin. Perinatol.,* **14**, 374–83.

12 Curnutte, J. T. and Boxer, L. A. (1987). Disorders of granulopoiesis and granulocyte function. In *Hematology of infancy and childhood* (ed. D. J. Nathan and F. A. Oski). W. B. Saunders, Philadelphia.

13 Sickles, E. A. and Greene, W. H. (1975). Clinical presentation of infection in granulocytic patients. *Arch. Int. Med.*, **135**, 715–19.
14 Kostmann, R. R. O. (1956). Infantile genetic agranulocytosis. *Acta Paediatr. Scand.*, **45 (Suppl. 105)**, 1–78.
15 Kostmann, R. (1975). Infantile genetic agranulocytosis: a review with presentation of ten new cases. *Acta Paediatr. Scand.*, **64**, 362–8.
16 Alter, B. P. (1987). The bone marrow failure syndromes. In *Hematology of infancy and childhood* (ed. D. J. Nathan and F. A. Oski). W. B. Saunders, Philadelphia.
17 Rappeport, J. M., Parkman, R., Newburger, P., Camitta, B. M., and Chusid, M. J. (1980). Correction of infantile agranulocytosis (Kostmann's syndrome) by allogeneic bone marrow transplantation. *Am. J. Med.*, **68**, 605–9.
18 Bonilla, M. A., Gillio, A. P., Ruggeiro, M., Kernan, N. A. Brochstein, J. A., Abboud, M. *et al.* (1989). Effects of recombinant human granulocyte colony-stimulating factor on neutropenia in patients with congenital agranulocytosis. *N. Engl. J. Med.*, **320**, 1574–80.
19 Welte, K., Zeidler, C., Reiter, A., Müller, W., Odenwald, E., Souza, L., and Riehm, H. (1990). Differential effects of granulocyte-macrophage colony-stimulating factor in children with severe congenital neutropenia. *Blood*, **75**, 1056–63.
20 Weston, B., Todd, R. F., III, Axtell, R., Balazovich, K., Stewart, J., Mayo-Bond, L., *et al.* (1991). Severe congenital neutropenia: clinical effects and neutrophil function during treatment with granulocyte colony-stimulating factor. *J. Lab. Clin. Med.*, **117**, 282–90.
21 Glasser, L., Duncan, B. R., and Corrigan, J. J. (1991). Measurement of serum granulocyte colony-stimulating factor in a patient with congenital agranulocytosis (Kostmann's syndrome). *Am. J. Dis. Child.*, **145**, 925–8.
22 Coulombel, L., Morardet, N., Veber, F., Leroy, C., Mielot, F., Fischer, A., *et al.* (1988). Granulopoietic differentiation in long-term bone marrow cultures from children with congenital neutropenia. *Am. J. Hematol.*, **27**, 93–8.
23 Daghistani, D., Jimenez, J. J., Toledano, S. R., Cirocco, R. E., and Yunis, A. A. (1990). Congenital neutropenia: a case study. *Am. J. Pediatr. Hematol. Oncol.*, **12**, 210–14.
24 Chang, J., Craft, A. W., Reid, M. M., Coutinho, L. H., and Dexter, M. (1990). Lack of response of bone marrow, in vitro, to growth factors in congenital neutropenia. *Am. J. Hematol.*, **35**, 125–6.
25 Kobayashi, M., Yumiba, C., Kawaguchi, Y., Tanaka, Y., Ueda, K., Komazawa, Y., and Okada, K. (1990). Abnormal responses of myeloid progenitor cells to recombinant human colony-stimulating factors in congenital neutropenia. *Blood*, **75**, 2143–9.
26 Mizuno, Y., Hara, T., Nagata, M., Omori, F., Shimoda, K.,

Okamura, S., *et al.* (1990). Serum granulocyte colony-stimulating factors levels in chronic neutropenia of infancy. *Pediatr. Hematol. Oncol.*, **7**, 377–81.

27 Pietsch, T., Bührer, C., Mepel, K., Menzel, K., Steffens, U., Schrader, C., *et al.* (1991). Blood mononuclear cells from patients with severe congenital neutropenia are capable of producing granulocyte colony-stimulating factor. *Blood*, **77**, 1234–7.

28 Mempel, K., Pietsch, T., Menzel, T., Zeidler, C., and Welte, K. (1991). Increased serum levels of granulocyte colony-stimulating factor in patients with severe congenital neutropenia. *Blood*, **77**, 1919–22.

29 Gabrilove, J., Jakubowski, A., Scher, H., Sternberg, C., Wong, G., Grous, J. *et al.* (1988). Effects of granulocyte colony-stimulating factor on neutropenia and associated morbidity due to chemotherapy for transitional-cell carcinoma of the urothelium. *N. Engl. J. Med.*, **318**, 1414–22.

30 Weetman, R. M. and Boxer, L. A. (1980). Childhood neutropenia. *Pediatr. Clin. North Am.*, **27**, 361–75.

31 Dale, D. C., Guerry, D., Wewerka, J. R., Bull, J. M., and Chusid, M. J. (1979). Chronic neutropenia. *Medicine*, **58**, 128–44.

32 Espanol, T., Compte, J., Alvarez, C., Tallada, N., Laverde, R., and Peguero, G. (1979). Reticular dysgenesis: report of two brothers. *Clin. Exp. Immunol.*, **38**, 615–20.

33 Levinsky, R. J. and Tiedeman, K. (1983). Successful bone marrow transplantation for reticular dysgenesis. *Lancet*, **i**, 671–3.

34 Wright, D. G., Dale, D. C., Fauci, A. S., and Wolff, S. M. (1981). Cyclic neutropenia: a clinical review. *Medicine*, **60**, 1–13.

35 Hammond, W. P., Price, T. H., Souza, L. M., and Dale, D. C. (1989). Treatment of cyclic neutropenia with granulocyte colony-stimulating factor. *N. Engl. J. Med.*, **320**, 1306–11.

36 Wright, D. G., LaRussa, V. F., Salvado, A. J., and Knight, R. D. (1989). Abnormal responses of myeloid progenitor cells to granulocyte-macrophage colony-stimulating factor in human cyclic neutropenia. *J. Clin. Invest.*, **83**, 1414–18.

37 Loughran, T. P., Clark, E. A., Price, T. H., and Hammond, W. P. (1986). Adult-onset cyclic neutropenia is associated with increased large granular lymphocytes. *Blood*, **68**, 1082–7.

38 Hammond, W. P., Boone, T. C., Donahue, R. E., Souza, L. M., and Dale, D. C. (1990). A comparison of treatment of canine cyclic hematopoiesis with recombinant human granulocyte-macrophage colony-stimulating factor (GM-CSF), G-CSF, interleukin-3, and canine G-CSF. *Blood*, **76**, 523–32.

39 Dale, D. C. and Hammond, W. P. (1988). Cyclic neutropenia: a clinical review. *Blood Rev.*, **2**, 178–85.

40 Sugimoto, K., Togawa, A., Miyazono, K., Itoh, K., Amano, M., Chiba, S., *et al.* (1990). Treatment of childhood-onset cyclic neutropenia with recombinant human granulocyte colony-stimulating factor. *Eur. J. Haematol.,* **45,** 110–11.

41 Misago, M., Kikuchi, M., Tsukada, J., Hanamura, T., Kamachi, S., and Eto, S. (1991). Serum levels of G-CSF, M-CSF, and GM-CSF in a patient with cyclic neutropenia. *Eur. J. Haematol.,* **46,** 312–13.

42 Watari, K., Asano, S., Shirafuji, N., Kodo, H., Ozawa, K., Takaku, F., and Kamachi, S. (1989). Serum granulocyte colony-stimulating factor levels in healthy volunteers and patients with various disorders as estimated by enzyme immunoassay. *Blood,* **73,** 117–22.

43 Hammond, W. P., Chatta, G., Andrews, R. G., Bernstein, I. D., and Dale, D. C. (1989). Human cyclic neutropenia: abnormal progenitor cell response to G-CSF and GM-CSF. *Blood,* **74,** 48 (abstr.).

44 Freund, M. R. F., Luft, S., Schöber, C., Heussner, P., Schrezenmaier, H., Porzsolt, F., and Welte, K. (1990). Differential effect of GM-CSF and G-CSF in cyclic neutropenia. *Lancet,* **336,** 313.

45 Hanada, T., Ono, I., and Nagasawa, T. (1990). Childhood cyclic neutropenia treated with recombinant human granulocyte colonystimulating factor. *Br. J. Haematol.,* **75,** 135–7.

46 Zuelzer, W. W. (1964). 'Myelokathesis': a new form of chronic granulocytopenia. *N. Engl. J. Med.,* **270,** 699–704.

47 Ganser, A., Ottman, O. G., Erdmann, H., Schulz, G., and Hoelzer, D. (1989). The effect of recombinant human granulocyte-macrophage colony-stimulating factor on neutropenia and related morbidity in chronic severe neutropenia. *Ann. Intern. Med.,* **111,** 887–92.

48 Ochs, H. D. and Wedgwood, R. J. (1989). Disorders of the B-cell system. In *Immunological disorders in infants and children* (ed. E. R. Stiehm). W. B. Saunders, Philadelphia.

49 Scriver, C. R., Beaudet, A. L., Sly, W. S., and Valle, D. (ed.) (1989). *The metabolic basis of inherited disease.* McGraw Hill, New York.

50 Gallin, J. I., Buescher, E. S., and Seligmann, B. E. (1983). Recent advances in chronic granulomatous disease. *Ann. Intern. Med.,* **99,** 657–74.

51 Babior, B. M. (1988). The respiratory burst oxidase. *Hematol. Oncol. Clin. North. Am.,* **2,** 201–12.

52 Segal, A. W. (1988). The molecular and cellular pathology of chronic granulomatous disease. *Eur. J. Clin. Invest.,* **18,** 433–43.

53 Smith, R. M. and Curnutte, J. T. (1991). Molecular basis of chronic granulomatous disease. *Blood,* **77,** 673–86.

54 Mills, E. L. and Quie, P. H. (1983). Inheritance of chronic granulomatous disease. In *Advances in host defense mechanisms* (ed. J. I. Gallin and A. S. Fauci). Raven Press, New York.

55 Schapiro, B. L., Newburger, P. E., Klempner, M. S., and Dinauer,

M. C. (1991). Chronic granulomatous disease presenting in a 69-year-old man. *N. Engl. J. Med.*, **325**, 1786–90.

56 Regelmann, W., Hays, N., and Quie, P. G. (1983). Chronic granulomatous disease: Historical perspective and clinical experience at the University of Minnesota Hospitals. In *Advances in host defense mechanisms* (ed. J. I. Gallin, and A. S. Fauci). Raven Press, New York.

57 Forrest, C. B., Forehand, J. R., Axtell, R. A., Roberts, R. L., and Johnston, R. B. (1988). Clinical features and current management of chronic granulomatous disease. *Hematol. Oncol. Clin. North Am.*, **2**, 253–66.

58 Lazarus, G. M. and Neu, H. C. (1975). Agents responsible for infection in chronic granulomatous disease of childhood. *J. Pediatr.*, **86**, 415–17.

59 Quie, P. G., White, J. G., Holmes, B., and Good, R. A. (1967). In vitro bactericidal capacity of human polymorphonuclear leucocytes: Diminished activity in chronic granulomatous disease of childhood. *J. Clin. Invest.*, **46**, 668–79.

60 Allen, R. C., Mills, E. L., McNitt, T. R., and Quie, P. G. (1981). Role of myeloperoxidase and bacterial metabolism in chemiluminescence of granulocytes from patients with chronic granulomatous disease. *J. Infect. Dis.*, **144**, 344–8.

61 Ochs, H. D. and Igo, R. P. (1973). The NBT slide test: A simple screening method for detecting chronic granulomatous disease and female carriers. *J. Pediatr.*, **83**, 77.

62 Roesler, J. and Emmendorffer, A. (1991). Diagnoses of chronic granulomatous disease. (Letter) *Blood*, **78**, 1387–8.

63 Curnutte, J. T. and Smith, R. M. (1991). Response. *Blood*, **78**, 1388–9.

64 Mills, E. L., Rholl, K. S., and Quie, P. G. (1980). X-linked inheritance in females with chronic granulomatous disease. *J. Clin. Invest.*, **66**, 332–40.

65 Newburger, P. E., Cohen, H. J., Rothchild, S. B., Hobbins, J. C., Malawista, S. E., and Mahoney, M. J. (1979). Prenatal diagnosis of chronic granulomatous disease. *N. Engl. J. Med.*, **300**, 178–81.

66 Stjernholm, R. L., Allen, R. C., Steele, R. H., Waring, W. W., and Harris, J. (1973). Impaired chemiluminescence during phagocytosis of opsonized bacteria. *Infect. Immun.*, **7**, 313–14.

67 Mills, E. L., Rholl, K. S., and Quie, P. G. (1980). Luminol amplified chemiluminescence: a sensitive method for detecting the carrier state in chronic granulomatous disease. *J. Clin. Microbiol.*, **12**, 52–6.

68 Allen, R. C., Stjernholm, R. L., and Steele, R. H. (1972). Evidence for the generation of an electronic excitation state(s) in human polymorphonuclear leucocytes and its participation in bactericidal activity. *Biochem. Biophys. Res. Commun.*, **47**, 679–84.

69 Stevens, P., Winston, D. J., and Van Dyke, K. (1978). In vitro circulation of opsonic and granulocyte function by luminol-dependent chemiluminescence. Utility in patients with severe neutropenia and cellular deficiency states. *Infect. Immun.,* **22,** 41–51.

70 Curnutte, J. T., Whitten, D. M., and Babior, B. M. (1974). Defective superoxide production by granulocytes from patients with chronic granulomatous disease. *N. Engl. J. Med.,* **290,** 593–7.

71 Curnutte, J. T. (1988). Classification of chronic granulomatous disease. *Hematol. Oncol. Clin. North Am.,* **2,** 241–52.

72 Bohler, M. C., Seger, R. A., Mouy, R., Vilmer, E., Fischer, A., and Griscelli, C. (1988). A study of 25 patients with chronic granulomatous disease: A new classification by correlating respiratory burst, cytochrome b, and flavoprotein. *J. Clin. Immunol.,* **6,** 136–45.

73 Janeway, C. A., Craig, J., Davidson, M., Downey, W., Gittin, D., and Sullivan, J. C. (1954). Hypergammaglobulinemia associated with severe recurrent and chronic nonspecific infection. *Am. J. Dis. Child.,* **88,** 388–91.

74 Carson, M. L., Chadwick, D. L., Brubaker, C. A., Cleland, R. S., and Landing, B. H. (1965). Thirteen boys with progressive septic granulomatosis. *Pediatrics,* **35,** 405–12.

75 Johnston, R. B. Jr and McMurray, J. S. (1967). Chronic familial granulomatosis. *Pediatrics,* **40,** 808–15.

76 Holmes, B., Page, A. R., and Good, R. A. (1967). Studies of the metabolic activity of leucocytes from patients with a genetic abnormality of phagocytic function. *J. Clin. Invest.,* **46,** 1422–32.

77 Segal, A. W. and Jones, O. T. G. (1978). Novel cytochrome b system in phagocytic vacuoles from human granulocytes. *Nature,* **276,** 515–17.

78 Segal, A. W., Cross, A. R., and Garcia, R. C., Borregaard, N., Valerius, N. H., Soothill, J. F., and Jones, O. T. G. (1983). Absence of cytochrome b_{-245} in chronic granulomatous disease. A multicentre European evaluation of its incidence and relevance. *N. Engl. J. Med.,* **308,** 245–51.

79 Borregaard, N., Johansen, K. S., Taudorff, E., and Wandall, J. H. (1979). Cytochrome b is present in neutrophils from patients with chronic granulomatous disease. *Lancet,* **i,** 949–51.

80 Borregaard, N., Cross, A. R., Herlin, T., Jones, O. T. G., Segal, A. W., and Valerius, N. H. (1983). A variant form of X-linked chronic granulomatous disease with normal nitroblue tetrazolium slide test and cytochrome b. *Eur. J. Clin. Invest.,* **13,** 243–8.

81 Weening, R. S., Corbeil, L., de Boer, M., Lutter, R., van Zwieten, R., Hamers, M. N., and Roos, D. (1985). Cytochrome b deficiency in an autosomal form of chronic granulomatous disease. A third form of chronic granulomatous disease recognized by monocyte hybridization. *J. Clin. Invest.,* **75,** 915–20.

82 Ohno, Y., Buescher, E. S., Roberts, R., Metcalf, J. A., and Gallin, J. I. (1986). Reevaluation of cytochrome b and flavin adenine dinucleotide in neutrophils from patients with chronic granulomatous disease and description of a family with probable autosomal recessive inheritance of cytochrome b deficiency. *Blood*, **67**, 1132–8.

83 Parkos, C. A., Allen, R. A., Cochrane, C. G., and Jesaitis, A. J. (1987). Purified cytochrome b from human granulocyte plasma membrane is comprised of two polypeptides with relative molecular weights of 91 000 and 22 000. *J. Clin. Invest.*, **80**, 732–42.

84 Royer-Pokora, B., Kunkel, L. M., Monaco, A. P., Goff, S. C., Newberger, P. E., Baehner, R. L., *et al.* (1986). Cloning the gene for an inherited human disorder—chronic granulomatous disease—on the basis of its chromosomal location. *Nature*, **322**, 32–8.

85 Dinauer, M. C., Orkin, S. H., Brown, R., Jesaitis, A. J., and Parkos, C. A. (1987). The glycoprotein encoded by the X-liked chronic granulomatous disease locus is a component of the neutrophil cytochrome b complex. *Nature*, **327**, 717–20.

86 Teahan, C., Rowe, P., Parker, P., Totty, N., and Segal, A. W. (1987). The X-linked chronic granulomatous disease gene codes for the beta chain of cytochrome b_{-245}. *Nature*, **327**, 720–1.

87 Parkos, C. A., Dinauer, M. C., Walker, L. E., Allen, R. A., Jesaitis, A. J., and Orkin, S. H. (1988). Primary structure and unique expression of the 22-kilodalton light chain of human neutrophil cytochrome b. *Proc. Natl Acad. Sci. USA*, **85**, 3319–23.

88 Parkos, C. A., Allen, R. A., Cochrane, C. G., and Jesaitis, A. J. (1988). The quaternary structure of the plasma membrane b-type cytochrome of human granulocytes. *Biochim. Biophys. Acta*, **392**, 71–83.

89 Quinn, M. T., Parkos, C. A., Walker, L. E., Orkin, S. H., Dinauer, M. C., and Jesaitis, A. J. (1989). Association of a ras-related protein with cytochrome b of human neutrophils. *Nature*, **342**, 198–200.

90 Curnutte, J. T., Scott, P. J., and Mayo, L. A. (1989). The cytosolic components of the respiratory burst oxidase: Resolution of four components, two of which are missing in complementing forms of chronic granulomatous disease. *Proc. Natl Acad. Sci. USA*, **86**, 825–9.

91 Curnutte, J. T., Kuver, R., and Scott, P. J. (1987). Activation of neutrophil NADPH oxidase in a cell-free system. Partial purification of components and characterization of the activation process. *J. Biol. Chem.*, **262**, 5563–9.

92 McPhail, L. C., Shirley, P. S., Clayton, C. C., and Snyderman, R. (1985). Activation of the respiratory burst enzyme from human neutrophils in a cell-free system. *J. Clin. Invest.*, **75**, 1735–9.

93 Curnutte, J. T., Kuver, R., and Babior, B. M. (1987). Activation of the respiratory burst oxidase in a fully soluble system from human neutrophils. *J. Biol. Chem.*, **262**, 6450–2.

94 Dinauer, M. C., Pierce, E. A., Bruns, B. A. P., Curnutte, J. T., and Orkin, S. H. (1990). Human neutrophil cytochrome-b light chain (p22-phox): Gene structure, chromosomal location, and mutations in cytochrome negative autosomal recessive chronic granulomatous disease. *J. Clin. Invest.*, **86**, 1729–37.

95 Clark, R. A., Malech, H. L., Gallin, J. I., Nunoi, H., Volpp, B. D., Pearson, D. W., *et al.* (1989). Genetic variants of chronic granulomatous disease: Prevalence of deficiencies of two cytosolic components of the NADPH oxidase system. *N. Engl. J. Med.*, **321**, 647–52.

96 Parkos, C. A., Dinauer, M. C., Jesaitis, A. J., Orkin, S. H., and Curnutte, J. T. (1989). Absence of both the 91kD and 22kD subunits of human neutrophil cytochrome b in two genetic forms of chronic granulomatous disease. *Blood,* **73**, 1416–20.

97 Baehner, R. L., Kunkel, L. M., Monaco, A. P., Haines, J. L., Coneally, P. M., Palmer, C., *et al.* (1986). DNA linkage analysis of X chromosome-linked chronic granulomatous disease. *Proc. Natl Acad. Sci. USA,* **83**, 3398–401.

98 Segal, A. W. (1987). Absence of both cytochrome b_{-245} subunits from neutrophils in X-linked chronic granulomatous disease. *Nature,* **326**, 88–91.

99 Orkin, S. H. (1989). Molecular genetics of chronic granulomatous disease. *Annu. Rev. Immunol.,* **7**, 277–307.

100 Royer-Pokora, B., Kunkel, L. M., Monaco, A. P., Goff, S. C., Leuburger, P. E., Biehner, R. L., *et al.* (1986). Cloning the gene for the inherited disorder chronic granulomatous disease on the basis of its chromosomal location. *Cold Spring Harbor Symp. Quant. Biol.,* **51**, 177–83.

101 Lomax, K. J., Malech, H. L., and Gallin, J. I. (1989). The molecular biology of selected phagocyte defects. *Blood Rev.,* **3**, 94–104.

102 Dinauer, M. C., Curnutte, J. T., Rosen, H., and Orkin, S. H. (1989). A missense mutation in the neutrophil cytochrome b heavy chain in cytochrome-positive X-linked chronic granulomatous disease. *J. Clin. Invest.,* **84**, 2012–16.

103 Bolscher, B.H.J.M., de Boer, M., de Klein, A., Weening, R. S., and Roos, D. (1991). Point mutations in the β-subunit of cytochrome b_{558} leading to X-linked chronic granulomatous disease. *Blood,* **77**, 2482–7.

104 Lew, P. D., Southwick, R. S., Stossel, T. P., Whitin, J. C., Simons, E., and Cohen, H. J. (1981). A variant of chronic granulomatous disease: Deficient oxidative metabolism due to a low-affinity NADPH oxidase. *N. Engl. J. Med.,* **305**, 1329–33.

105 Seger, R. A., Tiefenauer, L., Matsunagal, T., Wildfeuer, A., and Newburger, P. E. (1983). Chronic granulomatous disease due to granulocytes with abnormal NADPH oxidase activity and deficient cytochrome-b. *Blood,* **61**, 423–8.

106 Newburger, P. E., Luscinskas, F. W., Ryan, T., Beard, C. J., Wright, J., Platt, O. S., *et al.* (1986). Variant chronic granulomatous disease: Modulation of the neutrophil defect by severe infection. *Blood,* **68,** 914–19.
107 Ezekowitx, R. A. B., Orkin, S. H., and Newburger, P. E. (1987). Recombinant interferon gamma augments phagocyte superoxide production and X-chronic granulomatous disease gene expression in X-linked variant chronic granulomatous disease. *J. Clin. Invest.,* **80,** 1009–16.
108 Ezekowitz, R. A. B., Dinauer, M. C., Jaffe, H. S., Orkin, S. H., and Newburger, P. E. (1988). Partial correction of the phagocyte defect in patients with X-linked chronic granulomatous disease by subcutaneous interferon gamma. *N. Engl. J. Med.,* **319,** 146–51.
109 Dinauer, M. C., Muhlebach, T., Erickson, R. W., Pierce, E., Messner, H., Orkin, S. H., *et al.* (1990). A missense mutation in the p22-phox subunit of cytochrome b associated with a nonfunctional cytochrome b and chronic granulomatous disease. *Blood,* **76,** 179a (abstr.).
110 Curnutte, J. T., Berkow, R. L., Roberts, R. L., Shurin, S. B., and Scott, P. J. (1988). Chronic granulomatous disease due to a defect in the cytosolic factor required for nicotinamide adenine dinucleotide phosphate oxidase activation. *J. Clin. Invest.,* **81,** 606–10.
111 Lomax, K. J., Leto, T. L., Nunoi, H., Gallin, J. I., and Malech, H. L. (1989). Recombinant 47-kilodalton cytosol factor restores NADPH oxidase in chronic granulomatous disease. *Science,* **245,** 409–12 (published erratum appears in *Science,* **246,** 987, 1989).
112 Nunoi, I. I., Rotrosen, D., Gillin, J. I., and Malech, H. L. (1988). Two forms of autosomal chronic granulomatous disease lacks distinct neutrophil cytosol factors. *Science,* **242,** 1298–301.
113 Volpp, B. D., Nauseef, V. M., Donelson, J. E., Moser, D. R., and Clark, R. A. (1989). Cloning of the cDNA and functional expression of the 47-kilodalton cytosolic component of human neutrophil respiratory burst oxidase. *Proc. Natl Acad. Sci. USA,* **86,** 7195–9 (published erratum appears in *Proc. Natl Acad. Sci. USA,* **86,** 9563, 1989).
114 Bolscher, B.S.J.M., van Zwieten, R., Kramer, I. M., Weening, R. S., Verhoeven, A. J., and Roos, D. (1989). A phosphoprotein of Mr 47 000, defective in autosomal chronic granulomatous disease, copurifies with one of two soluble components required for NADPH: O_2 oxidoreductase activity in human neutrophils. *J. Clin. Invest.,* **83,** 757–63.
115 Teahan, C. G., Totty, N., Casimir, C. M., and Segal, A. W. (1990). Purification of the 47kDa phosphoprotein associated with the NADPH oxidase of human neutrophils. *Biochem. J.,* **267,** 485–9.
116 Leto, T. L., Lomax, K. J., Volpp, B. D., Nunoi, H., Sechler, J.M.G.,

Nauseef, W. M., *et al.* (1990). Cloning of a 67-kD neutrophil oxidase factor with similarity to a non-catalytic region of p60$^{c\text{-src}}$. *Science,* **248,** 727–30.

117 Weening, R. S., Adriaansz, L. H., Weemaes, C. M., Lutter, R., and Roos, D. (1985). Clinical differences in chronic granulomatous disease in patients with cytochrome b-negative or cytochrome b-positive neutrophils. *J. Pediatr.,* **107,** 102–4.

118 Rappaport, J. M., Newburger, P. E., Goldblum, R. M., Goldman, A. S., Nathan, D. G., and Parkman, R. (1982). Allogeneic bone marrow transplantation for chronic granulomatous disease. *J. Pediatr.,* **101,** 952–7.

119 Kamani, N., August, C. S., Campbell, D. E., Hassan, N. F., and Douglas, S. D. (1988). Marrow transplantation in chronic granulomatous disease: An update, with 6-year follow-up. *J. Pediatr.,* **113,** 697–700.

120 Schettini, F., De Mattia, D., Manzionna, M. M., Seger, R., Jumarulo, R., Torlontano, G., and Iacone, A. (1987). Bone marrow transplantation for chronic granulomatous disease associated with cytochrome b deficiency. *Pediatr. Hematol. Oncol.,* **4,** 277–9.

121 The International Chronic Granulomatous Disease Cooperative Study Group. (1991). The controlled trial of interferon gamma to prevent infection in chronic granulomatous disease. *N. Engl. J. Med.,* **324,** 509–16.

122 Nauseef, W. M. (1990). Myeloperoxidase deficiency. *Hematol. Pathol.,* **4,** 165–78.

123 Nauseef, W. M. (1988). Myeloperoxidase deficiency. *Hematol. Oncol. Clin. North Am.,* **2,** 135–58.

124 Mansberg, H. P., Saunders, A. M., and Groner, W. (1974). The hemalog-D differential system. *J. Histochem. Cytochem.,* **22,** 711–24.

125 Kitahara, M., Eyre, H. J., Simonian, Y., Atkin, C. L., and Hasstedt, S. J. (1981). Hereditary myeloperoxidase deficiency. *Blood,* **57,** 888–93.

126 Cech, P., Papathanassiou, A., Boreaux, G., Roth, P., and Mieschler, D. A. (1979). Hereditary myeloperoxidase deficiency. *Blood,* **53,** 403–11.

127 Tobler, A., Selsted, M. E., Miller, C. W., Johnson, K. R., Novotny, M. J., Rovera, G., and Koeffler, H. P. (1989). Evidence for a pretranslational defect in hereditary and acquired myeloperoxidase deficiency. *Blood,* **73,** 1980–6.

128 Nauseef, W. M. (1989). Aberrant restriction endonuclease digests of DNA from subjects with hereditary myeloperoxidase deficiency. *Blood,* **3,** 290–5.

129 Nauseef, W. M., Root, R. K., and Malech, H. L. (1983). Biochemical

and immunologic analysis of hereditary myeloperoxidase deficiency. *J. Clin. Invest.*, **71**, 1297–307.

130 Anderson, D. C. and Springer, T. A. (1987). Leucocyte adhesion deficiency: An inherited defect in the Mac-1, LFA-1, and p150,95 glycoproteins. *Annu. Rev. Med.*, **38**, 175–94.

131 Todd III, R. F. and Fryer, D. R. (1988). The CD11/CD18 leucocyte glycoprotein deficiency. *Hematol. Oncol. Clin. North Am.*, **2**, 13–31.

132 Fischer, A., Lisowska-Grospierre, B., Anderson, D. C., and Springer, T. A. (1988). Leucocyte adhesion deficiency: Molecular basis and functional consequences. *Immunodefic. Rev.*, **1**, 39–54.

133 Abramson, J. S., Mills, E. L., Sawyer, M. K., Regelman, W. R., Nelson, J. D., and Quie, P. G. (1981). Recurrent infections and delayed separation of the umbilical cord in an infant with abnormal phagocytic cell locomotion and oxidative response during particle phagocytosis. *J. Pediatr.*, **99**, 887–94.

134 Dana, N., Clayton, L. K., Tennen, D. G., Pierce, M. W., Lachmann, P. J., Law, S. A., and Arnaout, M. A. (1987). Leucocytes from four patients with complete or partial Leu-CAM deficiency contain the common β-subunit precursor and β-subunit messenger RNA. *J. Clin. Invest.*, **79**, 1010–15.

135 Kishimoto, T. K., Hollander, N., Roberts, T. M., Anderson, D. C., and Springer, T. A. (1987). Heterogeneous mutations in the β subunit common to the LFA-1, Mac-1, and p150,95 glycoproteins cause leucocyte adhesion deficiency. *Cell*, **50**, 193–202.

136 Kishimoto, T. K., O'Connor, K., and Springer, T. A. (1989). Leucocyte adhesion deficiency: Aberrant splicing of a conserved integrin sequence causes a moderate deficiency phenotype. *J. Biol. Chem.*, **264**, 3588–95.

137 Dimanche-Boitrel, M. T., Guyot, A., De Sainte-Basile, G., Fischer, A., Griscelli, C., and Lisowska-Grospierre, B. (1988). Heterogeneity in the molecular defect leading to the leucocyte adhesion deficiency. *Eur. J. Immunol.*, **18**, 1575–9.

138 Arnaout, M. A., Dana, N., Gupta, S. K., Tenen, D. G., and Fathallah, D. M. (1990). Point mutations impairing cell surface expression of the commmon β subunit (CD18) in a patient with leucocyte adhesion molecule (Leu-CAM) deficiency. *J. Clin. Invest.*, **85**, 977–81.

139 Wardlaw, A. J., Hibbs, M. L., Stacker, S. A., and Springer, T. A. (1990). Distinct mutations in two patients with leucocyte adhesion deficiency and their functional correlates. *J. Exp. Med.*, **172**, 335–45.

140 Springer, T. A., Thompson, W. S., Miller, L. J., Schmalstieg, F. C., and Anderson, D. C. (1984). Inherited deficiency of the Mac-1, LFA-1, p150,95 glycoprotein family and its molecular basis. *J. Exp. Med.*, **160**, 1901–18.

141 Lisowska-Grospierre, B., Bohler, M. C., Fischer, A., Mawas, C.,

Springer, T. A., and Griscelli, C. (1986). Defective membrane expression of the LFA-1 complex may be secondary to the absence of the β chain in a child with recurrent bacterial infection. *Eur. J. Immunol.*, **16**, 205–8.

142 Marlin, S. D., Morton, C. C., Anderson, D. C., and Springer, T. A. (1986). LFA-1 immunodeficiency disease: Definition of the genetic defect and chromosomal mapping of α and β subunits of the lymphocyte function-associated antigen 1 (LFA-1) by complementation in hybrid cells. *J. Exp. Med.*, **164**, 855–67.

143 Corbi, A. L., Larson, R. S., Kishimoto, T. K., Springer, T. A., and Morton, C. C. (1988). Chromosomal location of the genes encoding the leucocyte adhesion receptors LFA-1, Mac-1, and p150,95. *J. Exp. Med.*, **167**, 1597–607.

144 Baehner, R. L. (1989). Disorders of granulocyte function. In *Blood diseases of infancy and childhood* (ed. D. R. Miller and R. L. Baehner), C. V. Mosby, St Louis.

145 Blume, R. S. and Wolff, S. M. (1972). The Chédiak–Higashi syndrome: Studies in four patients and a review of the literature. *Medicine,* **51**, 247–80.

146 Bejaoui, M., Veber, F., Girault, D., Gaud, C., Blanche, S., and Griscelli, C. (1989). The accelerated phase of Chédiak–Higashi syndrome. *Arch. Fr. Pédiatr.*, **46**, 733–6.

147 Bainton, D. F. (1988). Phagocytic cells: Developmental biology of PMNs and eosinophils. In *Inflammation: basic principles and clinical correlates* (ed. J. I. Gallin, I. M. Goldstein, and R. Snyderman). Raven Press, New York.

148 Haak, R. A., Ingraham, L. M., Baehner, R. L., and Boxer, L. A. (1979). Membrane fluidity in human and mouse Chédiak–Higashi leucocytes. *J. Clin. Invest.*, **64**, 138–44.

149 Wolff, S. M., Dale, D. C., Clark, R. A., Root, R. K., and Kimball, H. R. (1972). The Chédiak–Higashi syndrome: Studies of host defense. *Ann. Intern. Med.*, **76**, 293–306.

150 Gallin, J. I. (1985). Neutrophil specific granule deficiency. *Annu. Rev. Med.*, **36**, 263–74.

151 Spitznagel, J. K., Cooper, M. R., McCall, A. E., DeChatelet, L. R., and Welsh, I. R. H. (1972). Selective deficiency of granules associated with lysozyme and lactoferrin in human polymorphonuclear leucocytes with reduced microbicidal capacity. *J. Clin. Invest.*, **51**, 93a.

152 Ganz, T., Metcalf, J. A., Gallin, J. I., Boxer, L. A., and Lehrer, R. I. (1988). Microbicidal/cytotoxic proteins of neutrophils are deficient in two disorders: Chédiak–Higashi syndrome and 'specific' granule deficiency. *J. Clin. Invest.*, **82**, 552–6.

153 Parmley, R. T., Gilbert, C. S., and Boxer, L. A. (1989). Abnormal

peroxidase-positive granules in 'specific granule' deficiency. *Blood,* **73,** 838–44.

154 Lomax, K. J., Gallin, J. I., Rotrosen, D., Raphael, G. D., Kaliner, M. A., Benz, E. J., *et al.* (1989). Selective defect in myeloid cell lactoferrin gene expression in PMN specific granule deficiency. *J. Clin. Invest.,* **83,** 514–19.

155 Raphael, G. D., Davis, J. L., Fox, P. C., Malex, H. L., Gallin, J. I., Baraniuk, J. N., and Kaliner, M. A. (1989). Glandular secretion of lactoferrin in a patient with neutrophil lactoferrin deficiency. *J. Allergy Clin. Immunol.,* **84,** 914–19.

7 Neutrophil-mediated tissue injury

J. A. LEFF and J. E. REPINE

1 Clinical case: adult respiratory distress syndrome (ARDS)

A 47-year-old alcoholic woman with a 30-year history of smoking was admitted to the intensive care unit with progressive shortness of breath. She was well until 24 h prior to admission when she developed fever, chills, vomiting, pleuritic chest pain, cough productive of rusty sputum, and worsening dyspnoea. Physical examination revealed a plethoric, ill-appearing woman in respiratory distress. Temperature was 37.2 °C, respirations 28/min, pulse 128/min, and blood pressure 102/48 mm Hg. Lung examination revealed egophony in the right lower lobe, with decreased breath sounds in the left lower lobe and right lung. There were rare expiratory wheezes and tactile fremitus in the right middle lobe. Heart examination revealed tachycardia with no murmurs, gallops, or rubs. The abdomen was benign and extremities were without cyanosis, clubbing or oedema. Neurological examination revealed a resting tremor but was otherwise non-focal. Abnormal admission laboratories included white blood cell count of 15 000 cells/mm^3 (12 per cent polys, 32 per cent bands, 37 per cent lymphs, 10 per cent metamyelocytes, 3 per cent myelocytes, 6 per cent monocytes), potassium 3.2 meq/l, bicarbonate 14 meq/l, ethanol level 264 mg/dl, and a decreased magnesium level. Sputum examination revealed no predominant organism on Gram stain. Chest radiograph revealed diffuse alveolar infiltrates sparing the left upper lobe. Broad spectrum antibiotics, fluids, multivitamins, folate, thiamine, and antacids were administered. After 2 h in the ICU, her fatigue and oxygenation worsened; she was intubated and mechanical ventilation was begun with a high FiO$_2$. Her oxygenation and infiltrates worsened during her second day in the ICU. A pulmonary artery catheter was placed which revealed a low cardiac output and dobutamine was begun. Admission blood cultures grew *Streptococcus pneumoniae*. Her oxygenation continued to deteriorate and based on poor oxygenation, diffuse pulmonary infiltrates, very low pulmonary compliance, and a normal pulmonary capillary wedge pressure, a diagnosis of adult respiratory distress syndrome (ARDS) was made. Positive end expiratory pressure was added with moderate improvement. Over the next 2 weeks, the FiO$_2$ could not be weaned below 50–60 per cent and the lungs remained very stiff. Solumedrol was added in an attempt to hasten the recovery/ repair phase with moderate improvement in compliance (from 15 to 35 ml/cm H_2O) and chest radiograph; however, there was no improvement in oxygen requirement. Her ICU course was complicated by a perforated superior venae cavae during i.v. line placement, two episodes of pneumothorax due to high ventilator-induced airway pressures, alcohol withdrawal seizures and sepsis treated with an anti-endotoxin monoclonal antibody. After 3 weeks, a tracheostomy was performed, and after 5 weeks, a long, slow weaning process was begun. Weaning was eventually successful and she was discharged on oxygen.

2   Introduction

Neutrophils are well appreciated for their beneficial effects on human health. The potent antimicrobial activity of the neutrophil is now well recognized and has been reviewed in detail in Chapters 2, 3, and 4. Reduction in the numbers or defects in the function of neutrophils cause a number of devastating diseases characterized by more frequent and/or more severe infection (1) (see Chapter 6). More recently, however, the detrimental potential of neutrophils has been increasingly realized and has become a part of the analysis of the pathophysiology and treatment of a variety of common diseases. Accordingly, a better understanding of the nature of this process and ways of interfering with neutrophil-mediated injury are the subject of intense investigation. Neutrophils have been implicated, at least in part, in a number of diseases including ARDS, as presented in the case above, myocardial infarction, rheumatoid arthritis, gout, emphysema, glomerulonephritis, inflammatory bowel disease, asthma, immune vasculitis, neutrophil dermatoses, and thermal injury (1, 2) (Table 7.1).

Several experimental strategies have evolved to address the question of whether neutrophils are important in tissue injury. First, if neutrophils are to be implicated in tissue injury they should be present, usually in increased numbers, at the site of injury as assessed morphometrically or by other means. Second, the timing of neutrophil influx should be consistent with a causal participation of neutrophils. That is, neutrophil influx should precede measurable injury. It should be noted that non-neutrophil related injury could also incite an inflammatory response which could then recruit neutrophils as a secondary phenomenon. Third, if tissue injury is abrogated by rendering animals neutropenic, then a causal role for neutrophils may be inferred from protection seen following neutrophil depletion. These are difficult experiments, however, since methods of inducing neutropenia are somewhat non-specific and may affect other cell lines or bodily functions. Nevertheless, many valuable observations have

Table 7.1 Human inflammatory diseases in which the neutrophil is implicated as a mediator of tissue destruction[a]

---

 1. Adult respiratory distress syndrome
 2. Ischaemia–reperfusion injury (myocardial infarction)
 3. Emphysema
 4. Rheumatoid arthritis
 5. Immune vasculitis
 6. Gout
 7. Glomerulonephritis
 8. Inflammatory bowel disease
 9. Asthma
10. Neutrophil dermatosis
11. Thermal injury
12. Chronic bronchitis
13. Bronchiectasis
14. Cystic fibrosis
15. Atherosclerosis
16. Psoriasis
17. Malignant neoplasms at sites of chronic inflammation

---

[a] Modified from reference 1.

been made using strategies involving nitrogen mustard, vinblastine and/or anti-neutrophil antibodies. Fourth, drugs antagonizing neutrophil functions have been utilized to implicate neutrophils in tissue damage; however, these studies suffer from the same limitations, again mainly the non-specificity of the reagents.

The goal of this chapter is to review briefly some of the basic mechanisms which have been purported to be involved in neutrophil-induced tissue injury, and to consider some of the clinical syndromes in which neutrophils are thought to contribute in adverse ways.

3   Theoretical mechanisms of neutrophil-induced tissue injury

Several ways exist in which neutrophils might induce tissue injury (Table 7.2). The major possibilities include production and release of toxic oxygen metabolites [also called reactive oxygen species (ROS)], granular components, or products of arachidonic acid metabolism. Neutrophils may contain as many as 50 toxins (2). Thus, when the neutrophil is exposed to one or various stimuli, a process occurs which is similar to the reaction

Table 7.2   Theoretical mechanisms through which
neutrophils may mediate tissue destruction

1. Toxic oxygen metabolites
2. Granular enzymes
3. Arachidonic acid metabolism products
4. Hypochlorous acid and/or its metabolites

following ingestion of bacteria, except that the reactions appear to be directed extracellularly into surrounding tissues rather than internally into phagocytic vacuoles. Briefly, following activation, the membrane-bound NADPH oxidase system begins to generate large quantities of superoxide anion (O_2^-). Almost simultaneously, neutrophil granules fuse with the external membrane at sites of activation and toxins are released into the extracellular medium. As a result, host tissues are directly attacked by neutrophil-derived toxins (Fig. 7.1). A popular proposal has been the concept of a 'frustrated phagocyte'—a condition in which a neutrophil can not phagocytose impossibly large substances, such as damaged epithelial surfaces (3), and accordingly, generates increasing amounts of toxins continually. This may be another mechanism through which the neutrophil might then release toxic products into the extracellular space. Even though various stimuli may be relatively selective for enhancing production of toxins (e.g. oxygen radicals or proteinases), it is unlikely that a single class of neutrophil toxins causes the majority of tissue injury. In addition to the individual toxicities of toxic oxygen metabolites, granular substances, and arachidonic acid derivatives, synergistic interactions between these toxins are likely and capable of greatly potentiating the damaging effects of neutrophils.

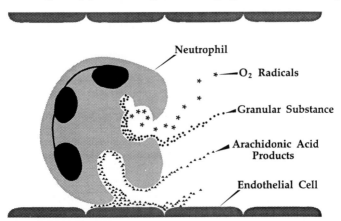

Fig. 7.1   Schematic diagram of a neutrophil releasing toxins which could injure tissue.

The neutrophil's two major granule types (specific and azurophilic) contain numerous toxic peptides, proteins, and enzymes, including myeloperoxidase, elastase, cathepsins, collagenase, cationic proteins, lysozyme, lactoferrin, among others. The potential role of these peptides in tissue injury is described below.

3.1   The myeloperoxidase system

Myeloperoxidase (MPO) is an enzyme, which together with H_2O_2 can oxidize a number of halides into their corresponding hypohalous acids. The neutrophil has been shown to produce primarily hypochlorous acid (HOCl) (2). HOCl in turn, is an extremely potent oxidant which can attack many biological substances including amines, amino acids, thiols, thioethers, nucleotides, haemoproteins, and polyenoic acids (4). MPO can also kill tumour cells (5). HOCl appears to be one of the major toxic species produced by neutrophils (2). HOCl is highly reactive and disappears rapidly by virtue of its reactions with various substances. When HOCl reacts with amines, the reaction products are toxic chloramines—an example of a specific target is taurine and the product is taurochloramine. Chlorinated oxidants are longer lived and toxic to tissue *in vitro* and possibly *in vivo*. However, *in vitro* studies rely on several indirect interventions. If injury is reduced following the addition of the H_2O_2 scavenger, catalase, thereby removing a needed substrate for MPO-derived products (HOCl), then a role for HOCl can be hypothesized. Similarly, if injury is reduced in the presence of a MPO inhibitor such as sodium azide, then a role for HOCl is strengthened. A chloride-free buffer system also limits the amount of HOCl that is produced. Finally, scavengers of HOCl, such as methionine and dimethylthiourea, can be used to infer a role for HOCl in tissue injury. Whether the final mediator of tissue injury is HOCl or a derivative chlorinated oxidant remains controversial (2).

3.2   Proteolytic enzymes

Neutrophil granules contain more than 20 different proteolytic enzymes. Their actions are also in sharp contrast to oxygen radicals which are non-specific, highly reactive and short-lived toxins. Granular enzymes have relatively specific substrates and toxicity, catalyse many reactions at exceptional speed, and are long-lived in tissue. Their role in tissue injury has been less studied than that of oxygen radicals primarily due to the lack of specific inhibitors to use as probes. The system seems more controlled than that of oxidants in some ways. For example, the extracellular space is bathed in potent antiproteinases which irreversibly inactivate the serine proteases; in addition, the metalloproteinases are secreted in an inactive, latent form. The importance of proteinases, directly or indirectly, in the bactericidal actions of neutrophils may be as important as oxygen radicals as evidenced by the infections incurred by patients with chronic granulomatous disease and specific granule deficiency (see Chapter 6). Nevertheless, the relatively benign nature of the clinical symptoms in patients with MPO deficiency points out, however, the relative toxicities of different granule constituents. Recent information seems to confirm this concept. Granular enzymes have received the greatest attention with respect to their ability to induce tissue injury: specifically, the serine protease, elastase, and two metalloproteinases, collagenase and gelatinase. These enzymes attack and digest the extracellular matrix containing elastin, collagen, proteoglycans, and glycoproteins. Once thought to be an inert backbone of the extracellular space, the extracellular matrix has since been recognized to serve many other functions as well including the regulation of cell shape, migration, growth and differentiation, and repair of tissue (6, 7).

3.2.1   Elastase

Neutrophil azurophilic granules contain large quantities of the serine protease, elastase. Elastase is named for its substrate, elastin, which it readily degrades. However, elastase has many substrates including types III and IV collagen, immunoglobulins, complement components, clotting factors, proteoglycans, fibronectin, and even intact cells (8, 9). The physiologic role of elastase is unclear. It putatively contributes to the degradation of micro-organisms within the phagocytic vacuole and may also be important for neutrophil locomotion and tissue penetration. There are several extracellular inhibitors of elastase, should the enzyme escape from the neutrophil. However, this inactivation system is not perfect. Indeed, there is evidence that elastase can escape, and induce tissue injury, despite the antiproteinase shield in the extracellular space. The three most important antiproteinases include α_1-proteinase inhibitor (A1PI, formerly called α_1-anti-trypsin), α_2-macroglobulin, and secretory leukoproteinase inhibitor. The most crucial elastase inhibitor appears to be A1PI, a 52 kDa glycoprotein which irreversibly inactivates elastase by forming a complex with the enzyme. This reaction is exceptionally fast making the active half-life of elastase roughly 0.6 ms *in vivo* (10).

Given the seemingly powerful antiproteinase defence in the interstitial fluids, it would appear unlikely that elastase could cause tissue injury. However, observations of free, active elastase at sites of inflammation (9), indicate that elastase can at times escape destruction, and is, at least, theoretically, able to mediate tissue damage. Most likely this occurs because antiproteinases have been inactivated at sites of inflammation, precisely the location where one would want them to remain intact. With no impairment by antiproteinases, elastase could freely digest extracelllular tissue. Of interest, the observation of antiproteinase inactivation was made at the turn of the century (2) and its implications lay dormant for over 50 years. The importance of the interaction between oxidants, proteinases, and antiproteinases *in vivo* was largely ignored until recently. In the early 1980s, the fascinating story of A1PI's susceptibility to oxidative inactivation was unravelled. Structural studies of the molecule revealed that A1PI contained a crucial methionine residue in its active site, position 358. Due to its thiol bond, methionine is very sensitive to oxidation either by chemicals or neutrophil-derived oxidants. In fact, oxidation of Met-358 causes a dramatic slowing of the association between elastase and A1PI, enhancing the half-life of elastase *in vivo* 200-fold from 0.6 ms to 1.2 s (9, 10). To study this in a controlled manner, we used the isolated perfused lung approach (Fig. 7.2) to investigate the anti-elastolytic properties of the lung with and without exposure to oxidants. The isolated lung approach offers great simplicity and control in that many of the factors usually circulating in blood can be removed (and added back individually) before the experiment. We found that lung perfusate inhibited human neutrophil elastase activity by about 60 per cent (11). Furthermore, when glucose oxidase-generated hydrogen peroxide (H_2O_2) was added to the perfusate, the ability of the perfusate to inhibit elastase activity decreased (Fig. 7.3). To study the interactions between oxidants and elastase, both H_2O_2 and human elastase were added to the perfusate. Subinjurious doses of H_2O_2

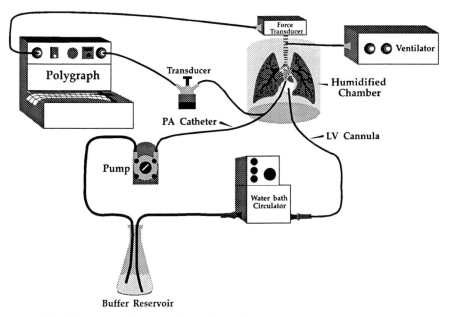

Fig. 7.2 Schematic diagram of the isolated perfused rat lung apparatus. PA, pulmonary artery; LV, left ventricle.

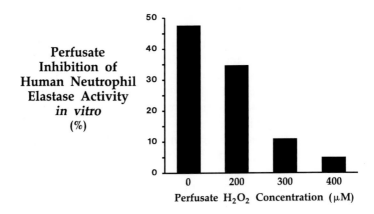

Fig. 7.3 The ability of samples of perfusates from isolated saline-perfused rat lungs to inhibit neutrophil elastase activity *in vitro* decreased ($P < 0.05$) as a function of increases in perfusate H_2O_2 concentrations following addition of glucose oxidase. Modified from reference 11.

and elastase were determined and when added individually produced no injury. In contrast, when the same doses of H_2O_2 and elastase were added together, we found marked lung injury as measured by lung weight gain, increases in lung permeability (lavage ficoll), and pulmonary artery perfusion pressure increases (Fig. 7.4). This synergistic injury is consistent with H_2O_2 (oxidatively) inactivating lung-associated A1PI activity.

If neutrophil elastase manages to escape from A1PI, it must still contend with α_2-macroglobulin and secretory leukoprotease inhibitor. The α_2-macroglobulin is a large, 725 kDa plasma protein, with broad specificity, that can inhibit almost all mammalian proteinases, although its specificity appears to be greater for tissue proteinases as opposed to the neutrophil-derived proteinases (8, 12).

Secretory leukoproteinase inhibitor (SLPI) is a small, 14 kDa antiproteinase found in mucous secretions and interstitial fluids. It can inhibit both free and tissue-bound elastase. Interestingly, both α_2-macroglobulin and SLPI can be oxidatively inactivated, similar to A1PI (2, 13). Thus, all three antiproteinases are susceptible to oxidative inactivation. This suggests that oxidant inactivation of antiproteases may be a key control mechanism in the normal and abnormal function of neutrophils.

3.2.2   The metalloproteinases

Two metalloproteinases, collagenase and gelatinase can also degrade the extracellular matrix. Collagenase can cleave the interstitial collagens (types I, II, and III) while gelatinase cleaves types V, XI, and possibly IV collagens (12). Initially, the tissue destructive potential of these enzymes was not fully recognized since they are released in latent, inactive forms.

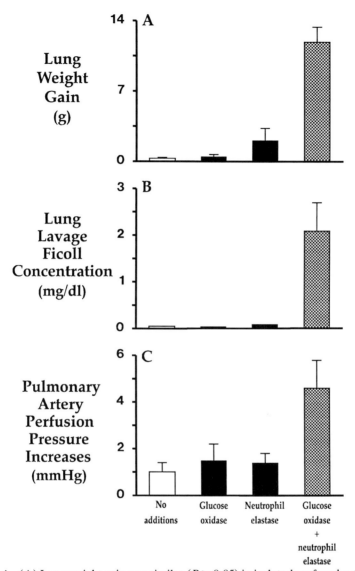

Fig. 7.4 (A) Lung weight gain was similar ($P \geq 0.05$) in isolated perfused rat lungs exposed to no additions, glucose oxidase alone, and neutrophil elastase alone. In contrast, lung weight gain increased ($P \leq 0.05$) when rat lungs were exposed to glucose oxidase and neutrophil elastase together. (B) Lung lavage ficoll concentration was similar ($P \geq 0.05$) in isolated perfused rat lungs exposed to no additions, glucose oxidase alone, and neutrophil elastase alone. In contrast, lung lavage ficoll concentration increased ($P \leq 0.05$) when rat lungs were exposed to glucose oxidase and neutrophil elastase together. (C) Pulmonary artery perfusion pressure increases were similar ($P \geq 0.05$) in isolated perfused rat lungs exposed to no additions, glucose oxidase alone, and neutrophil elastase alone. In contrast, the increase in perfusion pressure was greater ($P \leq 0.05$) when rat lungs were exposed to glucose oxidase and neutrophil elastase together. Modified from reference 11.

However, recent evidence has enhanced their role by elucidating mechanisms for their activation. Although neutrophil collagenase can be activated *in vitro* by trypsin, as well as by certain chemicals (alkylating agents, organomercurials, and heavy metals), an *in vivo* activator of collagenase has not been found and other neutrophil-derived proteases, elastase and cathepsin G seem to destroy, rather than activate, collagenase (12). Recent work, however, has demonstrated that the neutrophil can activate its own latent collagenase utilizing self-derived oxygen radicals (probably HOCl) (14). Neutrophils from CGD patients contain normal amounts of proteolytic enzymes, but contain a defective NADPH oxidase, and thus, produce only minute quantities of oxygen radicals (including O_2^-, H_2O_2, and HOCl). Normal, but not CGD, neutrophils could activate their own collagenase *in vitro* (14). Interestingly, it now appears that oxygen radicals can serve a prodigestive function by not only inactivating antiproteases (e.g. A1PI) but also by activating proteases. A similar autoactivation has since been shown for gelatinase as well (15).

Once activated, the regulation of the metalloenzyme proteinases is unclear. The α_2-macroglobulin and tissue inhibitor of metalloproteinases (TIMP), while powerful inhibitors of other tissue collagenases, do not appear to be potent inhibitors of neutrophil enzymes (12). These inhibitors can be inactivated; α_2-macroglobulin by oxidants, and TIMP by neutrophil elastase (12, 16).

Elastase and collagenase can digest glomerular basement membrane, articular cartilage, elastic tissue in arterial walls, and elastin in lung tissue (17). Cathepsins D and E have been shown to attack native proteins and degrade purified glomerular basement membrane (18). In addition to degrading tissue directly, neutrophil-derived proteases could amplify the inflammatory process by cleaving complement components, fibrinogen, and Hageman factor (19, 20). Lactoferrin might enhance hydroxyl radical formation as well (21).

3.3   Oxygen radical-induced tissue injury

Toxic oxygen metabolites induce tissue injury in many experimental models. Oxidants can damage fibroblasts (22), lung parenchymal cells (23), rat lungs (24, 25), endothelial cells (26, 27), red blood cells (28), and hyaluronic acid (29). Potential mechanisms of injury from oxygen radicals include damage to proteins (extracellular or intracellular), membrane lipids, and nucleic acids. Specifically, oxygen radicals may cause lipid peroxidation of cell membranes altering their structural integrity. Alternatively, lipid peroxidation in a localized membrane segment may perturb the microenvironment of membrane-bound proteins altering their function. Membrane lipids which are most susceptible to attack include those containing unsaturated double bonds which are most oxidizable. Lipid peroxides and aldehydes result from oxidation. Once a lipid peroxide is produced by an inciting free radical, it may quickly propagate through the membrane in a chain reaction. Downstream metabolites of the AA cascade such as prostaglandins, thromboxanes, and leukotrienes may lead to additional toxic effects (30–34).

Oxygen radicals may also directly attack membrane proteins involved with ion transport or other important functions. Those proteins with cysteinyl residues are particularly susceptible to inactivation, especially proteins with cysteinyl residues in their active site. There are several theoretical ways in which free radicals might alter protein function (35). First, oxygen radicals may affect specific amino acid residues leading to conformational changes. Second, oxygen radicals might induce denaturation. Finally, oxygen radicals may render the protein more susceptible to hydrolysis. In addition, oxygen radicals may alter the structure and function of RNA and DNA. Although all mammalian tissues contain the antioxidant enzymes superoxide dismutase and catalase (which detoxify superoxide anion and hydrogen peroxide, respectively), these enzyme systems may be overwhelmed during the intense local production of toxic oxygen metabolites. Furthermore, there is no known enzyme which detoxifies the highly potent hydroxyl radical.

4 Evidence implicating neutrophils in tissue injury *in vivo*

Many animal models have convincingly implicated neutrophils in tissue injury. Similarly, many animal models have conclusively shown a role of oxygen radicals in tissue injury. However, whether neutrophil-derived oxygen radicals act directly, or perhaps in part via proteinases (e.g. by activating proteinases or inactivating antiproteases) is less well understood. Furthermore, caution must be applied in extrapolating animal data to the human situation as there are important differences. Differences in neutrophil proteinases, as well as the antiproteinases have been noted in different species. For example, unlike the human protein, A1PI obtained from rabbits and sheep is highly resistant to oxidative inactivation (36, 37).

The role of oxygen radicals, granular enzymes and lipid products in causing various diseases and tissue injury is discussed below. Emphasis is given to ARDS and ischaemia-reperfusion syndromes where oxygen radicals play a central role. Brief discussions with appropriate review references have been added for other clinical diseases in which neutrophils appear to play a role.

4.1   Adult respiratory distress syndrome (ARDS)

ARDS is an acute, inflammatory process altering structure and function of lung tissue. ARDS is a poorly understood response to a variety of apparently diverse insults (38). It is not reliably known but it appears that ARDS afflicts roughly 150 000 patients yearly in the USA, if it is diagnosed by strict criteria (39). There may be many more mild cases of ARDS. The mortality rate remains at approximately 60 per cent and is unchanged since its original description in 1967 (40, 41). This is most likely due to our lack of understanding of the mechanisms of initiation, modulation, and termination of the syndrome.

Early descriptions of ARDS revealed neutrophils in interstitial and alveolar spaces as prominent findings (42–44). However, the pathogenic importance of this was not appreciated until other observations were made. Jacob and colleagues observed that pulmonary dysfunction occurred during haemodialysis that was associated with complement activation, leukopenia, and pulmonary vascular leukocyte sequestration. This response developed in both humans (45) and in animals (46). At the same time, leukopenia associated with respiratory insufficiency was noted in septic patients (43). Although the pulmonary dysfunction associated with dialysis was subclinical, mild, and transient, it led to the formulation of an important hypothesis which stated that various inciting events caused an abnormal accumulation of neutrophils in the lung, possibly via complement-mediated mechanisms, and that subsequent neutrophil stimulation and release of toxic products contributed to the development of ARDS (the 'neutrophil hypothesis') (47).

Neutrophils are usually present in small numbers in lung interstitium and alveolar spaces. However, there are a large number of circulating neutrophils and marginating pools, especially in the lung. Even though much is known about neutrophil chemotaxis, less is known about the presumed first step in neutrophil recruitment to the lung—adherence to the vascular endothelium (discussion of the biomolecular basis of adhesion and chemotaxis can be found in Chapters 2 and 3). Whether adherence is initiated by endothelial damge, changes in adhesion molecules or receptors, and/or responses to tissue factors is unknown. No clear ultrastructural abnormalities have been identified on endothelial cell surfaces during ARDS. The important role of adhesion molecules in neutrophil adhesion to endothelial cells is becoming increasingly appreciated.

4.1.1   *Clinical evidence supporting a role for neutrophils in ARDS*

The clinical evidence to support the neutrophil hypothesis is somewhat limited and indirect at this time. However, several lines of evidence are consistent with neutrophils playing an important role in ARDS; (i) neutrophils are abundant in lung biopsies and bronchoalveolar lavage (BAL) of ARDS patients; (ii) there is an accumulation of neutrophil products in the BAL and plasma of ARDS patients including elastase (48–52); (iii) neutrophils are present at very early time points in ARDS consistent with a potential pathogenic role as opposed to simply a response to injury; (iv) ARDS is only rarely reported in neutropenic patients (53, 54) and, interestingly, has been noted to worsen in neutropenic patients upon recovery of their peripheral neutrophil counts (55); (v) neutrophil-aggregating activity (probably C5a) has been found in plasma of ARDS patients (56); and (vi) alterations in the activity of blood neutrophils have been noted in ARDS patients (57–59). These latter studies are complicated by the apparently different levels of stimulation of neutrophils depending on their source (e.g. peripheral arterial versus pulmonary arterial). Nevertheless, the finding that neutrophils are either more or less active (exhausted) suggests their involvement. Obviously, these neutrophils from blood may not be representative of neutrophils that have marginated or already invaded tissues.

4.1.2 Experimental evidence supporting a role for neutrophils in ARDS

The greater support for the neutrophil hypothesis comes from a wealth of experimental data in animals, isolated lung preparations, and tissue culture experiments. Some of these experiments have focused on mechanisms of neutrophil recruitment to the lung. Others have depleted animals of neutrophils to determine if the absence of neutrophils protects them from an otherwise injurious insult. Finally, the advent of isolated lung techniques has enabled investigators to remove the complicating factors of nervous innervation and hormonal effects, and to add back isolated blood components in the perfusing buffer to ascertain the contribution of individual cell types better.

If neutrophils are to participate in acute lung injury, then it is reasonable to assume the presence of chemotactic factors that elicit neutrophil migration into lung tissue. Much evidence has been garnered to support this concept. Advances in endothelial cell culture techniques have allowed many questions to be answered relating to neutrophil–endothelial cell interactions. For example, pre-treatment of neutrophils or endothelial cells with chemotactic factors increases adherence *in vitro* (60). Similarly, alveolar macrophages exposed to hyperoxia release a factor(s) that increases neutrophil adherence to endothelium (61) as well as a chemotactic factor(s) for neutrophils (62). To study this phenomenon, alveolar macrophages were isolated from rabbits and then exposed to hyperoxia which was found to be toxic to the cells. With increasing duration of exposure, cultured alveolar macrophages released factors which were chemotactic for neutrophils *in vitro* (Fig. 7.5).

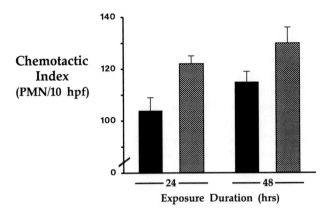

Fig. 7.5 Alveolar macrophages were isolated from rabbits and then exposed to hyperoxia. Macrophages exposed to hyperoxia for 24 and 48 h (cross-hatched bars) *in vitro* released more ($P \leq 0.05$) chemotaxins for PMN than macrophages exposed to normoxia (black bars). Modified from reference 62.

Other studies have confirmed that alveolar macrophages can secrete chemotactic factors for neutrophils (63–65). In addition, hyperoxia-exposed alveolar macrophages produce factors that increase neutrophil adhesion (61) and superoxide anion generation (O_2^-) (66). Intratracheal administration of complement-derived factors, most notably C5a, causes neutrophil recruitment, changes in the alveolar epithelium, and a protein-rich alveolar fluid indicative of increased capillary permeability (67). Rabbits depleted of neutrophils did not show these changes (68). From the vascular side, i.v. injection of two complement activators [zymosan and cobra venom factor (CVF)], as well as purified C5a, causes pulmonary leukocyte sequestration (69). However, neutrophil migration into airspaces and increased permeability to labelled albumin only occurred when complement activation was combined with an additional stress such as surgical manipulation, hypoxia, or infusion of PGE_2 (70).

Intravenous administration of CVF alone leads to neutrophil accumulation and subsequent lung injury in rats (71). Patients at risk for ARDS often have circulating activated complement components yet no obvious lung injury (72). Thus, controversy continues about whether complement activation alone can lead to lung injury. Nevertheless, it appears clear that both complement components and factors secreted by alveolar macrophages can cause neutrophil accumulation in the lung.

To assess the mechanisms of tissue damage further, we studied a model of acute lung injury in rabbits precipitated by i.v. injection of phorbol myristate acetate (PMA) (73). PMA is a potent neutrophil stimulant (74) causing increased neutrophil adherence as well as abrupt generation and release of oxygen radicals. Some rabbits were treated with nitrogen mustard to deplete them of circulating neutrophils. Following injection of PMA, circulating neutrophil counts decreased from approximately 2000 cells/mm^3 to less than 100 cells/mm^3 in control rabbits. PMA treatment resulted in a severe acute oedematous lung injury as measured by albumin in lung lavage and lung weight gains in control rabbits but not in nitrogen mustard (neutropenic) rabbits. Histological examination confirmed large numbers of neutrophils present in PMA-treated lungs as well as morphologic and histologic evidence of lung injury. Neutrophil depletion was so protective that there were no differences between the neutrophil-depleted rabbits given PMA and control rabbits. Neutrophils were further implicated in the tissue damage since lung injury, as assessed by increases in lung weights and lung lavage albumin concentrations, correlated with concentrations of circulating and lavage neutrophils.

These studies, and many other similar studies by other investigators, provide compelling evidence of neutrophil-mediated injury; however, since whole animal models are necessarily complex with many variables we chose to study the problem in a simpler, better defined system, namely the isolated perfused lung model (Fig. 7.2). The advantage of this approach is that it removes the effects of other circulating factors, cells, and the influence of neural pathways. In addition, the isolated saline-perfused lung can be mechanically ventilated in a temperature-controlled environment, perfused through cannulas that enter the pulmonary artery and exit through the left ventricle. Pressure and weight transducers can continuously monitor changes in pulmonary artery pressure and lung weight. We found that the addition of normal human neutrophils stimulated by PMA caused significant damage whereas unstimulated neutrophils did not. The damaging species appeared to be oxygen radical-dependent, since when neutrophils isolated from patients with CGD were used, no injury was seen when neutrophils were stimulated with PMA (Fig. 7.6). These experiments provide more direct evidence that neutrophils are capable of inducing tissue damage, and further suggest oxygen radicals as key mediators of this event. It is possible that the deleterious effects of oxygen radicals may be mediated through proteinases, if oxidant inactivation of antiproteinases occurs.

Further data supporting a role for the neutrophil in lung injury has emerged from the chronically catheterized unanaesthetized sheep model first described by Staub and colleagues (75). In this model, lung lymph is collected without the confounding effects on anaesthesia. In this system increased flow of protein-rich lymph in the absence of major haemodynamic changes and persistence of normal or increased lymph/plasma protein concentration ratio is considered to represent increased vascular permeability. Increased permeability has been demonstrated after administration of i.v. Gram-negative bacteria (65–78) and microemboli (79). These studies have shown attenuation of lung injury by rendering

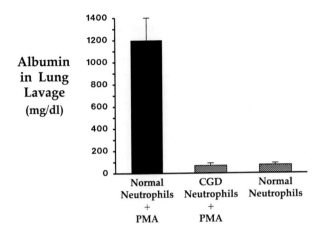

Fig. 7.6 Addition of normal human neutrophils stimulated with PMA increased ($P \leq 0.05$) lavage albumin concentration in isolated perfused rabbit lungs compared to the addition of unstimulated neutrophils. In contrast, addition of neutrophils from patients with chronic granulomatous diseases (CGD) stimulated by PMA did not increase lavage albumin concentration. Modified from reference 138.

sheep neutropenic with the use of bone marrow-suppressing drugs. Some questions have arisen, however, concerning the validity of using such non-specific means to deplete sheep of neutrophils.

Similar findings have been observed in other animal models of lung injury. Glass bead microemboli in dogs lead to an increased extravascular lung water content that can be attenuated by rendering the animals neutropenic (80). Similarly, hyperoxic lung injury in rabbits is decreased by neutrophil depletion (81).

Based on these and other studies the neutrophil hypothesis was refined to state that neutrophils might injure lungs by activation and subsequent release of toxic products that might include proteases, arachidonate products, and/or ROS. In support of ROS playing an important role, dimethylthiourea (DMTU), a potent ·OH, H_2O_2, and HOCl scavenger, inhibited PMA-stimulated neutrophil-induced lung oedema in isolated perfused rabbit lungs (73). Furthermore, neutrophils isolated from patients with CGD did not cause lung injury. The inability of CGD neutrophils to confer injury even when activated argues strongly for a major role for oxygen radicals in acute lung injury in these experimental models.

To explore the ability of ROS to induce lung injury further, isolated rabbit lungs were perfused with xanthine/xanthine oxidase (a generator of superoxide anion) and glucose/glucose oxidase (a generator of H_2O_2). Both manoeuvres caused lung injury. DMTU and catalase conferred protection while SOD did not, suggesting a central role for H_2O_2 in the pathogenesis of injury. The direct intratracheal instillation of ROS has also been shown to induce lung injury. In these studies O_2^-, H_2O_2, and MPO-derived species appeared to be most toxic (24).

To remove confounding variables encountered in whole animal or isolated organ preparations, a series of experiments has been performed on homogeneous populations of cultured cells, most notably endothelial cells. ROS have been shown directly to injure cultured endothelial cells (26, 27) and lung parenchymal cells *in vitro* (23). In addition to direct injury, oxygen radicals can amplify the inflammatory response (82, 83).

Further evidence supporting a role for neutrophils in injury to lung tissue concerns a role for neutrophil-derived proteases. Proteolytic enzymes have been shown to cause haemorrhagic pulmonary oedema and emphysema in animal models (84). Intratracheal neutrophil elastase also causes a low-pressure pulmonary oedema in isolated perfused rabbit lungs (85). In addition, neutrophil-derived proteases cause vascular injury and endo-thelial cell detachment (86, 87). As noted above, ARDS patients have detectable elastolytic activity in BAL. Furthermore, neutrophil-derived proteases may interact with oxygen radicals to further the damage (see Section 3.3). This synergistic interplay between proteases and oxygen radicals may be far more prevalent than currently recognized.

Another potential mechanism of neutrophil-induced lung injury may be through products of AA (prostaglandins, thromboxanes, and leuko-trienes). These compounds affect pulmonary vascular and airway smooth muscle as well as vascular permeability. Infusion of AA or its products has caused increases in pulmonary vascular resistance (88–91). In addition, endotoxin-induced haemodynamic changes in sheep and dogs apparently involve AA production because vasoconstriction is blocked by cyclo-oxygenase inhibitors (92, 93). Furthermore, increased pulmonary vascular resistance in sheep is associated with elevated thromboxane B_2 levels in lung lymph (94–96).

4.2   Ischaemia–reperfusion (I/R)

4.2.1   *I/R-mediated cardiac injury*

There is growing evidence that the syndrome of myocardial infarction is largely due to injury sustained from ischaemia followed by reperfusion (97). ROS are increasingly recognized for their important contribution to this I/R-induced injury, particularly during the reperfusion phase. The potential sources of these ROS include mitochondrial electron transport, purine catabolism by xanthine oxidase, prostaglandin biosynthesis, and tissue infiltration by neutrophils and/or monocytes. Indeed, there is strong evidence that neutrophils are an important source of injury in myocardial infarction (98).

Several lines of evidence suggest a role for free radicals in myocardial

I/R injury. Many indirect studies have utilized free radical scavengers to reduce damage in experimental animal models of I/R (99–102). This reduction infers a role for free radicals in the I/R-induced injury. However, studies using scavengers suffer from their indirect nature and possible non-specificity of the scavengers. More direct evidence comes from recent studies using electron paramagnetic resonance spectroscopy where free radicals may be directly measured in biological systems. Using isolated-perfused rabbit hearts subjected to global ischaemia, Zweier *et al.* (103, 104) demonstrated a rapid increase in free radical production upon reperfusion.

Recent investigations have begun to address the source of myocardial-damaging free radicals. Associated with I/R injury of the myocardium is an intense cellular inflammatory response which includes large numbers of neutrophils. It is reasonable to hypothesize that these neutrophils may extend the injury. In fact, several studies have noted a correlation between myocardial infarct size and the degree of neutrophil infiltration (105–108). Neutrophils infiltrate early and progressively with evolution of myocardial infarction (109, 110). These indirect data do not prove a causal relationship between the neutrophil influx and tissue injury, even though neutrophil influx precedes myocardial cell necrosis (107). Further, albeit indirect, evidence has emerged from studies demonstrating the presence of chemotactic factors generated during tissue injury and myocardial reperfusion in particular. These include complement fragments, leukotriene B_4, and plasma proteins (82, 111).

More direct evidence for the role of the neutrophil in I/R myocardial injury has been accumulating. Romson *et al.* (106) demonstrated in a dog model of myocardial infarction that prior neutrophil depletion reduced infarct size by 43 per cent compared to control animals replete with neutrophils. Using different techniques other laboratories have corroborated the importance of the neutrophil (107, 112, 113). Furthermore, studies utilizing monoclonal antibodies that block neutrophil adhesion (anti-Mo-1, anti-CD11b) also dramatically reduce infarct size in a dog model (114) (see Chapter 8, Section 2.2). Finally, numerous pharmacologic interventions which either affect neutrophil function or scavenge oxygen radicals have been investigated in I/R myocardial injury (111, 115–117).

Human studies have also demonstrated a reduction in reperfusion arrythmias after intracoronary streptokinase in patients rendered locally neutrophil-dependent with a leukocyte-removal filter (118). Dinerman *et al.* (119) have shown evidence of neutrophil elastase release during acute myocardial infarction and unstable angina (119).

In contrast to the deleterious effects of neutrophils in cardiac I/R alluded to above, there is evidence that neutrophils may also be beneficial. We utilized the isolated rat heart model to study this phenomenon (120). We found that hearts isolated from rats treated 36 h before with interleukin-1

(IL-1) had increased glucose-6-phosphate dehydrogenase (G6PD) activity and decreased H_2O_2 levels and injury after I/R (ischaemia = 20 min, reperfusion = 40 min), compared with hearts from untreated rats (Fig. 7.7). Hearts isolated from rats treated 6 h earlier with IL-1 had increased neutrophils, H_2O_2 levels and oxidized glutathione (GSSG) contents compared with hearts from control rats. Depletion of circulating blood neutrophils by prior treatment with vinblastine prevented both the early (6 h) IL-1-induced increases in myocardial neutrophil accumulation, H_2O_2 levels and GSSG contents, as well as the late (36 h) increases in myocardial G6PD activity and protection from I/R (Fig. 7.8). It appeared that a limited, early, neutrophil-derived oxidant stress caused compensatory responses which contributed to protection from I/R.

4.2.2 I/R-mediated renal injury

It appears clear that oxygen radicals are contributing factors to renal injury following I/R (121). This conclusion is based largely on the protection seen in I/R models following the administration of oxygen radical scavengers, such as superoxide dismutase and catalase. Since the role of neutrophils in renal I/R injury was less clear, we again used an isolated perfused rat organ (kidney) model. We measured glomerular filtration rate (GFR) as an index of injury. Ischaemia for 20 min followed by reperfusion for 60 min caused a marked decrease in GFR (Fig. 7.9) (122). Addition of unstimulated neutrophils isolated from healthy subjects caused further deterioration of GFR compared to ischaemic kidneys reperfused without neutrophils. In

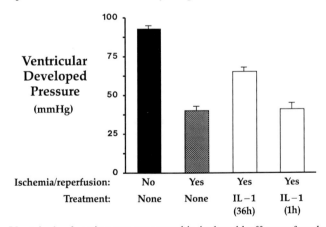

Fig. 7.7 Ventricular function was measured in isolated buffer-perfused rat hearts. Ventricular developed pressure was decreased ($P \leqslant 0.05$) after 20 min ischaemia followed by 40 min of reperfusion (I/R) compared with control hearts not exposed to I/R. In contrast, after I/R, hearts from rats treated 36 h prior with IL-1 (30 µg/kg i.p.) before heart isolation had increased ($P \leqslant 0.05$) developed pressure compared with I/R hearts not treated with IL-1. IL-1 given 1 h prior to heart isolation did not protect from I/R injury. Modified from reference 120.

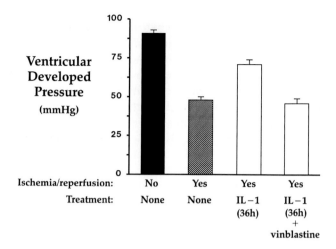

Fig. 7.8 Ventricular function was measured in isolated buffer-perfused rat hearts. Ventricular developed pressure was decreased ($P \le 0.05$) after 20 min ischaemia followed by 40 min reperfusion (I/R) compared to control hearts not exposed to I/R. In contrast, after I/R, hearts from rats treated 36 h prior with IL-1 (30 μg/kg i.p.) before heart isolation had increased ($P \le 0.05$) developed pressure compared with I/R hearts not treated with IL-1. The induction of neutropenia with vinblastine blocked the protection seen after IL-1 administration. Vinblastine treatment alone (without IL-1) had no effect on developed pressure after I/R. Modified from reference 120.

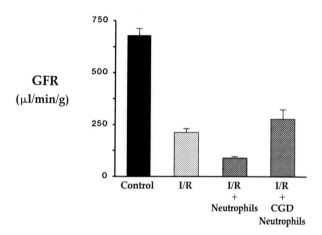

Fig. 7.9 Isolated perfused rat kidneys were prepared. Exposure to ischaemia for 20 min followed by reperfusion for 60 min (I/R) caused a marked decrease in GFR. Exposure to unstimulated normal human neutrophils with reperfusion caused a further decrease in GFR. In contrast, exposure to unstimulated neutrophils from CGD patients did not cause a further reduction in GFR compared with treatment with I/R alone. Modified from reference 122.

contast to ischaemic kidneys, addition of unstimulated neutrophils to non-ischaemic (control) kidneys did not cause functional alterations. Two further experiments suggested that oxygen radicals contributed to renal injury. First, reperfusion of I/R-treated kidneys with neutrophils isolated from a patient with CGD did not augment the injury from I/R compared with reperfusion with buffer alone. Second, the addition of the H_2O_2 scavenger, catalase, to the reperfusion buffer decreased the neutrophil-mediated injury. Thus, the findings for I/R were very similar to the findings for ARDS.

4.2.3   I/R-mediated skeletal muscle injury

Oxygen metabolites contribute to skeletal muscle injury following I/R (123). We investigated the possibility that neutrophils might contribute to the oxidant burden in skeletal muscle I/R (124). A model of rat hindlimb I/R was developed whereby the hindlimb was rendered ischaemic by application of a tight-fitting band and then blood flow was reintroduced. The gastrocnemius muscle was then isolated by dissection and muscle viability was determined by the amount of force generated during tetanic contraction (after electrical stimulation). The contralateral limb was used as a control. We found that I/R-treated hindlimbs generated approximately 14 per cent of the force compared with the untreated contralateral hindlimb (Fig. 7.10). Rats were then rendered neutropenic by treatment with vinblastine 4 days prior, resulting in only 6 per cent of the number of neutrophils found in control rats. When neutropenic rats were subjected to hindlimb I/R, recovered function was significantly greater compared with

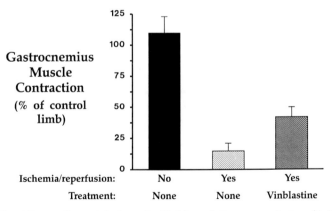

Fig. 7.10 After unilateral ischaemia (3 h) and then reperfusion (4 h) (I/R), gastrocnemius muscles from untreated rats had markedly decreased ($P \leq 0.05$) contraction compared with rat hindlimbs not exposed to I/R. In contrast, rats treated with vinblastine to induce neutropenia had increased ($P \leq 0.05$) muscle contraction after I/R compared with I/R-exposed rats not treated with vinblastine. Modified from reference 124.

control rats subjected to I/R. These data suggest that neutrophils contribute to muscle injury following I/R. By comparison, rats treated only 1 day prior with vinblastine (so that they still had normal neutrophil numbers), then subjected to I/R had similar muscle damage to control rats subjected to I/R. This last observation provides strong evidence that the ability of vinblastine to decrease I/R-induced injury was due to its ability to deplete neutrophils rather than non-specific effects of the drug.

4.3   Rheumatoid arthritis

Neutrophils account for more than 90 per cent of cells seen within the synovial fluid of rheumatoid arthritis patients. It has been suggested that lysosomal enzymes and other mediators of inflammation released by neutrophils after uptake of immune complexes are responsible for a large portion of the inflammation in rheumatoid joints (3, 125).

4.4   Inflammatory bowel disease

Animal studies have suggested that neutrophils may play a role in the pathogenesis of inflammatory bowel disease (126). Human studies have suggested alterations in neutrophil metabolism in patients with Crohn's disease and ulcerative colitis (127).

4.5   Asthma

Asthma is a common clinical syndrome characterized by bronchial hyperreactivity, excessive mucous secretion, and bronchoconstriction. Attention has focused recently on inflammation as an important pathogenic factor because the airway in asthmatics contains many neutrophils. Whether the neutrophil is merely responding to a site of inflammation or participating in the genesis of the inflammation is less clear. However, a pathogenic role for neutrophils has been explored in animal models. Neutrophil depletion attenuates the late phase asthmatic response and airway obstruction in a rabbit model of the late asthmatic response (128). Others have shown that the rat late phase cutaneous response is attenuated when the animals are rendered neutropenic by either vinblastine treatment (129) or anti-neutrophil antibodies (130). Of interest, peripheral blood neutrophils isolated from asthmatic patients demonstrate enhanced superoxide anion (O_2^-) compared with control patients (131), suggesting a possible role of neutrophil-derived free radicals in asthma. Further studies are needed to define the extent that neutrophils participate in human asthma.

4.6 Gout

The pathogenesis of acute gouty arthritis has been well delineated and it involves neutrophils. Briefly, after neutrophils phagocytose insoluble uric acid crystals, the neutrophil is destroyed releasing toxic substances which perpetuate the gout attack. The effectiveness of anti-inflammatory drugs, such as colchicine, in gouty arthritis is due in large part to their anti-neutrophil effects (132).

4.7 Neutrophilic dermatoses

A number of dermatologic diseases involve neutrophil infiltration of the skin which have been thought to augment the inflammatory response and lead to perpetuation of tissue injury. These include neutrophilic dermatoses such as Sweet's syndrome (133) and Behçet's disease (134), pyoderma gangrenosum (135), and psoriasis (136, 137).

5 Conclusions

Neutrophils are now considered to be both beneficial and detrimental in human health, or friendly and angry as depicted in the cartoon (Fig. 7.11). The mechanisms responsible for either behaviour of the neutrophil seem to be the same in many respects so we are now challenged with learning the difference in these intricate pathways that makes the cell good or bad. As we learn these mechanisms, we will hopefully be in a position to maximize

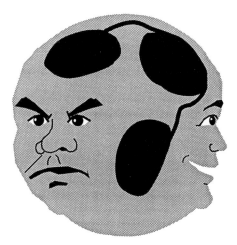

Fig. 7.11 Schematic diagram portraying the potential beneficial and deleterious effects of a neutrophil.

the beneficial features of neutrophils while minimizing their negative effects. Many new and increasingly specific ways of limiting the actions of neutrophils are on the horizon, so our knowledge of the role of neutrophils in health and disease will expand rapidly in the coming years. This knowledge should lead to a better opportunity to help these patients like the one described in our case report.

References

1 Malech, H. L. and Gallin, J. I. (1987). Neutrophils in human diseases. *N. Engl. J. Med.,* **317,** 687–94.
2 Weiss, S. J. (1989). Tissue destruction by neutrophils. *N. Engl. J. Med.,* **320,** 365–76.
3 Henson, P. M. (1972). Pathologic mechanisms in neutrophil-mediated injury. *Am. J. Pathol.,* **68,** 593–605.
4 Test, S. T. and Weiss, S. J. (1986). The generation and utilization of chlorinated oxidants by human neutrophils. *Adv. Free Radical Biol. Med.,* **2,** 91–116.
5 Clark, R. A. and Klebanoff, S. J. (1975). Neutrophil mediated tumor cell cytotoxicity: Role of the peroxide system. *J. Exp. Med.,* **141,** 1442–7.
6 Hay, E. D. (1981). *Cell biology of the extracellular matrix.* Plenum Press, New York.
7 Vracko, R. (1974). Basal lamina scaffold-anatomy and significance for maintenance of orderly tissue structure. *Am. J. Pathol.,* **77,** 314–46.
8 Henson, P. M., Henson, J. E., Fitlschen, C., Kimani, G., Bratton, D. L., and Riches, D. W. H. (1988). Phagocytic cells: degranulation and secretion. In *Inflammation: basic principles and clinical correlates* (ed. J. I. Gallin, I. M. Goldstein, and R. Snyderman), pp. 363–80. Raven Press, New York.
9 Janoff, A. (1985). Elastase in tissue injury. *Annu. Rev. Med.,* **36,** 207–16.
10 Travis, J. and Salveson, G. S. (1983). Human plasma proteinase inhibitors. *Annu. Rev. Biochem.,* **52,** 655–709.
11 Baird, B. R., Cheronis, J. C., Sandhaus, R. A., Berger, E. A., White, C. W., and Repine, J. E. (1986). O_2 metabolites and neutrophil elastase synergistically cause edematous injury in isolated rat lungs. *J. Appl. Physiol.,* **61,** 2224–9.
12 Weiss, S. J. and Peppin, G. J. (1986). Collagenolytic metalloenzymes of the human neutrophil: characteristics, regulation and potential function in vivo. *Biochem. Pharmacol.,* **35,** 3189–97.
13 Kramps, J. A., Van Twisk, C., and Dijkman, J. H. (1987). Oxidative

inactivation of bronchial antileukoprotease by triggered polymorphonuclear leukocytes. *Am. Rev. Resp. Dis.,* **135,** 290 (abstr.).

14 Weiss, S. J., Peppin, G., Ortiz, X., Ragsdale, C., and Test, S. T.
(1985). Oxidative autoactivation of latent collagenase by human
neutrophils. *Science,* **227,** 747–9.

15 Peppin, G. J. and Weiss, S. J. (1986). Activation of the endogenous
metalloproteinase, gelatinase, by triggered human neutrophils. *Proc.
Natl Acad. Sci. USA,* **83,** 4322–6.

16 Okada, Y., Watanabe, S., Nakanishi, I., Kishi, J., Hayakawa, T.,
Watorek, W., Travis, J., and Nagase, H. (1988). Inactivation of tissue
inhibitor of metalloproteinases by neutrophil elastase and other serine
proteinases. *FEBS Lett.,* **229,** 157–60.

17 Janoff, A. (1972). Human granulocyte elastase: Further delineation of
its role in connective tissue damage. *Am. J. Pathol.,* **68,** 579–92.

18 Cochrane, C. G. and Aiken, B. S. (1966). Polymorphonuclear leukocytes in immunologic reactions. The destruction of vascular basement
membrane in vivo and in vitro. *J. Exp. Med.,* **124,** 733–52.

19 Plow, E. F. (1978). Comparative immunochemical characterization of
products of plasmin and leukocyte protease cleavage of human fibrinogen. *Thromb. Res.,* **12,** 473–90.

20 Snyderman, R., Shin, H. S., and Dannenberg, A. M. (1972).
Macrophage proteinase and inflammation: The production of chemotactic activity from the fifth component of complement by macrophage
proteinase. *J. Immunol.,* **109,** 896–8.

21 Ambruso, D. R. and Johnston, R. B. Jr (1981). Lactoferrin enhances
hydroxyl radical production by human neutrophils, neutrophil particulate fractions, and an enzymatic generating system. *J. Clin. Invest.,* **67,**
352–60.

22 Simon, R. H., Scoggin, C. H., and Patterson, D. (1981). Hydrogen
peroxide causes the fatal injury to human fibroblasts exposed to
oxygen radicals. *J. Biol. Chem.,* **256,** 7181–6.

23 Martin, W. J., Gadek, J. E., Hunninghake, G. W., and Crystal, R. G.
(1981). Oxidant injury of lung parenchymal cells. *J. Clin. Invest.,* **68,**
1277–88.

24 Johnson, K. J., Fantone, J. C., Kaplan, J., and Ward, P. A. (1981). In
vivo damage of rat lungs by oxygen metabolites. *J. Clin. Invest.,* **67,**
983–93.

25 Johnson, K. J. and Ward, P. A. (1981). Role of oxygen metabolites in
immune complex injury of lung. *J. Immunol.,* **126,** 2365–9.

26 Weiss, S. J., Young, J., LoBuglio, A. F., Slivka, A., and Nimeh, N.
F. (1981). Role of hydrogen peroxide in neutrophil-mediated destruction of cultured endothelial cells. *J. Clin. Invest.,* **68,** 714–21.

27 Sacks, T., Moldow, C. F., Craddock, P. R., Bowers, T. K.,
and Jacob, H. S. (1978). Oxygen radicals mediate endothelial cell

damage by complement-stimulated granulocytes. *J. Clin. Invest.*, **61**, 1161–7.

28 Weiss, S. J. (1980). The role of superoxide in the destruction of erythrocyte targets by human neutrophils. *J. Biol. Chem.*, **255**, 9912–17.

29 McCord, J. M. (1974). Free radicals and inflammation: Protection of synovial fluid by superoxide dismutase. *Science*, **185**, 529–31.

30 Smith, M. J. H. (1979). Prostaglandins and the polymorphonuclear leukocyte. *Agents Actions*, **6**, 91–103.

31 Zurier, R. B. and Sayadoff, D. M. (1975). Release of prostaglandins from human polymorphonuclear leukocytes. *Inflammation*, **1**, 93–101.

32 Goldstein, I. M., Malmsten, C. L., Kindahl, H., Kaplan, H. B., Radmark, O., Samuelsson, B., and Weissmann, G. (1978). Thromboxane generation by human peripheral blood polymorphonuclear leukocytes. *J. Exp. Med.*, **148**, 787–92.

33 Ford-Hutchison, A. W., Bray, M. A., Doig, M. N., Shipley, M. E., and Smith, M. J. H. (1980). Leukotriene B, a potent chemokinetic and aggregating substance released from polymorphonuclear leukocytes. *Nature*, **286**, 264–5.

34 Weissmann, G. (1982). Activation of neutrophils and the lesions of rheumatoid arthritis. *J. Lab. Clin. Med.*, **100**, 322–33.

35 Wolff, S. P., Garner, A., and Dean, R. T. (1986). Free radicals, lipids and protein degradation. *Trends Biochem. Sci.*, **11**, 27–31.

36 Schraufstatter, I. U., Revak, S. D., and Cochrane, C. G. (1984). Proteases and oxidants in experimental pulmonary inflammatory injury. *J. Clin. Invest.*, **73**, 1175–84.

37 Sinha, U., Sinha, S., and Janoff, A. (1988). Characterization of sheep alpha-1-proteinase inhibitor: important differences from the human protein. *Am. Rev. Resp. Dis.*, **137**, 558–63.

38 Fowler, A. A., Hamman, R. F., Good, J. T., Benson, K. N., Baird, M., Eberle, D. J., *et al.* (1983). Adult respiratory distress syndrome: Risk with common predispositions. *Ann. Intern. Med.*, **98**, 593–7.

39 Repine, J. E. (1992). Scientific perspectives on adult respiratory distress syndrome. *Lancet*, **339**, 466–9.

40 Ashbaugh, D. G., Bigelow, D. B., Petty, T. L., and Levine, B. E. (1967). Acute respiratory distress in adults. *Lancet*, **ii**, 319–23.

41 Bernard, G. R., Luce, J. M., Sprung, C. L., Rinaldo, J. E., Tate, R. M., Sibbald, W. J., *et al.* (1987). High-dose corticosteroids in patients with the adult respiratory distress syndrome. *N. Engl. J. Med.*, **317**, 1565–70.

42 Ratliff, N. B., Wilson, J. W., Mikat, E., Hackel, D. B., and Graham, T. C. (1971). The lung in hemorrhagic shock. IV. The role of the polymorphonuclear leukocyte. *Am. J. Pathol.*, **65**, 325–34.

43 Bachofen, M. and Weibel, E. R. (1977). Alterations of the gas ex-

change apparatus in adult respiratory insufficiency associated with septicemia. *Am. Rev. Resp. Dis.,* **116,** 589–615.

44 Pratt, P. C. (1978). Pathology of adult respiratory distress syndrome. In *The lung: structure, function and disease* (ed. W. M. Thurlbeck and M. R. Abell), pp. 43–57. The Williams and Wilkins Company, Baltimore.

45 Craddock, P. R., Fehr, J., Brigham, K. L., Kronenberg, R. S., and Jacob, H. S. (1977). Complement and leukocyte-mediated pulmonary dysfunction in hemodialysis. *N. Engl. J. Med.,* **296,** 769–74.

46 Craddock, P. R., Fehr, J., Dalmasso, A. P., Brigham, K. L., and Jacob, H. S. (1977). Hemodialysis leukopenia. Pulmonary vascular leukostasis resulting from complement activation by dialyzer cellophane membranes. *J. Clin. Invest.,* **59,** 879–88.

47 Tate, R. M. and Repine, J. E. (1983). Neutrophils and the adult respiratory distress syndrome. *Am. Rev. Respir. Dis.,* **128,** 552–9.

48 Lee, C. T., Fein, A. M., Lippmann, M., Holtzman, H., Kimbel, P., and Weinbaum, G. (1981). Elastolytic activity in pulmonary lavage fluid from patients with adult respiratory distress syndrome. *N. Engl. J. Med.,* **304,** 192–6.

49 McGuire, W. W., Spragg, R. G., Cohen, A. B., and Cochrane, C. G. (1982). Studies on the pathogenesis of the adult respiratory distress syndrome. *J. Clin. Invest.,* **69,** 543–53.

50 Fowler, A. A., Walchak, S., Giclas, P. C., Henson, P. M., and Hyers, T. M. (1982). Characterization of antiproteinase activity in the adult respiratory distress syndrome. *Chest,* **81 (Suppl),** 50S–1S.

51 Zheutlin, L. M., Thonor, E. J., Jacobs, E. R., Hanley, M. E., Balk, R. A., and Bone, R. C. (1986). Plasma elastase levels in the adult respiratory distress syndrome. *J. Crit. Care,* **1,** 39–44.

52 Rocker, G. M., Pearson, D., Wiseman, M. S., and Shale, D. J. (1989). Diagnostic criteria for adult respiratory distress syndrome: Time for reappraisal. *Lancet,* **i,** 120–3.

53 Laufe, M. D., Simon, R. H., Flint, A., and Keller, J. B. (1986). Adult respiratory distress syndrome in neutropenic patients. *Am. J. Med.,* **80,** 1022–6.

54 Ognibene, F. P., Martin, S. E., Parker, M. M., Schlesinger, T., Roach, P., Burch, C., *et al.* (1986). Adult respiratory distress syndrome in patients with severe neutropenia. *N. Engl. J. Med.,* **315,** 547–51.

55 Rinaldo, J. E. and Borovetz, H. (1985). Deterioration of oxygenation and abnormal lung microvascular permeability during resolution of leukopenia in patients with diffuse lung injury. *Am. Rev. Respir. Dis.,* **131,** 579–83.

56 Hammerschmidt, D. E., Weaver, L. J., Hudson, L. D., Craddock, P. R., and Jacob, H. S. (1980). Association of complement activation

and elevated plasma-C5a with adult respiratory distress syndrome. Pathophysiological relevance and possible prognostic value. *Lancet, 3,* 947–9.

57 Zimmerman, G. A., Renzetti, A. D., and Hill, H. R. (1983). Functional and metabolic activity of granulocytes from patients with adult respiratory distress syndrome. *Am. Rev. Respir. Dis.,* **127,** 290–300.

58 Parsons, P. E., Worthen, G. S., Moore, F. A., Moore, E. E., and Henson, P. M. (1990). Activity levels of circulating neutrophils in acute lung injury. *Am. Rev. Respir. Dis.,* **141,** A511 (abstr.).

59 Martin, T. R., Pistorese, B. P., Hudson, L. D., and Maunder, R. J. (1991). The function of lung and blood neutrophils in patients with the adult respiratory distress syndrome. *Am. Rev. Respir. Dis.,* **144,** 254–62.

60 Hoover, R. L., Briggs, R. T., and Karnovsky, M. J. (1978). The adhesive interaction between polymorphonuclear leukocytes and endothelial cells in vitro. *Cell,* **14,** 423–8.

61 Bowman, C. M., Harada, R. N., and Repine, J. E. (1983). Hyperoxia stimulates alveolar macrophages to produce and release a factor which increases neutrophil adherence. *Inflammation, 7,* 331–8.

62 Harada, R. N., Vatter, A. E., and Repine, J. E. (1984). Macrophage effector function in pulmonary oxygen toxicity: hyperoxia damages and stimulates alveolar macrophages to make and release chemotaxins for polymorphonuclear leukocytes. *J. Leukocyte Biol.,* **35,** 373–83.

63 Kazmierowski, J. A., Gallin, J. I., and Reynolds, H. Y. (1978). Mechanism for the inflammatory response in primate lungs: Demonstration and partial characterization of an alveolar macrophage derived chemotactic factor with preferential activity for polymorphonuclear leukocytes. *J. Clin. Invest.,* **59,** 273–81.

64 Hunninghake, G. W., Gallin, J. I., and Fauci, A. S. (1978). Immunologic reactivity of the lung: The in vivo and in vitro generation of a neutrophil chemotactic factor by alveolar macrophages. *Am. Rev. Respir. Dis.,* **117,** 15–23.

65 Fox, R. B., Hoidal, J. R., Brown, D. M., and Repine, J. E. (1981). Pulmonary inflammation due to oxygen toxicity: involvement of chemotactic factors and polymorphonuclear leukocytes. *Am. Rev. Respir. Dis.,* **123,** 521–3.

66 Harada, R. N., Bowman, C. M., Fox, R. B., and Repine, J. E. (1982). Alveolar macrophage secretions: Initiators of inflammation in pulmonary oxygen toxicity. *Chest, 81,* 52S–3S.

67 Larsen, G. L., McCarthy, K., Webster, R. O., Henson, J. E., and Henson, P. M. (1980). A differential effect of C5a and C5a des arg in the induction of pulmonary inflammation. *Am. J. Pathol.,* **100,** 179–92.

68 Shaw, J. O., Henson, P. M., Henson, J. E., and Webster, R. O.

(1980). Lung inflammation induced by complement-derived chemotactic fragments in the alveolus. *Lab. Invest.,* **42,** 547–8.

69 Worthen, G. S., Goins, A., Mitchell, B., Larsen, G., Reeves, J., and Henson, P. M. (1982). Effects of intravascular C5 fragments and platelet activating factor on lung injury and neutrophil accumulation in the rabbit. *Am. Rev. Respir. Dis.,* **125,** 274 (abstr.).

70 Henson, P. M., Larsen, G. L., Webster, R. O., Mitchell, B. C., Goins, A. J., and Henson, J. E. (1982). Pulmonary microvascular alterations and injury induced by complement fragments: Synergistic effect of complement activation, neutrophil sequestration, and prostaglandins. *Ann. N.Y. Acad. Sci.,* **384,** 287–99.

71 Till, G. O., Johnson, K. J., Kunkel, R., and Ward, P. A. (1982). Intravascular activation of complement and acute lung injury. Dependency on neutrophils and toxic oxygen metabolites. *J. Clin. Invest.,* **69,** 1126–35.

72 Parsons, P. E. and Giglas, P. C. (1990). The terminal complement complex (sC5b-9) is not specifically associated with the development of the adult respiratory distress syndrome. *Am. Rev. Respir. Dis.,* **141,** 98–103.

73 Shasby, D. M., Vanbenthuysen, K. M., Tate, R. M., Shasby, S. S., McMurtry, I. F., and Repine, J. E. (1982). Granulocytes mediate acute edematous lung injury in rabbits and isolated rabbit lungs perfused with phorbol myristate acetate: Role of oxygen radicals. *Am. Rev. Respir. Dis.,* **125,** 443–7.

74 Repine, J. E., White, J. G., Clawson, C. C., and Holmes, B. M. (1974). Effect of phorbol myristate acetate on the metabolism and ultrastructure of neutrophils in chronic granulomatous disease. *J. Clin. Invest.,* **54,** 83–90.

75 Staub, N., Bland, R., Brigham, K., Demling, R., Erdmann, J., and Woolverton, W. (1975). Preparation of chronic lung lymph fistula in sheep. *J. Surg. Res.,* **19,** 315–20.

76 Brigham, K. L., Bowers, R., and Haynes, J. (1979). Increased sheep lung vascular permeability caused by *E. coli* endotoxin. *Circ. Res.,* **45,** 292–7.

77 Brigham, K. L., Woolverton, W., Blake, I., and Staub, N. (1974). Increased sheep lung vascular permeability caused by *Pseudomonas* bacteria. *J. Clin. Invest.,* **54,** 792–804.

78 Heflin, A. J. and Brigham, K. L. (1981). Prevention by granulocyte depletion of increased vascular permeability of sheep lung following endotoxemia. *J. Clin. Invest.,* **68,** 1253–60.

79 Flick, M. R., Perel, G., and Staub, N. C. (1981). Leukocytes are required for increased lung microvascular permeability after microembolism in sheep. *Circ. Res.,* **48,** 344–51.

80 Johnson, A. and Malik, A. B. (1980). Effect of granulocytopenia on

extravascular lung water content after microembolization. *Am. Rev. Respir. Dis.*, **122**, 561–6.

81 Shasby, D. M., Fox, R. B., Harada, R. N., and Repine, J. E. (1982). Reduction of the edema of acute hyperoxic lung injury by granulocyte depletion. *J. Appl. Physiol.*, **52**, 1237–44.

82 Petrone, W. F., English, D. K., Wong, K., and McCord, J. M. (1980). Free radicals and inflammation: Superoxide-dependent activation of a neutrophil chemotactic factor in plasma. *Proc. Natl Acad. Sci. USA*, **77**, 1159–63.

83 Perez, H. D., Weksler, B. B., and Goldstein, I. M. (1980). Generation of a chemotactic lipid from arachidonic acid by exposure to a superoxide generating system. *Inflammation*, **4**, 313–28.

84 Senior, R. M., Tegner, H., Kuhn, C., Ohlsson, K., Starcher, B. C., and Pierce, J. A. (1977). The induction of pulmonary emphysema with human leukocyte elastase. *Am. Rev. Respir. Dis.*, **116**, 469–75.

85 Spragg, R. J., Lonkey, S. A., Loomis, W. H., Marsh, J., and Abraham, J. L. (1982). Human neutrophil elastase causes acute high permeability pulmonary edema in the isolated perfused rabbit lung. *Am. Rev. Respir. Dis.*, **125**, 276.

86 Janoff, A. (1970). Mediators of tissue damage in leukocyte lysosomes. Further studies on human granulocyte elastase. *Lab. Invest.*, **22**, 228–36.

87 Harlan, J. M., Killen, P. D., Harker, L. A., Striker, G. E., and Wright, D. G. (1981). Neutrophil-mediated endothelial injury in vitro. Mechanisms of cell detachment. *J. Clin. Invest.*, **68**, 1394–405.

88 Ogletree, M. L. and Brigham, K. L. (1980). Arachidonate raises vascular resistance but not permeability in lungs of awake sheep. *J. Appl. Physiol.*, **48**, 581–6.

89 Kadowitz, P. J., Gruetter, C. A., Spannhake, E. W., and Hyman, A. L. (1981). Pulmonary vascular responses to prostaglandins. *Fed. Proc.*, **40**, 1991–6.

90 Bowers, R. E., Ellis, E. F., Brigham, K. L., and Oates, J. A. (1979). Effects of prostaglandin cyclic endoperoxides on the lung circulation of unanesthetized sheep. *J. Clin. Invest.*, **63**, 131–7.

91 Wicks, T. C., Rose, J. C., Johnson, M., Ramwell, P. W., and Kot, P. A. (1976). Vascular responses to arachidonic acid in the perfused canine lung. *Circ. Res.*, **38**, 167–71.

92 Brigham, K. L. and Ogletree, M. L. (1981). Effects of prostaglandins and related compounds on lung vascular permeability. *Bull. Eur. Physiopathol. Respir.*, **17**, 703–22.

93 Ogletree, M. L. and Brigham, K. L. (1982). Effects of cyclooxygenase inhibitors on pulmonary vascular responses to endotoxin in unanesthetized sheep. *Prostaglandins Leukotrienes Med.*, **8**, 489–502.

94 Huttmeier, P. C., Watkins, W. D., Peterson, M. B. and Zapol, W. M.

(1982). Acute pulmonary hypertension and lung thromboxane release after endotoxin infusion in normal and leukopenic sheep. *Circ. Res.,* **50,** 688–94.

95 Smith, M. E., Gunther, R., Gee, M., Flynn, J., and Demling, R. H. (1981). Leukocytes, platelets, and thromboxane A2 in endotoxin-induced lung injury. *Surgery,* **90,** 102–7.

96 Demling, R. H. (1982). Role of prostaglandins in acute pulmonary microvascular injury. *Ann. N.Y. Acad. Sci.,* **384,** 517–34.

97 McCord, J. M. (1985). Oxygen-derived free radicals in post-ischemic tissue injury. *N. Engl. J. Med.,* **312,** 159–63.

98 Lucchesi, B. R. and Mullane, K. M. (1986). Leukocytes and ischemia-induced myocardial injury. *Annu. Rev. Pharmacol. Toxicol.,* **26,** 201–24.

99 Shlafer, M., Kane, P. F., and Kirsh, M. M. (1982). Superoxide dismutase plus catalase enhances the efficacy of hypothermic cardioplegia to protect the globally ischemic, reperfused heart. *J. Thorac. Cardiovasc. Surg.,* **83,** 830–9.

100 Shlafer, M., Kane, P. F., Wiggins, V. Y., and Kirsh, M. M. (1982). Possible role for cytotoxic oxygen metabolites in the pathogenesis of cardiac ischemic injury. *Circulation,* **66 (suppl I),** 85–92.

101 Jolly, S. R., Kane, W. J., Bailie, M. B., Abrams, G. D., and Lucchesi, B. R. (1984). Canine myocardial reperfusion injury. Its reduction by the combined administration of superoxide dismutase and catalase. *Circ. Res.,* **54,** 277–85.

102 Werns, S. W., Shea, M. J., Driscoll, E. M., Cohen, C., Abrams, G. D., Pitt, B., and Lucchesi, B. R. (1985). The independent effects of oxygen radical scavengers on canine infarct size. Reduction by superoxide dismutase but not catalase. *Circ. Res.,* **56,** 895–8.

103 Zweier, J. L., Flaherty, J. T., and Weisfeldt, M. L. (1987). Direct measurement of free radical generation following reperfusion of ischemic myocardium. *Proc. Natl Acad. Sci. USA.,* **84,** 1404–7.

104 Zweier, J. L., Kuppusamy, P., Williams, R., Rayburn, B. K., Smith, D., Weisfeldt, M. L., and Flaherty, J. T. (1989). Measurement and characterization of postischemic free radical generation in the isolated perfused heart. *J. Biol. Chem.,* **264,** 18890–5.

105 Jolly, S. R., Kane, W. J., Hook, B. G., Abrams, G. D., Kunkel, S. L., and Lucchesi, B. R. (1986). Reduction of myocardial infarct size by neutrophil depletion: Effect of duration of occlusion. *Am. Heart J.,* **112,** 682–90.

106 Romson, J. L., Hook, B. G., Kunkel, S. L., Abrams, G. D., Schork, M. A., and Lucchesi, B. R. (1983). Reduction of the extent of ischemic myocardial injury by neutrophil depletion in the dog. *Circulation,* **67,** 1016–23.

107 Mullane, K. M., Read, N., Salmon, J. A., and Moncada, S. (1984).

Role of leukocytes in acute myocardial infarction in anesthetized dogs: Relationship to myocardial salvage by anti-inflammatory drugs. *J. Pharmacol. Exp. Ther.*, **228**, 510–22.

108 Romson, J. L., Hook, B. G., Rigot, V. H., Schork, M. A., Swanson, D. P., and Lucchesi, B. R. (1982). The effect of ibuprofen on accumulation of indium-111-labeled platelets and leukocytes in experimental myocardial infarction. *Circulation*, **66**, 1002–11.

109 Mallory, G., White, P., and Salcedo-Salgar, J. (1939). The speed of healing myocardial infarction: a study of the pathologic anatomy in seventy-two cases. *Am. Heart J.*, **18**, 647–71.

110 Fishbein, M. C., Maclean, D., and Maroko, P. R. (1978). Histopathologic evolution of myocardial infarction. *Chest*, **73**, 843–9.

111 Simpson, P. J., Fantone, J. C., and Lucchesi, B. R. (1988). Myocardial ischemia and reperfusion injury: oxygen radicals and the role of the neutrophil. In *Oxygen radicals and tissue injury: proceedings of an Upjohn symposium* (ed. B. Halliwell), pp. 63–77. FASEB, Bethesda.

112 Schmid-Schoenbein, G. W. and Engler, R. L. (1982). Leukocyte capillary plugging in myocardial ischemia and during reperfusion in the dog. *Microvasc. Res.*, **23**, 273.

113 Litt, M. R., Jeremy, R. W., Weisman, H. F., Winkelstein, J. A., and Becker, L. C. (1989). Neutrophil depletion limited to reperfusion reduces myocardial infarct size after 90 minutes of ischemia: Evidence for neutrophil-mediated reperfusion injury. *Circulation*, **80**, 1816–27.

114 Simpson, P. J., Todd, R. F., Fantone, J. C., Mickelson, J. K., Griffin, J. D., and Lucchesi, B. R. (1988). Reduction of experimental canine myocardial reperfusion injury by a monoclonal antibody (anti-Mo1, anti-CD11b) that inhibits leukocyte adhesion. *J. Clin. Invest.*, **81**, 624–9.

115 Wargovich, T. J., Mehta, J., Nichols, W. W., Ward, M. B., Lawson, D., Franzini, D., and Conti, C. R. (1987). Reduction in myocardial neutrophil accumulation and infarct size following administration of thromboxane inhibitor U-63, 557A. *Am. Heart J.*, **114**, 1078–85.

116 Simpson, P. J., Mickelson, J., Fantone, J. C., Gallagher, K. P., and Lucchesi, B. R. (1988). Reduction of experimental canine myocardial infarct size with prostaglandin E1: inhibition of neutrophil migration and activation. *J. Pharmacol. Exp. Ther.*, **244**, 619–24.

117 Jacob, H. S. (1983). Neutrophil activation as a mechanism of tissue injury. *Semin. Arthritis Rheum.*, **13**, 144–7.

118 Kutsumi, Y., Misawa, T., Tada, H., Kim, S. S., Nakai, T., Miyabo, S., *et al.* (1989). The effect of neutrophil depletion on reperfusion arrhythmias during intracoronary thrombolysis using the leukocyte removal filter. *ASAIO Trans.*, **35**, 265–7.

119 Dinerman, J. L., Mehta, J. L., Saldeen, T. G., Emerson, S., Wallin, R., Davda, R., and Davidson, A. (1990). Increased neutrophil elastase

release in unstable angina pectoris and acute myocardial infarction. *J. Am. Coll. Cardiol.*, **15**, 1559–63.

120 Brown, J. M., White, C. W., Terada, L. S., Grosso, M. A., Shanley, P. F., Mulvin, D. W., *et al.* (1990). Interleukin 1 pretreatment decreases ischemia/reperfusion injury. *Proc. Natl Acad. Sci. USA*, **87**, 5026–30.

121 Linas, S. L., Whittenburg, D., and Repine, J. E. (1987). O_2 metabolites cause reperfusion injury after short but not prolonged renal ischemia. *Am. J. Physiol.*, **253**, F685–91.

122 Linas, S. L., Shanley, P. F., Whittenburg, D., Berger, E., and Repine, J. E. (1988). Neutrophils accentuate ischemia–reperfusion injury in isolated perfused rat kidneys. *Am. J. Physiol.*, **255**, F728–35.

123 McCutchan, H. J., Schwappach, J. R., Enquist, E. G., Walden, D. L., Terada, L. S., Reiss, O. K., *et al.* (1990). Xanthine oxidase derived H_2O_2 contributes to reperfusion injury of ischemic skeletal muscle. *Am. J. Physiol.*, **258**, H1415–19.

124 Walden, D. L., McCutchan, H. J., Enquist, E. G., Schwappach, J. R., Shanley, P. F., Reiss, O. K., *et al.* (1990). Neutrophils accumulate and contribute to skeletal muscle dysfunction after ischemia–reperfusion. *Am. J. Physiol.*, **259**, H1809–12.

125 Weismann, G. and Korchak, H. (1984). Rheumatoid arthritis. The role of neutrophil activation. *Inflammation*, **8**, S3–14.

126 Chester, J. F., Ross, J. S., Malt, R. A., and Weitzman, S. A. (1985). Acute colitis produced by chemotactic peptides in rats and mice. *Am. J. Pathol.*, **121**, 284–90.

127 Wandall, J. H. (1985). Function of exudative neutrophilic granulocytes in patients with Crohn's disease or ulcerative colitis. *Scand. J. Gastroenterol.*, **20**, 1151–6.

128 Murphy, K. R., Wilson, M. C., Irvin, C. G., Glezen, L. S., Marsh, W. R., Haslett, C., *et al.* (1986). The requirement for polymorphonuclear leukocytes in the late asthmatic response and heightened airway reactivity in an animal model. *Am. Rev. Respir. Dis.*, **134**, 62–8.

129 Lemanske, R. F., Guthman, D. A., Oertel, H., Barr, L., and Kaliner, M. (1983). The biological activity of mast cell granules. VI. The effect of vinblastine-induced neutropenia on rat cutaneous late phase reactions. *J. Immunol.*, **130**, 2837–42.

130 Lemanske, R. F., Guthman, D. A., and Kaliner, M. (1983). The biological activity of mast cell granules. VII. The effect of anti-neutrophil antibody-induced neutropenia on rat cutaneous late phase reactions. *J. Immunol.*, **131**, 929–33.

131 Kanazawa, H., Kurihara, N., Hirata, K., and Takeda, T. (1991). The role of free radicals in airway obstruction in asthmatic patients. *Chest*, **100**, 1319–22.

132 Malawista, S. E. (1975). The action of colchicine in acute gouty arthritis. *Arthritis Rheum.*, **18**, 835–46.

133 Cooper, P. H., Frierson, H. F., and Greer, K. E. (1983). Subcutaneous neutrophilic infiltrates in acute febrile neutrophilic dermatosis. *Arch. Dermatol.*, **119**, 610–11.

134 Jorizzo, J. L., Hudson, R. D., Schmalstieg, F. C., Daniels, J. C., Apisarnthanarax, P., Henry, J. C., *et al.* (1984). Behçet's syndrome: immune regulation, circulating immune complexes, neutrophil migration, and colchicine therapy. *J. Am. Acad. Dermatol.*, **10**, 205–14.

135 Hickman, J. G. (1983). Pyoderma gangrenosum. *Clin. Dermatol.*, **1**, 102–13.

136 Ragaz, A. and Ackerman, A. B. (1979). Evolution, maturation, and regression of lesions of psoriasis. New observations and correlation of clinical and histologic findings. *Am. J. Dermatopathol.*, **1**, 199–214.

137 Glinski, W. and Mansbridge, J. (1985). Polymorphonuclear leukocytes in psoriasis. *Cutis*, **35**, 441–2.

138 Repine, J. E. (1985). Neutrophils, oxygen radicals, and the adult respiratory distress syndrome. In *The pulmonary circulation and acute lung injury* (ed. S. I. Said), pp. 249–81. York: Futura Publishing Co., Mount Kisco, NY.

8 Therapeutic modulation of neutrophil number and function

L. A. BOXER and R. F. TODD III

1 Clinical case: leukocyte adhesion deficiency (LAD)

H.M. was a 20-month-old Hispanic baby girl admitted for evaluation and therapy of a recurrent respiratory and cutaneous infection.

She was born by spontaneous vaginal delivery in March 1986, at 42 weeks gestation to a $G_5P_5AB_0$ 36-year-old mother. The initial course was complicated by meconium aspiration versus 'respiratory distress syndrome'. The post-delivery cord blood had a white blood cell count of 30×10^9 cells/l. Her postpartum course was uneventful, and she was discharged on day 5 postpartum. She remained at the 50th percentile for height and weight until the time of admission. However, she was afflicted with recurrent infections associated with a marked leukocytosis: at 7 weeks of age, she was diagnosed with a pneumonia. A white blood cell count on admission was 30×10^9 cells/l. A sepsis evaluation was negative and her pneumonia responded to i.v. antibiotics. At 3 months of age, she was hospitalized with pneumonia and marked leukocytosis. She again responded to antibiotic therapy and no pathogenic organisms were isolated. She was hospitalized at 7 months of age for otitis media secondary to *Pseudomonas* with a leukocytosis of 35×10^9 cells/l. She again did well on i.v. antibiotics and was discharged within 1 week of admission. Upon discharge, she was placed on Bactrim prophylaxis in an attempt to prevent bacterial infections and remained free of infection until 18 months of age, when she was hospitalized for fever, leukocytosis, and a *Pseudomonas* folliculitis which resolved on a third generation cephalosporin. At 20 months of age, the skin infections reoccurred and her white blood cell count increased to 42×10^9 cells/l. She was transferred to the University of Michigan Medical Center for further evaluation and treatment.

Her past medical history was significant for her lack of immunization due to her recurrent infections. Her umbilical remnant fell off at 10 days of life. Her only medication on transfer was Ceftazidime. Her five siblings were alive and well. Both of her parents were free of medical problems. There was no family history of recurrent infections.

A physical examination revealed a chubby, well-developed toddler in no acute distress. Positive findings on admission included multiple scattered pustules on her abdomen and legs, scattered rhonchi, and tachycardia without murmurs or rubs. The rest of her examination was normal.

Laboratory evaluation on admission demonstrated a white blood cell count of 29.5×10^9 cells/l with 45 per cent segmented neutrophils, 5 per cent bands, 45 per cent lymphocytes, and 1 per cent monocytes. Her haemoglobin was 12.7 g/dl and her platelet count was 60.5×10^9/l. Her urinalysis was unremarkable. A Gram stain of her skin lesions demonstrated numerous Gram-negative rods. A flow cytometric analysis of β_2 integrin expression by her peripheral blood neutrophils demonstrated a significant reduction in the surface expression of LFA-1, Mo-1/MAC-1, and p150,95 (as determined by immunofluorescent staining using monoclonal antibodies specific for CD11a, CD11b, CD11c, and CD18). Upon *in vitro* stimulation of her neutrophils with formyl-Met-Leu-Phe (FMLP) reduced but detectable levels of surface integrin expression were observed. Nitroblue tetrazolium stain of her peripheral blood neutrophils was normal. Serum immunoglobulins levels were normal.

Based upon her history of recurrent bacterial infections and her reduced leukocyte β_2 integrin expression, she was given the diagnosis of leukocyte adhesion deficiency of the 'moderate' phenotype.

2   Introduction

Neutrophils are the most important of the phagocytic cells that defend the host against acute bacterial infection. Neutrophils have a particularly important role in protecting the skin, mucous membrane and lining of the respiratory and gastrointestinal tracks. As such, they form the first line of defence against microbial invasion. Therefore it is not surprising when neutrophil function is severely compromised, as illustrated in our patient with leukocyte adhesion deficiency (LAD), or when numbers are limited as discussed later in the chapter in patients with various causes of neutropenia, that the host is predisposed to cutaneous and mucous membrane infections. Disorders of phagocyte and microbicidal activity as observed in chronic granulomatous disease (CGD) is also associated with cutaneous abscesses, pulmonary infections, and gastrointestinal problems such as antral obstruction. This chapter will discuss the potential of gene replacement for therapy of LAD and detail newer approaches to enhancing host defence in patients with CGD or restoration of neutrophil numbers in patients with neutropenia.

In some instances neutrophils have been implicated as mediators of tissue injury in several inflammatory diseases. Significant progress has been made in our understanding of the pathologic mechanisms underlying

neutrophil-mediated tissue damage. With this knowledge it has been possible to devise several strategies that might attenuate the destructive effects
of activated neutrophils. As discussed below it might be possible to modulate the inflammatory response at several points during the process of
neutrophil recruitment and activation.

3   Potential for gene therapy of phagocyte disorders

Recent advances in our understanding of the molecular basis for several
haematopoietic diseases have made it reasonable to consider the possibility
of somatic gene replacement as a therapeutic strategy. LAD is one example
of an inherited disorder of phagocyte function for which the underlying
genetic defect has been defined and normal leukocyte function restored
after genetic reconstitution *in vitro*. LAD is a rare (100 cases reported
world-wide) autosomal recessive disorder of leukocyte function that is
characterized by decreased or absent expression of the β_2 (leukocyte)
integrins, LFA-1 (CD11a/CD18), Mo-1 or MAC-1 (CD11b/CD18), and
p150,95 (CD11c/CD18) on the leukocytes of afflicted individuals (reviewed in 1–3). As described in Chapter 2, Section 3.2 and Chapter 6,
Section 6, the β_2 integrins function as adhesion-promoting molecules that
are important in many adherence-dependent interactions of leukocytes.
Absent or diminished expression of the β_2 integrins on the surface of LAD
leukocytes results in defective adherence-dependent lymphocyte and
phagocyte function as observed *in vitro* and is manifested clinically
by defective recruitment of effector cells (predominantly neutrophils) to
inflammatory sites as noted in the above case. The only known cure for
LAD is allogeneic bone marrow tansplantation, the success of which in
reconstituting normal inflammatory function in several treated patients
confirms the haematopoietic stem cell origin of this disorder (4).

Data demonstrating that LAD is caused by a defective CD18 gene (5–7)
provide a rational basis for contemplating somatic gene therapy as a form
of treatment (Table 8.1). In further support of this therapeutic strategy is
the fact that regulation of integrin gene function appears to take place at a
post-transcriptional level [as manifested by changes in receptor avidity (8–
10)] and that normal cellular levels of gene product expression are not
required for therapeutic benefit [i.e. the limited β_2 integrin expression (5–
7 per cent of normal) seen in patients with 'moderate' LAD is sufficient to
promote a rudimentary inflammatory response compatible with survival
beyond childhood (11)].

Considering that LAD is mainly a disorder of the short-lived neutrophil,
the only practical target of somatic gene therapy is a haematopoietic
progenitor cell capable of self renewal. To assess the potential for intro-
ducing the CD18 gene into haematopoietic stem cells in the hope of

Table 8.1   Leukocyte adhesion deficiency. Rationale for considering gene replacement therapy

---

1. Single autosomal recessive gene defect
2. Fatal disorder curable only by allogeneic bone marrow transplantation
3. High level of gene expression not required for clinical benefit
4. Post-transcriptional regulation of integrin function

---

reconstituting β_2 integrin expression in their progeny, an animal model for LAD is desirable. Whereas LAD has been reported in canine and bovine species (12, 13), there exist significant impediments to the application of CD18-directed gene therapy in these animals: in the canine system, only one such animal was documented and is now deceased; in the bovine system, the long gestation period and the significant expense of maintaining LAD calves makes this species less desirable as an experimental animal for gene therapy. Pending further progress in the current efforts to create LAD mice [by β_2 gene 'knockout' (14)], Krauss *et al.* (16) have taken advantage of the close homology between murine and human β_2 integrins in their attempts to demonstrate stable expression of human CD18 in the progeny of murine stem cells transduced with the human CD18 gene.

As initially reported by Marlan *et al.* (15), and confirmed by Krauss *et al.* (16), insertion of the human CD18 β_2 gene into murine lymphoid cell lines gives rise to the surface expression of inter-species hybrid LFA-1 molecules consisting of human β_2 CD18 subunits noncovalently associated with murine CD11a α_L subunits (in addition to the unaltered parallel expression of endogenous murine LFA-1 molecules). Having thus demonstrated the capacity of murine haematopoietic cells to express human CD18 stably, Krauss *et al.* (17) then performed similar retrovirus-mediated transduction experiments targeting murine bone marrow cells. Specifically, these investigators used recombinant retroviruses to transduce the human CD18 gene into bone marrow cells derived from C3H/HeJ mice; lethally irradiated syngeneic recipients were then reconstituted with the genetically modified bone marrow cells. Out of 80 transplanted mice, 60 demonstrated marrow engraftment and 25 of these 60 animals demonstrated detectable levels of human CD18 when their peripheral blood leukocytes were analysed by flow cytometry after immunofluorescence staining by human-specific anti-CD18 monoclonal antibodies.

Among the human CD18-expressing mice, there was considerable heterogeneity in the level of expression ranging from a few per cent of circulating cells to over 70 per cent expression of the total peripheral blood granulocytes. In every recipient in which human CD18 was detectable, the proportion of granulocytic cells expressing human CD18 was 5- to 10-fold higher than the proportion of lymphoid cells [most probably due to a lymphoid-specific block at the transcriptional or post-transcriptional levels (17)]. A similar disproportion between myeloid and lymphoid expression was seen in the organs of selected murine recipients subjected to immunofluorescence flow cytometric analysis (Table 8.2). On a per granulocyte basis, the basal surface density of human CD18-containing heterodimers was roughly similar to that of murine CD18-containing integrin molecules (and was also similar to the level of human CD18 expression displayed by human neutrophils), and responded to the same mechanism of post-transcriptional regulation; namely, an increase in the number of CD11b/CD18 integrin molecules on the granulocyte surface [recruited from cytoplasmic granular stores (18)] after exposure to activating stimuli such as PMA. Expression of human CD18 in transplanted mice was stable when last analysed at 12 months post-transplant and had no apparent effect on the number or differential of circulating leukocytes, no effect on the basal or stimulated expression of endogenous leukocyte CD11a, CD11b, or CD18, and produced no obvious gross or histopathologic abnormalities in haematopoietic or non-haematopoietic organs. Similarly, the proportion of animals successfully engrafted with transduced bone marrow cells (75 per cent) was comparable to that observed in recipients receiving bone marrow transduced with retroviral vectors containing other genes (J. C. Krauss, unpublished observations).

In summary, Krauss *et al.* (17) were able to demonstrate stable human CD18 gene expression in a significant proportion of bone marrow recipients with no apparent ill effects. In several engrafted animals, the magnitude of human CD18 expression by granulocytic cells was above the range (>5 per cent) that might be associated with therapeutic benefit in a β_2 integrin-deficient state, and the quantitative level of granulocyte human CD18 expression was subject to normal post-transcriptional control mechanisms.

The application of these positive results to somatic gene therapy of LAD awaits the outcome of additional *in vivo* experiments in animal models and *in vitro* experiments using human LAD bone marrow. If LAD mice can be constructed by CD18 gene knockout, it will be important to attempt murine CD18 genetic reconstitution [as outlined by Krauss *et al.* (17)] to determine the functional competency of transfected CD18 in promoting adhesion-dependent leukocyte functions *in vitro* and in alleviating the expected clinical manifestations of murine LAD *in vivo*. In parallel to definitive CD18 gene replacement experiments in the murine system, substantial progress must be made in defining the appropriate conditions for optimally transducing human CD18 into haematopoietic progenitor cells purified from human LAD bone marrow (with documentation of β_2 integrin expression and function in their differentiated progeny as propagated in short- and long-term bone marrow culture).

In addition to LAD, chronic granulomatous disease (CGD) is another disorder of phagocyte function for which somatic gene therapy is potentially

Table 8.2 Human CD18 expression by tissue leukocytes of a murine transplant recipient[a]

	Blood		Spleen		Bone marrow		Thymus	Lymph nodes
	Lymph.	Gran.	Lymph.	Gran.	Lymph.	Gran.		
Human CD18-positive	14[b]	75	11	15	16	74	24	7

[a] Modified from Krauss *et al.* (17).
[b] Per cent positive cells.

applicable (19). With the recent advances in our understanding of the genetic basis for CGD (see Chapter 3), the prospect for gene replacement therapy may become a reality in the not too distant future.

4   Therapeutic modulation of neutrophil inflammatory function

Neutrophils have been implicated as effector cells producing inappropriate tissue injury in several inflammatory diseases (20). Significant progress has been made in our understanding of the pathologic mechanisms that result in this neutrophil-mediated tissue destruction (see Chapters 2 and 7). With this knowledge, it has been possible to conceive of several strategies to circumvent the destructive effects of activated neutrophils. As discussed below, it should be possible to block the inflammatory response at several points during the process of neutrophil recruitment, priming, and activation leading to hyperadherence, diapedesis, and generation of tissue destructive factors. A comprehensive review of all investigative attempts to inhibit neutrophil-mediated tissue damage is beyond the scope of this chapter, but Tables 8.3–8.7 serve to highlight specific approaches that show promise of therapeutic benefit.

4.1   Inhibition at the level of neutrophil recruitment, priming, and activation by soluble stimuli

The development of therapeutic strategies to inhibit the inflammatory response by interfering with the receipt of pro-inflammatory signals by neutrophils and mononuclear phagocytes (Table 8.3) represents an area of intense pre-clinical and clinical investigation. TNFα, LPS, and IL-1 have all been implicated in the pathogenesis of the septic shock syndrome. Among the most promising approaches are the use of monoclonal antibodies that neutralize the stimulatory effects of LPS (30, 31) and TNFα (28, 29) or the use of soluble receptors [for TNFα (33, 34)] or other competitive antagonists of receptor-dependent binding of inflammatory cytokines [e.g. IL-1 receptor antagonist (35, 36)]. The first therapeutic tool to reach the clinic is an anti-LPS IgM monoclonal antibody, HA-1A, which was recently recommended for approval by the Food and Drug Administration (FDA) in the United States for use in the therapy of Gram-negative sepsis. FDA approval will be based, in part, upon the results of a randomized double-blind, placebo-controlled, phase II trial in which, among 196 patients with documented Gram-negative bacteraemia, those individuals randomized to receive HA-1A antibody demonstrated an improved survival relative to those individuals given placebo (63 per cent versus 48 per cent, $P < 0.038$)

Table 8.3 Inhibition at the level of neutrophil recruitment, priming, and activation by soluble inflammatory stimuli. Selected therapeutic approaches[a]

1. Inhibit the generation of activating factors,
   (b) Block complement activation at the level of C3a and C5a by soluble CR_1 (21)
   (b) Block lipoxygenase pathway of arachidonic acid metabolism with pharmacologic inhibitors of cyclooxygenase and/or lipoxygenase using dipyrdamole (22, 23), nafazatrom (24), or BW755C (25)
   (c) Block oxidant-dependent formation of chemotactic lipid by SOD (26)
2. Neutralize the stimulatory effect of priming or activating factors
   (a) Neutralize C5a by anti-C5 mAb (27)
   (b) Neutralize TNF by anti-TNF mAb (28, 29)
   (c) Neutralize endotoxin by anti-endotoxin mAb (30, 31)
3. Inhibit receptor-dependent binding of priming or activating factors
   (a) Block PAF binding by receptor antagonists BN52021, kedsurenone, or L-652 (32)
   (b) Block TNF binding by soluble $TNF\alpha$ receptor (33, 34)
   (c) Block IL-1 binding by IL-1 receptor antagonist, IL-1ra (35, 36)
   (d) Block LPS binding by LPS receptor antagonist, lipid IVa (37)

[a] Abbreviations: SOD, superoxide dismutase; mAb, monoclonal antibody; PAF, platelet-activating factor.

(30). Similar beneficial effects were observed in a recent trial involving the use of another anti-endotoxin antibody, E5 (31). Other inflammatory agents currently in human clinical trials include monoclonal antibodies specific for $TNF\alpha$ (28, 29) and an IL-1 receptor antagonist (35, 36). The sheer magnitude of septicaemia—an estimated 400 000 cases per year in the USA (30)—and the high mortality rate from septic shock despite antibiotics and other supportive measures have provided significant impetus to the biotechnology and pharmaceutical industries to expedite the development of this novel class of anti-inflammatory agents (38).

4.2   Inhibition at the level of neutrophil adhesion

Since neutrophil adhesion (either neutrophil aggregation or neutrophil adherence to vascular elements) is a prerequisite for subsequent events leading to tissue injury, agents that block neutrophil adhesive interactions are being tested for therapeutic efficacy (Table 8.4). While none of these (with the exception of anti-ICAM-1 monoclonal antibody) have reached clinical trials, it is likely that anti-integrin monoclonal antibodies will soon be tested in the setting of hypovolaemic shock after major trauma. The therapeutic potential of monoclonal antibodies that block LFA-1 and/or Mo1/MAC-1-dependent adhesion is based upon their efficacy in several

Table 8.4 Inhibition at the level of neutrophil adhesion (heterotypic and homotypic adhesive interactions). Selected therapeutic strategies

---

1. Competitive inhibition of selectin-dependent (low avidity) neutrophil–endothelial interactions using:
   (a) Anti-L-selectin mAb (39–41)
   (b) Anti-E-selectin mAb (42)
   (c) Anti-P-selectin (CD62) mAb (43)
   (d) Anti-Lewis X (CD15; P-selectin ligand) mAb (44)
   (e) Anti-sialyl Lewis X (E-selectin ligand) mAb (45)
   (f) Soluble E-selectin chimeric globulin (46)
   (g) Soluble L-selectin chimeric globulin (39, 40)
   (h) Soluble P-selectin (47)
2. Competitive inhibition of β_2 integrin-dependent (high avidity) neutrophil–endothelial interactions using:
   (a) Anti-CD11b (Mo1/MAC-1), CD11a (LFA-1), or CD18 (β2) mAb (48–61)
   (b) Anti-ICAM-1 (CD54; LFA-1, Mo1/MAC-1 ligand) mAb (49, 62–65)
   (c) Soluble CD11b/CD18 (Mo1/MAC-1) (66)
   (d) Soluble ICAM-1 (CD54) (67)
3. Competitive inhibition of Mo1/MAC-1-dependent neutrophil aggregation using:
   (a) Anti-CD11b (Mo1/MAC-1) or CD18 (β2) mAb (68, 48)

---

animal models of acute inflammatory injury (Table 8.5) (48–61). Most striking are the effects of anti-CD18 (β_2) and anti-CD11b reagents in inhibiting various forms of ischaemia–reperfusion injury (48–58). Of particular clinical relevance are the reports of Harlan *et al.* who demonstrated the efficacy of anti-CD18 mAb 60.3 in attenuating the severity and mortality of multi-organ failure resulting from hypovolaemic shock: antibody administered to rabbits (57) and primates (58) at the time of resuscitation (fluid repletion, etc.) significantly improved survival and reduced histopathologic evidence of neutrophil injury in liver and gut as compared to administration of vehicle alone. Anti-integrin antibodies have also been shown to reduce infarct size in animal models of myocardial ischaemia–reperfusion injury (48–52) suggesting their potential efficacy after thrombolytic therapy in humans. However, given the therapeutic benefit of thrombolytic therapy alone and the uncertain clinical significance of myocardial ischaemia–reperfusion injury in humans, hypovolaemic shock after trauma will likely be the clinical setting in which anti-integrin antibodies will first be evaluated.

Despite promising results of animal studies, concerns have been raised over the application of anti-integrin antibodies to other forms of shock (namely, septic shock) where temporary paralysis of phagocyte anti-

Table 8.5 Anti-inflammatory properties of monoclonal antibodies specific for β_2 (CD11/CD18) integrins. Animal models of acute inflammation in which anti-CD11/CD18 mAb attenuate leukocyte-mediated tissue injury

Model (species)	mAb	Reference
Myocardial ischaemia–reperfusion injury (dog, rabbit, ferret, monkey)	Anti-CD11b, CD11a, CD18	48–52
Intestinal ischaemia–reperfusion injury (cat)	Anti-CD18	53
Ear ischaemia–reperfusion injury (rabbit)	Anti-CD18	54
Brain ischaemia–reperfusion injury (rabbit)	Anti-CD18	55
Multi-organ failure after hypovolaemic shock (rabbit, monkey)	Anti-CD18	56–58
Bacterial meningitis (rabbit)	Anti-CD18	59
Endotoxin-induced pneumonia (rabbit)	Anti-CD18	60
Galactosamine/endotoxin hepatitis (mouse)	Anti-CD11b, CD18	61

bacterial function (in effect, creating a form of LAD) might have detrimental host effects (69). These concerns have, in part, led to another therapeutic strategy in which the ligand for neutrophil integrin-binding, endothelial cell ICAM-1, rather than neutrophil integrin molecules themselves, has been the target for competitive antibody binding (49, 62–65). Preclinical studies of anti-ICAM-1 monoclonal antibody have demonstrated its efficacy in thwarting β_2 integrin-dependent mediated cytotoxicity of renal and cardiac allografts (63, 64) and have led to phase I clinical trials of its capacity to block acute renal allograft rejection. However, animal experiments to assess the ability of anti-ICAM-1 antibodies to block neutrophil-mediated tissue damage have produced mixed results [efficacy in certain models (49, 62–65) but no benefit in others (R. Winn, unpublished data)], which suggests the importance of ICAM-1-independent neutrophil aggregation in causing the 'no reflow phenomenon' (distal ischaemia) in certain models of acute inflammatory injury (70, 71).

The selectins (neutrophil L-selectin; endothelial cell E- and P-selectin) represent other targets for anti-adhesion therapy. Whereas anti-selectin monoclonal antibodies have been shown to block integrin-dependent neutrophil endothelial cell binding *in vitro*, few *in vivo* preclinical trials have been conducted (39, 40–42). In one such study, however, an anti-ELAM-1 antibody was found to attenuate neutrophil recruitment significantly to an inflammatory focus in the peritoneal cavities of glycogen-injected rats and to reduce immune complex-induced pulmonary and cutaneous neutrophil-mediated injury (42). Additional preclinical animal experiments will need to be conducted to evaluate more fully the potential therapeutic benefit of anti-selectin reagents.

If clinical trials using monoclonal anti-integrin or anti-selectin monoclonal antibodies validate the therapeutic benefit of blocking neutrophil adhesion during the acute inflammatory response, it is likely that these results will pave the way for the development and testing of soluble receptors (or peptide fragments of receptors) that may accomplish the same end without the need for administration of potentially antigenic antibodies (66, 72). An even longer term goal is the synthesis of medicinal compounds that antagonize adhesion receptor function.

4.3   Inhibition at the level of neutrophil generation and secretion of toxic oxidants and proteases

Pharmacologic inhibition of neutrophil respiratory burst and secretion represents another strategy for limiting neutrophil-mediated tissue damage (Table 8.6). Prostacyclin and its stable analogue Iloprost, which have been shown to reduce the production of reactive oxygen species and the release of degradative lysosomal enzymes by neutrophils *in vitro* (73), represent candidate drugs of this type. Indeed, Prostacyclin and/or Iloprost have shown efficacy in reducing infarct size in canine models of myocardial ischaemia–reperfusion injury (74) and in an *ex vivo* rat model of adult respiratory distress syndrome (75). However, in the latter model, Iloprost had no inhibitory effect on neutrophil superoxide production, and attenuation of pulmonary injury was attributable to Iloprost inhibition of neutrophil adhesion to pulmonary endothelium (by a mechanism referable to Iloprost's ability to stimulate intracellular cAMP) (75).

Other drugs that have been shown to limit infarct size in animal models of myocardial ischaemia–reperfusion injury and which may act directly on neutrophils to inhibit superoxide anion generation in response to certain inflammatory stimuli *in vitro* include ibuprofen (76–78) and adenosine (79,

Table 8.6   Inhibition at the level of neutrophil generation and secretion of toxic oxidants and proteases. Selected therapeutic agents

1. Prostacyclin (Iloprost) (73–75)
2. Ibuprofen (76–78)
3. Adenosine (79, 80)

80). Adenosine is thought to bind to neutrophils via specific receptors which, when stimulated, inhibit NADPH oxidase-mediated superoxide production (79) that is triggered by receptor-dependent binding of inflammatory cytokines. Similarly, the anti-inflammatory properties of the widely used drug ibuprofen may include suppression of respiratory burst activity (76) as well as inhibition of neutrophil influx into inflammatory sites (including previously ischaemic myocardium) (77).

4.4   Inhibition at the level of oxidant and protease cytopathic effect

The mechanism of inflammatory injury caused by oxidants and proteases and the development and testing of agents to inhibit their cytopathic effects have been the focus of several recent comprehensive reviews (81–83) and will therefore only be summarized here (Table 8.7). It is now well recognized that oxidative metabolites and proteases work synergistically to produce local tissue destruction (81, 82, and Chapter 7). In fact, the major destructive effects of neutrophil oxidants *in vivo* may be indirect, that is, to activate latent metalloproteinases and to neutralize the local antiprotease defence screen (107–109), rather than to cause cellular cytotoxicity directly [that is most demonstrable *in vitro* (110)]. Among the agents that have been documented to neutralize the cytopathic effect of neutrophil oxidants *in vitro* and to reduce inflammatory tissue injury in certain animal models *in vivo* are the free radical scavengers superoxide dismutase (SOD) and catalase which act to catalyse O_2^- to H_2O_2 and H_2O_2 to H_2O, respectively (84–94). In addition, since iron released by inflammatory tissues may react with H_2O_2 to form the highly toxic HO·, the iron-chelating agent desferoxamine has also been shown to have anti-inflammatory properties *in vitro* and *in vivo* (95–97). Other drugs with antioxidant properties include the sulphydryl-containing thiol compounds, most notably *N*-acetylcysteine,

Table 8.7   Inhibition at the level of oxidant and protease cytopathic effect. Selected therapeutic strategies

---

1. Neutralization of oxidants by
    (a) SOD and/or catalase (84–94)
    (b) Deferoxamine (95–97)
    (c) Hemin (98)
    (d) N-Acetylcysteine (99–101)
    (e) N^G-Monomethyl-L-arginine (102)
2. Neutralization of proteases by
    (a) Recombinant α_1 antiproteinase (103, 104)
    (b) Recombinant secretory leukoproteinase inhibitor (rSLPI) (105, 106)

---

which may scavenge oxidants both directly via its reduced sulphydryl group and indirectly by its metabolism to glutathione (99). In the setting of myocardial ischaemia–reperfusion injury, the potential clinical utility of SOD and catalase was first suggested by Shlafer *et al.* (84) and Jolly *et al.* (89), who demonstrated a reduction in myocardial necrosis in the isolated perfused rabbit heart and in dogs, respectively, subjected to myocardial ischaemia followed by reperfusion. Several confirmatory reports have followed (90–92) as have additional animal studies that demonstrate the therapeutic efficacy of recombinant SOD (93). Similar cardioprotective effects have been observed in animals (and isolated perfused hearts) treated with *N*-acetylcysteine (100, 101). However, despite these positive results, the therapeutic benefit of antioxidant therapy has not been a uniform observation (111–113), possibly due to the short *in vivo* half-life of SOD and to differences in the experimental conditions employed (114, 115). An initial human trial of SOD demonstrated no adjunctive cardio-protective effect after acute angioplasty (113). More promising, albeit preliminary, findings have been seen with the use of *N*-acetylcysteine in phase I/II trials of antioxidant therapy of ARDS (99) and in patients recovering from coronary bypass grafting (101). In these clinical settings, *N*-acetylcysteine-treated patients demonstrated objective improvement in cardiopulmonary function including increases in cardiac output, and, in the case of ARDS patients, improvement in oxygen delivery and consumption.

Direct inhibition of neutrophil proteolysis represents another potential strategy for reducing neutrophil-mediated inflammatory injury (103–106). Among several non-toxic proteinase inhibitors that have been examined, recombinantly produced secretory leukoproteinase inhibitor (SLPI), a selective regulator of serine protease activity, is particularly promising (105, 106). In *in vitro* assays of neutrophil-mediated proteolysis, SLPI was a potent inhibitor of subjacent extracellular matrix degradation (105), and, in a canine model of acute myocardial ischaemia–reperfusion injury, SLPI-treated dogs demonstrated significant reduction in infarct size when compared with untreated controls (106). Additional *in vivo* experiments will be required to assess fully the potential clinical utility of SLPI in reducing neutrophil-mediated tissue damage.

5 The role of myeloid growth factors in the treatment of isolated neutropenia

5.1 The biology of the myeloid growth factors

The myeloid growth factors are glycoprotein hormones that regulate the proliferation and differentiation of myeloid progenitor cells and the function of mature blood cells (116, 117). Several of these factors have been molecularly characterized and produced for clinical application via recombinant DNA technology (Table 8.8). In particular, granulocyte-macrophage colony-stimulating factor (GM-CSF), granulocyte colony-stimulating factor (G-CSF), macrophge colony-stimulating factor (M-CSF), and interleukin-3 (IL-3) have been developed as potential therapeutic agents, and their effects on myelopoiesis in mature blood cells are currently under active investigation.

The major cellular sources of the myeloid colony-stimulating factors are activated T lymphocytes, monocytes, macrophages, endothelial cells, and fibroblasts. The biological effects of the colony-stimulating factors are mediated via binding to high affinity specific receptors on the surface of target cells which include the myeloid precursor cells (Tables 8.8, 8.9). The overlap in action of GM-CSF and IL-3 is paralleled by an overlap in the expression of the different receptors on target cells. Low numbers of high- and low-affinity GM-CSF receptors are expressed by neutrophils, eosinophils, and monocytes (118, 119). High affinity receptors for IL-3 are present on eosinophils, basophils, and monocytes but not on neutrophils (120, 121). Thus, these two factors have pleiotropic effects in terms of

Table 8.8 Characteristics of human haematopoietic growth factors[a]

Growth factor	Chromosomal location of gene	Cellular source	Progenitor cell target	Mature cell target
IL-3	5q23-31	T lymphocytes	CFU-Blast, CFU-GEMM, CFU-GM CFU-G, CFU-M, CFU-Eo, CFU-Meg, CFU-Baso BFU-E	Eosinophils, monocytes
GM-CSF	5q23-31	T lymphocytes, monocytes, fibroblasts, endothelial cells	CFU-Blast, CFU-GEMM, CFU-GM, CFU-G, CFU-M, CFU-Eo, CFU-Meg, BFU-E	Granulocytes, eosinophils, monocytes
G-CSF	17q11.2-21	Monocytes, fibroblasts, endothelial cells	CFU-G	Granulocytes
M-CSF	5q33.1	Monocytes, fibroblasts, endothelial cells	CFU-M	Monocytes

[a] Modified from reference 116.

Table 8.9 The human colony-stimulating factors and their receptors[a]

Factor	Molecular weight of core protein	Molecular weight of glycosylated protein	Molecular weight of receptor	Biochemical features
GM-CSF	14700	18000 to 30000	85000	Lacks tyrosine kinase domain
G-CSF	18600	20000	150000	Shares homology with GM-CSF, immunoglobin, and fibronectin
M-CSF	21000 (× 2 dimer)	70000 to 90000	165000	Has cytoplasmic tyrosine domain
IL-3	15400	15000 to 30000	95000	Shares homology to GM-CSF, IL-4, IL-6, erythropoietin receptors

[a] Modified from reference 117.

stimulating multiple cell lineages. In contrast, high affinity functional receptors for G-CSF are expressed mainly by neutrophils and to a much lesser extent by monocytes (122, 123). The M-CSF receptor has been identified as the product of the cellular proto-oncogene c-*fms* and is found on the cells in the mononuclear phagocyte series and placental cells (124). The *in vitro* observation that one colony-stimulating factor can affect the number and possibly the affinity of receptors for another may have implications for the proposed employment of these factors in combinations in the clinical setting (125). For instance, endothelial cells interact with GM-CSF via receptors as well as having the ability to produce colony-stimulating factors (126).

The myeloid growth factors hold great promise for numerous clinical applications. Clinical trials of GM-CSF and G-CSF have been conducted in the context of neutropenias associated with acquired immunodeficiency syndrome (AIDS), chemotherapy-induced neutropenia, autologous bone marrow transplantation, myelodysplasia, and aplastic anaemia (127–132). Additionally, G-CSF has been shown to benefit patients with congenital, idiopathic, and cyclic forms of neutropenia in phase I/II trials (133–136).

5.2   The clinical efficacy of recombinant G-CSF in the treatment of isolated neutropenia

The severe nature of infections in some patients with congenital neutropenia, as outlined in Chapter 6, Section 6, has led to vigorous efforts to develop therapies. In 1988 we began an open-labelled randomized phase III trial of recombinant-methionyl human G-CSF (r-metHUG-CSF) in which patients with various forms of severe chronic neutropenia were enrolled at the University of Michigan as part of a larger national study (137). Patients with diagnoses of congenital, cyclic, and idiopathic neutropenia with histories of recurrent infection were evaluated. Forty-one such patients had a prestudy ANC of less than 0.5×10^9 cells/l. The primary objective of the trial was to evaluate the ability of G-CSF to increase the ANC to more than 1.5×10^9 cells/l. A secondary objective was to evaluate the variables associated with infection-related morbidity in severe chronic neutropenia. G-CSF treatment consisted of 1 month of dose titration followed by 4 months of treatment at an optimal dose. Patients were randomized to either immediate treatment with G-CSF or 4 months of observation consisting of daily documentation of fever, infections, and antibiotic usage, followed by G-CSF treatment.

5.2.1   The use of G-CSF in the treatment of cyclic neutropenia

Cyclic neutropenia is estimated to affect approximately 300–400 patients in the United States. It is characterized by regular, periodic oscillation in the numbers of circulating neutrophils and is associated with cyclic clinical manifestations (138). These episodes occur approximately every 18–21 days and last 6–10 days. At the nadir, circulating neutrophil counts typically fall to below 0.2×10^9 cells/l. The clinical manifestations of this disease are described in Chapter 6, Section 3.

Prior treatment efforts including splenectomy, nutritional supplements, and androgens either failed or were at best marginally successful. The use of corticosteroids has produced some amelioration of the conditions in adults (138); however, in only one adult patient have corticosteroids completely obliterated the cycling (139). In contrast, in our study, when G-CSF was administered subcutaneously at 5 μg/kg in patients with cyclic neutropenia, marked benefit was noted. The duration of the neutropenia below 0.2×10^9 cells/l was reduced from 8 days to 1 day. Most importantly, the propensity for chronic gingivitis and pyogenic infections was markedly reduced. Interestingly, cycling was reduced from 18–20 days to 11–13 days. In contrast, use of GM-CSF has failed to induce neutrophilia but rather induces eosinophilia and monocytosis in this group of patients (140).

5.2.2   The use of G-CSF in the treatment of severe congenital agranulocytosis (Kostmann's syndrome)

In Scandinavia this disorder is inherited as an autosomal recessive disorder known as Kostmann's disease (141). In the United States it occurs in approximately 300–400 individuals and is inherited as a sporadic disorder. These patients chronically maintain an ANC of less than 0.2×10^9 cells/l (see Chapter 6, Section 6 for further details on pathogenesis and clinical manifestations).

At the University of Michigan, treatment of severe congenital neutropenia with 5 μg/kg of G-CSF subcutaneously twice daily began to correct the neutropenia within 8 days and decreased the occurrence of acute infections, antibiotic use, and hospitalization. Administration of G-CSF led to an increased size of the postmitotic pool, increased numbers of neutrophils and increased cellularity of the bone marrow (Fig. 8.1). The findings strongly suggest that the increased ANC was due to increased neutrophil production in the bone marrow. A direct action of G-CSF in the recruitment and maturation of the neutrophil precursor cells is the most likely explanation for these results as suggested by *in vitro* and *in vivo* animal studies (142, 143). Two patterns of neutrophil count responses were noted in patients receiving G-CSF with the diagnosis of severe congenital neutropenia (134). Some patients experienced full restoration of a normal neutrophil count. In other patients the ANC cycles were characterized by a periodicity varying from 7 to 22 days with peak responses observed at a mean of 11 ± 3 days. Treatment was associated with marked improvement in oral pathology, including elimination of gingivitis, aphthous ulcers, and bleeding gums. Over 10 months, the number of anaerobic micro-organisms

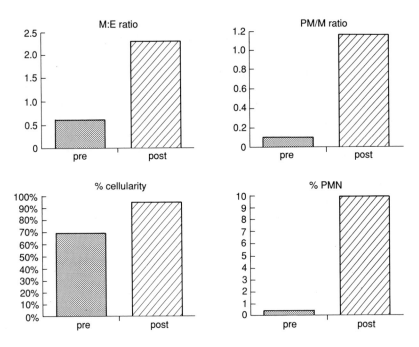

Fig. 8.1 Effects of G-CSF on bone marrows of patients with severe congenital agranulocytosis. M:E, myeloid:erythroid; PM/M post-mitotic/mitotic ratio: i.e. metamyelocytes, juvenile, bands, and segmented neutrophils divided by myeloblasts, promyelocytes, and myelocytes. PMN represents polymorphonuclear leukocytes or segmented neutrophils. Taken from reference 117.

in subgingival tissue also diminished. However in those patients showing evidence of varying degrees of interdental alveolar bone loss, G-CSF treatment did not reverse destructive changes in the alveolar bone. Neutrophils from patients with severe congenital neutropenia undergoing treatment with G-CSF have decreased surface expression of FcRIII (CD16) and subnormal upregulation of the β_2 integrin the CD11b/CD18 (134). All patients' neutrophils, however, had normal contents of both primary and specific granule constituents. In spite of the reduced expression of the FcRIII and CD11b/CD18 receptors, the clinical response to G-CSF was evident by the marked improvement in the degree of periodontitis. It is apparent that restoration of normal neutrophil number coincides with a protective role of the neutrophils suggesting that they are at least partially functional, which allows them to deal with localized bacterial infections within periodontal tissue. Furthermore, in those patients with documented liver abscesses, restoration of the circulating neutrophil count led to resolution of the liver abscesses.

5.2.3   The use of G-CSF in the treatment of severe chronic idiopathic neutropenia

Severe chronic neutropenic disorders are composed of a pot-pourri of congenital and acquired abnormalities associated with variable clinical presentations (Table 8.10). The pathophysiology and specific aetiology of many of these conditions are poorly understood. Patients with severe chronic idiopathic neutropenia, like those with severe congenital neutropenia, have neutrophil counts frequently less than 0.5×10^9 cells/l. Quite commonly a peripheral monocytosis is observed. Somewhat less often peripheral eosinophilia is present. In general, patients with the lowest neutrophil count ($<0.2 \times 10^9$ cells/l) tend to have the greatest number of problems and infections and are considered to have the most severe forms of neutropenia. In contrast to severe chronic idiopathic neutropenia, there is a disorder sometimes referred to as chronic benign neutropenia (144).

Table 8.10   Differential diagnosis of severe chronic neutropenia[a]

Acquired	Congenital
Idiopathic	Myelokathexis
Large granular lymphocyte-mediated neutropenia	Schwachman–Diamond syndrome
	X-linked agammaglobulinaemia
Vitamin B_{12} or folate deficiencies	Dysgammaglobulinaemia
Drug induced hypersplenism	Glycogenosis—type IB
	Cartilage-hair hypoplasia syndrome
	Dyskeratosis congenita
	'Lazy leukocyte' syndrome
	Chédiak–Higashi syndrome

[a] Adapted from reference 117.

This condition is characterized by a variable degree of neutropenia. Patients with chronic benign neutropenia may present in infancy and the condition may persist for months to years. Some patients demonstrate resolution over time. These patients are frequently found to have immune neutropenia of infancy (145). In the patients with chronic benign neutropenia the bone marrow typically reveals normal to increased numbers of neutrophils that appear normal by electron microscopic examination. In general, patients with chronic benign neutropenia when challenged with intravenous corticosteroids are usually able to mobilize neutrophils from the bone marrow reserve pool which likely accounts for their ability to mount an appropriate inflammatory response during infection (146).

Patients with chronic benign neutropenia do not require treatment with G-CSF.

Patients with chronic idiopathic neutropenia may have bone marrow containing variable numbers of myeloid precursors. For instance in myelokathexis the bone marrow aspiration reveals myeloid hyperplasia with binucleated myelocytes and hypersegmented neutrophils with strand-like intranuclear bridges, pyknotic nuclei and increased cytoplasmic vacuolization. In the 'lazy leukocyte' syndrome the bone marrow aspiration reveals myeloid hyperplasia with maturation through the band or segmented forms. Other acquired and congenital disorders may contain normal to increased numbers of promyelocytes with markedly increased numbers of bands and segmented cells or have reduced numbers of early myeloid precursors. In contrast to those patients with chronic benign neutropenia, patients with symptomatic infectious complications fail to raise their circulating neutrophil count upon challenge with intravenous corticosteroids.

Most patients with severe chronic neutropenia will respond to G-CSF with a dramatic rise in the peripheral neutrophil count. Administration of 3–5 μg/kg of G-CSF once per day subcutaneously is often sufficient to raise the circulating neutrophil count. In our own series at the University of Michigan, two patients with large granular lymphocyte-mediated neutropenia with evidence of monoclonal T cell gene rearrangement responded to the administration of G-CSF in spite of demonstrable suppressor activity *in vitro* to myeloid colony development mediated by their peripheral blood T lymphocytes (147). In a patient with myelokathexis in our series administration of G-CSF led to a rise in the circulating neutrophil count within 24 h suggesting that G-CSF serves as a neutrophil-releasing factor from the bone marrow as well as being able to induce proliferation and maturation of myeloid precursors (148). Results from the national trial revealed that 73 patients of 77 with severe chronic neutropenic showed normalization of their neutrophil count, defined as a median ANC of $\geqslant 1.5 \times 10^9$ cells/l (137). An additional three patients with a diagnosis of idiopathic neutropenia and two with a diagnosis of congenital neutropenia demonstrated a partial response, defined as a median ANC of less than 1.5×10^9 cells/l and more than 0.2×10^9 cells/l. Only one patient with an initial diagnosis of idiopathic neutropenia failed to show any response to G-CSF. Of note, even in those patients who showed a partial response to G-CSF, they largely remained free of bacterial infections. The beneficial response in the partial responders may relate to the ability of G-CSF to enhance the respiratory burst of neutrophils (134, 149).

5.2.4   The use of GM-CSF in the treatment of isolated neutropenias

Another haematopoietic growth factor, GM-CSF has been successfully used to treat neutropenias secondary to myelodysplastic syndromes (131), acquired immunodeficiency syndrome (127), chemotherapy (150), and in patients undergoing autologous bone marrow transplantation (129). Preliminary reports, however, have not demonstrated efficacy of GM-CSF in the treatment of severe chronic neutropenia. In one study, RhGM-CSF was administered to five patients with congenital neutropenia, only one of whom showed an increase in ANC (151). These same five patients were then treated with RhG-CSF and responded with an increase in ANC to 1 × 10^9 cells/l. A differential effect of these haematopoietic growth factors also has been confirmed in one patient with cyclic neutropenia (152).

5.2.5   Toxicity of G-CSF in the treatment of isolated neutropenias

Safety analysis from 77 patients in the national co-operative study were analysed (137). The patient-reported adverse events associated with G-CSF therapy were generally mild and consisted of bone pain, headache, and rash. Other reported events related to G-CSF therapy were mild splenomegaly, thrombocytopenia, and alopecia. Finally, serum samples from 77 patients were screened for G-CSF antibody reactivity and there was no evidence that G-CSF treatment elicited any antibodies to the drug.

The reduction in infection-related events with G-CSF treatment of patients with severe chronic neutropenia may have consequences on the long-term modality and morbidity associated with this group of diseases. The mortality rate of severe congenital agranulocytosis has been estimated to be greater than 70 per cent with only 30 per cent predicted to survive more than 5 years (153). Although morality is lower with other neutropenic syndromes, the morbidity rates from serious bacterial infections, recurring mouth sores and oral respiratory infections and the regular loss of days from work or school can affect quality of life. From phase I-II clinical trials, the long-term use of G-CSF up to 4 years has shown continued efficacy and minimal toxicity (137). There has been no evidence of bone marrow exhaustion or evidence of formation of neutralizing antibodies to G-CSF. Further evaluation however is required to determine long-term safety of G-CSF in the population of severe chronic neutropenic patients.

6   The role of interferon γ (INFγ) in the treatment of chronic granulomatous disease (CGD)

6.1   The clinical characteristics of CGD

CGD comprises a heterogeneous group of defects, which share in common, the failure of neutrophils, monocytes, macrophages, and eosinophils to undergo a respiratory burst and generate O_2^-. The disorder is relatively rare, approximately 1 in 1 million individuals being affected. Because of the central role of superoxide and other respiratory burst products in microbial killing, patients with CGD suffer from recurrent bacterial and fungal infections which are often severe. Although phagocytes from patients with CGD ingest micro-organisms, bacterial killing is impaired because the capacity of the phagocytes to produce superoxide and related microbicidal oxygen intermediates is compromised as a result of the defective NADPH oxidase (154). Detailed descriptions of the normal function of the oxidase system and the abnormalities in this system which results in the clinical syndrome of CGD are contained in Chapters 3, Sections 2 and 5 and Chapter 6, Section 4, respectively.

Therapy of CGD is dependent upon prevention and early treatment of infections, aggressive use of parental antibiotics for most infections, employment of prophylactic trimethoprim/sulphamethoxazole (5 mg/kg/day) or dicloxacillin (25–50 mg/kg/day) for sulpha-allergic patients, and the use of prophylactic recombinant human rINFγ (155). Patients with CGD should receive all their routine immunizations including influenza vaccine on a yearly basis. Frequent brushing, flossing, and professional cleaning of teeth can help ameliorate gingivitis. Use of corticosteroids should generally be avoided including extensive topical use except in cases of severe asthma, gastric or antral narrowing, or inflammatory bowel disease.

6.2   The biology of rINFγ

With the recent advances in the field of molecular biology there has been a rapid increase in the understanding of the function of many biological response modifiers including the interferon family and research has resulted in their application for treatment of various disease states. The interferon family is a group of species-specific proteins produced by eukaryotic cells in response to viruses and a variety of natural and synthetic stimuli (156). While the different interferons (α, β_1, and γ) have certain common properties, rINFγ alone possesses potent phagocyte activating effects, including the generation of toxic oxygen products to kill micro-organisms (157–160). INFγ is a recombinant protein prepared from genetically engineered *E. coli* containing DNA encoding the human protein. Purified rINFγ is obtained by conventional column chromatography. INFγ is a noncovalent dimer of two identical monomers, each a single chain polypeptide containing 140 amino acids identical to naturally occurring human rINFγ. Experiments in both humans and mice have shown that rINFγ is a principal macrophage-activating factor. Administration of rINFγ either *in vivo* or *in vitro* enhances both the production of reactive oxygen intermediates and the killing of bacteria and protozoan pathogens (157–160). Studies in patients treated with rINFγ demonstrate an enhancement of macrophage oxidative metabolism (161–163) which led to the rationale for using the drug in patients with CGD. Not only is rINFγ able to enhance oxidative metabolism of phagocytes but it has other pleiotrophic biological responses, which include enhancement of antibody-dependent cellular cytotoxicity and natural killer cell activity, as well as monocyte Fc receptor expression (164–167).

6.2.1   The use of INFγ in the treatment of CGD

In vitro and *in vivo* studies of phagocytes from some patients with CGD indicated that rINFγ could increase superoxide levels, normalize cytochrome *b* gene expression, and improve killing of micro-organisms such as *S. aureus* and *Aspergillus fumigatus* (168–173). *In vivo* correction of the functional defects was also observed following treatment in some patients with CGD with subcutaneous rINFγ. Those patients who responded best were the CGD patients who were capable of generating minimal amounts of superoxide variants (69, 170). INFγ was initially postulated to work by priming phagocytes (174). Others had shown that the level of NADPH oxidase activity, which was dormant in resting cells was affected by exposure to priming substances including cytokines and bacterial lipopolysaccharides (175, 176). These agents do not directly activate the oxidase but serve to enhance its level of activity following subsequent stimulation by exogenous particulate and soluble stimuli. Rather surprisingly rINFγ not only served to prime CGD phagocytes, but in CGD patients whose phagocytes were partially deficient in cytochrome *b* levels, rINFγ normalized the level of cytochrome *b* gene expression following *in vivo* treatment (169).

As the treatment was well tolerated with minimal side effects an international randomized double-blind, placebo-control trial involving 13 centres was designed to determine whether rINFγ could decrease the severity of serious infectious episodes, improve chronic infectious and inflammatory conditions in patients with all genetic types of CGD (155). A total of 128 eligible patients with X-linked or autosomal recessive CGD were involved in this double-blind parallel-controlled group trial (155). They were randomized to treatment with rINFγ or placebo after stratification on the basis and pattern of disease inheritance, study-centre institution, and use or non-use of prophylactic antibiotics and corticosteroids. The two groups were comparable at entry for demographic and clinical data. The median age of the patients was 15 years, and 37 patients were less than 9 years of age. The patients received rINFγ or placebo by subcutaneous injection three times weekly for up to 12 months. The dose was administered on the basis of body surface area, which had to be at least $0.5/m^2$. When body surface area was less than $0.5/m^2$, the dose was administered on the basis of body weight as 1.5 μ/kg. The study was terminated prematurely because of a statistically and clinically significant benefit gain with active therapy; the mean duration of treatment was 8.9 months, representing 95 patient years. Figure 8.2 is a Kaplan–Meier curve displaying the time to the first serious infection after randomization to rINFγ or placebo. Using the Kaplan–Meier estimates, 77 per cent in the treated group versus 30 per cent in the placebo were free of serious infections at 12 months. Corresponding values at 6 months were 89 per cent in the rINFγ group versus 72 per cent in the placebo, demonstrating a beneficial effect of rINFγ therapy during the first year. Twenty-two per cent of patients receiving rINFγ compared with 46 per cent of patients receiving placebo had at least one serious infection. Throughout the study, there were more infections in the group receiving placebo compared with the patients receiving rIFNγ (56 versus 20; $P < 0.0001$). INFγ appeared most effective in attenuating the incidence of adenitis, abscesses, cellulitis, and pulmonary infections. Those patients receiving placebo required about three times as many days of hospitalization for the treatment of clinical disease compared with those receiving rIFNγ. Moreover, the mean hospital stay was longer in the placebo recipients compared with those receiving rIFNγ (48 versus 32 days; $P = 0.02$). In all cases when patients were analysed for age, pattern of inheritance, prophylactic antibiotic use and sex, rINFγ was beneficial

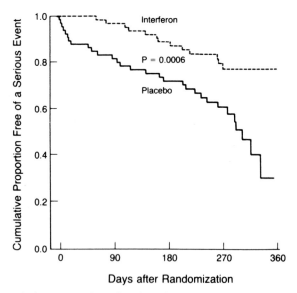

Fig. 8.2 Cumulative proportion of patients in each treatment group who were free of serious infections during the study. The Kaplan–Meier curves show the time to the first serious infection after randomization. In a Cox regression model in which treatment served as a covariate there was a 67% reduction in the relative risk of serious infection in the interferon group ($P = 0.0006$, by two-sided log-rank test). Taken from reference 155.

when compared to placebo. The greatest benefit of rINFγ, however, was found in patients younger than 10 years old. Additionally there were individual patients with pre-existing complications such as pulmonary nodules or gastrointestinal granulomas who improved on rINFγ treatment.

Despite the finding of a significant therapeutic benefit mediated by rINFγ for the prevention of severe infectious episodes in both the X-linked and autosomal recessive forms of CGD disease, complimentary *ex vivo* study of phagocyte function revealed no significant differences between the placebo group and rINFγ in terms of demonstrating enhanced superoxide production, bacterial killing or cytochrome *b* gene expression. The failure to demonstrate enhanced phagocyte function by rINFγ probably relates to the variability of biological studies performed by the heterogeneous group of laboratories. Alternatively, rINFγ may contribute to clinical improvement by enhancing non-oxidative means of bacterial killing by the CGD phagocyte, a hypothesis which requires verification. While rINFγ improved phagocyte function in a subset of rare patients with abnormal Michaelis kinetics, it may be that only those rare patients, unlike the majority of patients with CGD, are able to respond to rINFγ by increases in cytochrome *b* gene expression which in turn is associated with a normalized respiratory burst.

6.2.2 Toxicity of INFγ in CGD patients

The most frequent adverse reactions occurring at a statistically significant level in patients receiving rINFγ compared with the placebo were fever, headaches, chills, and erythema at the site of injection. The majority of these reactions were mild in intensity and relieved by the administration of acetaminophen. Adverse effects were most frequent with increasing age, with flu-like symptoms occurring twice as frequently in the patients aged 10 years or older compared with those younger than 10. Four patients receiving rINFγ had to be withdrawn from the study because of the following toxicities: rash, flu-like symptoms, and exacerbation of granulomatous colitis. It appears that rINFγ offers an effective and well-tolerated therapy for patients with CGD leading to significant clinical improvement in the propensity to develop infections as well as ameliorating obstructive complications secondary to granulomatous formation once they have occurred.

7 Conclusions

A better understanding of the molecular basis for several haematopoietic diseases have made it possible to consider different therapeutic strategies to attenuate inflammation. LAD is one example of an inherited disorder of phagocyte function in which the role of neutrophil integrins in terms of mediating neutrophil adhesion to target tissue has been demonstrated.

With the knowledge now of the role of neutrophil integrins in promoting neutrophil attachment to target tissue leading to an inflammatory response, it has been possible to conceive of several strategies to dampen neutrophil function through inhibition of neutrophil-mediated integrin activation. On the other hand, it is now possible to consider restoring neutrophil function in LAD by applying retrovirus-mediated CD18 gene transfer.

A better understanding of haematopoiesis has also led to the effective use of G-CSF in correcting the neutrophil count in patients with severe chronic neutropenias. The use of G-CSF provides a significant clinical advance in the treatment of the neutropenic disorders by not only improving the neutrophil count, but also by enhancing neutrophil function. In patients with CGD use of INFγ also improves the health of CGD patients by enhancing prognosis of the serious, life-threatening infections accompanying CGD. The mechanism by which INFγ enhances the health of patients in CGD currently remains unknown. Although significant studies have been made, future challenges remain in discovering even better means of regulating neutrophil function and number in clinical disease.

References

1 Anderson, D. C. and Springer, T. A. (1987). Leukocyte adhesion deficiency: an inherited defect in the Mac-1, LFA-1, and p150,95 glycoproteins. *Annu. Rev. Med., * **38,** 175–94.

2 Todd III, R. F. and Freyer, D. R. (1988). The CD11/CD18 leukocyte glycoprotein deficiency. *Hematol. Oncol. Clin. North Am., * **2,** 13–28.

3 Arnaout, M. A. (1990). Leukocyte adhesion molecule deficiency: Its structural basis, pathophysiology, and implications for modulating the inflammatory response. *Immunol. Rev., * **114,** 145–80.

4 Le Deist, F., Blanche, S., Keable, S., Gaud, C., Pham, H., Descamp-Latscha, B., *et al.* (1989). Successful HLA nonidentical bone marrow transplantation in three patients with the leukocyte adhesion deficiency. *Blood, * **74,** 512–16.

5 Hibbs, M. L., Wardlaw, A. J., Stacker, S. A., Anderson, D. C., Lee, A., Roberts, T. M., and Springer, T. A. (1990). Transfection of cells from patients with leukocyte adhesion deficiency with an integrin beta subunit (CD18) restores lymphocyte function-associated antigen-1 expression and function. *J. Clin. Invest., * **85,** 674–81.

6 Wilson, J. M., Ping, A. J., Krauss, J. C., Mayo-Bond, L., Rogers, C. E., Anderson, D. C., and Todd III, R. F. (1990). Correction of CD18-deficient lymphocytes by retrovirus-mediated gene transfer. *Science, * **248,** 1413–16.

7 Back, A. L., Kwok, W. W., Adam, M., Collins, S. J., and Hickstein,

D. D. (1990). Retroviral-mediated gene transfer of the leukocyte integrin CD18 subunit. *Biochem. Biophys. Res. Commun.*, **171**, 787–95.

8 Springer, T. A. (1990). Adhesion receptors of the immune system. *Nature*, **346**, 425–34.

9 Dustin, M. L. and Springer, T. A. (1989). T-cell receptor cross-linking transiently stimulates adhesiveness through LFA-1. *Nature*, **341**, 619–24.

10 Wright, S. D. and Meyer, B. C. (1986). Phorbol esters cause sequential activation and deactivation of complement receptors on polymorphonuclear leukocytes. *J. Immunol.*, **136**, 1759–64.

11 Anderson, D. C., Schmalstieg, F. C., Finegold, M. J., Hughes, B. J. Rothlein, R., Miller, L. J., *et al.* (1985). The severe and moderate phenotypes of heritable Mac-1, LFA-1, p150,95 deficiency: their quantitative definition and relation to leukocyte dysfunction and clinical features. *J. Infect. Dis.*, **152**, 668–89.

12 Giger, U., Boxer, L. A., Simpson, P. J., Lucchesi, B. R., and Todd III, R. F. (1987). Deficiency of leukocyte surface glycoproteins Mo1, LFA-1, and Leu-M5 in a dog with recurrent bacterial infections: an animal model. *Blood*, **69**, 1622–30.

13 Kehrli, M. E., Schmalstieg, F. C., Anderson, D. C., van der Maaten, M. J., Hughes, B. J., Ackermann, M. R., *et al.* (1990). Molecular definition of the bovine granulocytopathy syndrome: identification of deficiency of the Mac-1 (CD11b/CD18) glycoprotein. *Am. J. Vet. Res.*, **51**, 1826–36.

14 Wilson, R. W., Lorenzo, I., Bradley, A., O'Brien, W. E., Anderson, D. C., and Beaudet, A. L. (1991). Targeted mutation of the murine leukocyte integrin, CD18 and expression of CD18 using a retroviral vector. *Clin. Res.*, **39**, 337a (abstr.).

15 Marlin, S. D., Morton, C. C., Anderson, D. C., and Springer, T. A. (1986). LFA-1 immunodeficiency disease. Definition of the genetic defect and chromosomal mapping of alpha and beta subunits of the lymphocyte function-associated antigen 1 (LFA-1) by complementation in hybrid cells. *J. Exp. Med.*, **164**, 855–67.

16 Krauss, J. C., Mayo-Bond, L., Todd III, R. F., and Wilson, J. M. (1991). Expression of retroviral transduced human CD18 in murine cells: An *in vitro* model of gene therapy for the leukocyte adhesion deficiency. *Hum. Gene Ther.*, **2**, 221–8.

17 Krauss, J. C., Mayo-Bond, L., Rogers, C. E., Weber, K. L., Todd III, R. F., and Wilson, J. M. (1991). An *in vivo* animal model of gene therapy for leukocyte adhesion deficiency. *J. Clin. Invest.*, **88**, 1412–17.

18 Todd III, R. F., Arnaout, M. A., Rosin, R. E., Crowley, C. A., Peters, W. A., and Babior, B. M. (1984). The subcellular localization of Mo1 (Mo1α; formerly, gp 110) a surface glycoprotein associated with neutrophil adhesion. *J. Clin. Invest.*, **74**, 1280–90.

19 Williams, D. A. (1988). Gene transfer and the prospects for somatic gene therapy. *Hematol. Oncol. Clin. North Am.*, **2**, 277–87.

20 Malech, H. L. and Gallin, J. I. (1987). Current concepts: immunology. Neutrophils in human diseases. *N. Engl. J. Med.*, **317**, 687–93.

21 Weisman, H. F., Bartow, T., Leppo, M. K., Marsh, H. C. Jr, Carson, G. R., Concino, M. F., et al. (1990). Soluble human complement receptor type I: *In vivo* inhibitor of complement suppressing post-ischemic myocardial inflammation and necrosis. *Science*, **249**, 146–51.

22 Carter, G. W., Dyer, R., and Young, P. (1985). Dipyridamole: a potent and specific 5-lipoxygenase inhibitor. *Fed. Proc.*, **44**, 904 (abstr.).

23 Blumenthal, D. S., Hutchins, G. M., Jugdutt, B. I., and Becker, L. C. (1981). Salvage of ischemic myocardium by dipyridamole in the conscious dog. *Circulation*, **64**, 915–23.

24 Bednar, M., Smith, B., Pinto, A., and Mullane, K. M. (1985). Nafazatrom-induced salvage of ischemic myocardium in anesthetized dogs as mediated through inhibition of neutrophil function. *Circ. Res.*, **57**, 131–41.

25 Jolly, S. R. and Lucchesi, B. R. (1983). Effective BW755C in an occlusion reperfusion model of ischemic myocardial injury. *Am. Heart J.*, **106**, 8–13.

26 Petrone, W. F., English, D. K., Wong, K., and McCord, J. M. (1980). Free radicals in inflammation: superoxide-dependent activation of a neutrophil chemotactic factor in plasma. *Proc. Natl Acad. Sci. USA*, **77**, 1159–63.

27 Stevens, J. H., O'Hanley, P., Shapiro, J. M., Mihm, F. G., Satoh, P. S., Collins, J. A., and Raffin, T. A. (1986). Effects of anti-C5a antibodies on the adult respiratory distress syndrome in septic primates. *J. Clin. Invest.*, **77**, 1812–16.

28 Mathison, J. C., Wolfson, E., and Ulevitch, R. J. (1988). Participation of tumor necrosis factor in the mediation of gram-negative bacterial lipopolysaccharide induced injury in rabbits. *J. Clin. Invest.*, **81**, 1925–37.

29 Tracy, K., Fong, Y., Hesse, D. G., Manogue, K. R., Lee, A. T., Kuo, G. C., Lowry, S. F., and Cerami, A. (1987). Anti-cachectin/TNF monoclonal antibodies prevent septic shock during lethal bacteremia. *Nature*, **330**, 662–4.

30 Zeigler, E. J., Fisher, C. J., Sprung, C. L., Straube, R. C., Sadoff, J. C., Foulke, G. E., et al. (1991). Treatment of gram-negative bacteremia and septic shock with HA-1A human monoclonal antibody against endotoxin. *N. Engl. J. Med.*, **324**, 429–36.

31 Greenman, R. L., Schein, R. M., Martin, M. A., Wenzel, R. P., MacIntyre, N. R., Emmanuel, G., et al. (1991). A controlled clinical trial of E5 murine monoclonal IgM antibody to endotoxin in the

treatment of gram-negative sepsis. The XOMA Sepsis Study Group. *J. Am. Med. Assoc.,* **266,** 1097–102.

32 Jacob, H. S. and Vercellotti, G. M. (1987). Granulocyte-mediated endothelial injury. Oxidant damage amplified by lactoferrin and platelet-activating factor. In *Oxygen radicals and tissue injury. Proceedings of an Upjohn Symposium* (ed. B. Halliwel), pp. 57–62. FASEB, Bethesda.

33 Gray, P. W., Barrett, K., Chantry, D., Turner, M., and Feldmann, M. (1990). Cloning of human tumor necrosis factor (TNF) receptor cDNA and expression of recombinant soluble TNF-binding protein. *Proc. Natl Acad. Sci. USA,* **87,** 7380–4.

34 Seckinger, P., Vey, E., Turcatti, G., Wingfield, P., and Dayer, J. M. (1990). Tumor necrosis factor inhibitor: purification, NH_2-terminal amino acid sequence and evidence for anti-inflammatory and immunomodulatory activities. *Eur. J. Immunol.,* **20,** 1167–74.

35 Ohlsson, K., Bjork, P., Bergenfeldt, M., Hageman, R., and Thompson, R. C. (1990). Interleukin-1 receptor antagonist reduces mortality from endotoxin shock. *Nature,* **348,** 550–2.

36 Wakabayashi, G., Gelfand, J. A., Burke, J. F., Thompson, R. C., and Dinarello, C. A. (1991). A specific receptor antagonist for interleukin-1 prevents *Escherichia coli*-induced shock in rabbits. *FASEB J.,* **5,** 338–43.

37 Kovach, N. L., Yee, E., Munford, R. S., Raetz, C. R. H., and Harlan, J. M. (1990). Lipid IVa inhibits synthesis and release of tumor necrosis factor induced by lipopolysaccharide in human whole blood *ex vivo. J. Exp. Med.,* **172,** 77–84.

38 Johnston, J. (1991). Molecular science sets its sites on septic shock. *J. Natl Inst. Health Res.,* **3,** 61–5.

39 Ley, K., Gaehtgens, P., Fennie, C., Singer, M. S., Lasky, L. A., and Rosen, S. D. (1991). Lectin-like cell adhesion molecule-1 mediates leukocyte rolling in mesenteric venules *in vivo. Blood,* **77,** 2553–5.

40 Watson, S. R., Fennie, C., and Lasky, L. A. (1991). Neutrophil influx into an inflammatory site inhibited by a soluble homing receptor-IgG chimaera. *Nature,* **349,** 164–7.

41 Jutila, M. A., Rott, L., Berg, E. L., and Butcher, E. C. (1989). Function and regulation of the neutrophil MEL-14 antigen *in vivo*: comparison with a LFA-1 and Mac-1. *J. Immunol.,* **143,** 3318–24.

42 Mulligan, M. S., Varani, J., Dame, M. K., Lane, C. L., Smith, C. W., Anderson, D. C., and Ward, P. A. (1991). Role of endothelial-leukocyte adhesion molecule-1 (ELAM-1) in neutrophil-mediated lung injury in rats. *J. Clin. Invest.,* **88,** 1396–406.

43 Geng, J. G., Bevilacqua, M. P., Moore, K. L., McIntyre, T. M., Prescott, S. M., Kim, J. M., *et al.* (1990). Rapid neutrophil adhesion to activated endothelium mediated by GMP-140. *Nature,* **343,** 757–60.

44 Larsen, E. T., Palabrica, T., Sajer, S., Gilbert, G. E., Wagner, D. D., Furie, B. C., and Furie, B. (1990). PADGEM-dependent adhesion of platelets to monocytes and neutrophils is mediated by a lineage-specific carbohydrate, LNF III (CD15). *Cell,* **63,** 467–74.

45 Phillips, M. L., Nudelman, E., Gaeta, F. C., Perez, M., Singhal, A. K., Hakomori, S., and Paulson, J. C. (1990). ELAM-1 mediates cell adhesion by recognition of a carbohydrate ligand, sialyl-Le[x]. *Science,* **250,** 1130–2.

46 Walz, G., Aruffo, A., Kolanus, W., Bevilacqua, M., and Seed, B. (1990). Recognition by ELAM-1 of the sialyl-Le[x] determinant on myeloid and tumor cells. *Science,* **250,** 1132–5.

47 Lorant, D. E., Patell, K. D., McIntyre, T. M., Prescott, S. M., McEver, R. P., and Zimmerman, G. A. (1991). Fluid phase granule membrane protein-140 (GMP-140) inhibits neutrophil (PMN) binding to activated endothelium. *Clin. Res.,* **39,** 285a (abstr.).

48 Simpson, P. J., Todd III, R. F., Mickelson, J. K., Fantone, J. C., Gallagher, K. P., Lee, K. A., *et al.* (1990). Sustained limitation of myocardial reperfusion injury by a monoclonal antibody that alters leukocyte function. *Circulation,* **81,** 226–37.

49 Seewaldt-Becker, E., Rothlein, R., and Dammgen, J. W. (1989). CDw18-dependent adhesion of leukocytes to endothelium and its relevance for cardiac reperfusion. In *Leukocyte adhesion molecules. Structure, function, and regulation* (ed. T. A. Springer, D. C. Anderson, A. Rosenthal, and R. Rothlein), pp. 138–48. Springer-Verlag, New York.

50 Gomoll, A. W., Lekich, R. F., and Grove, R. I. (1991). Efficacy of a monoclonal antibody (MoAb 60.3) in reducing myocardial injury resulting from ischemia/reperfusion in the ferret. *J. Cardiovasc. Pharm.,* **17,** 873–8.

51 Winquist, R., Frei, P., Harrison, M., McFarlen, D. G., Letts, G., Van, G., *et al.* (1990). An anti-CD18 mAb limits infarct size in primates following ischemia and reperfusion. *Circulation,* **82,** III–701a (abstr.).

52 Ma, X.-L., Tsao, P. S., and Lefer, A. M. (1991). Antibody to CD18 exerts endothelial and cardiac protective effects in myocardial ischemia and reperfusion. *J. Clin. Invest.,* **88,** 1237–43.

53 Hernandez, L. A., Grisham, M. B., Twohig, B., Arfors, K.-E., Harlan, J. M., and Granger, D. N. (1987). Role of neutrophils in ischemia–reperfusion-induced microvascular injury. *Am. J. Physiol.,* **253,** H699–703.

54 Vedder, N. B., Winn, R. K., Rice, C. L., Chi, E. Y. Arfors, K.-E., and Harlan, J. M. (1990). Inhibition of leukocyte adherence by anti-CD18 monoclonal antibody attenuates reperfusion injury in the rabbit ear. *Proc. Natl Acad. Sci. USA,* **87,** 2643–6.

55 Clark, W. M., Madden, K. P., Rothlein, R., and Zivin, J. A. (1991). Reduction of central nervous system ischemic injury in rabbits using leukocyte adhesion antibody treatment. *Stroke*, **22**, 877–83.

56 Vedder, N. B., Winn, R. K., Rice, C. L., Chi, E. Y., Arfors, K.-E., and Harlan, J. M. (1988). A monoclonal antibody to the adherence-promoting leukocyte glycoprotein, CD18, reduces organ injury and improves survival from hemorrhagic shock and resuscitation in rabbits. *J. Clin. Invest.*, **81**, 939–44.

57 Vedder, N. B., Fouty, B. W., Winn, R. K., Harlan, J. M., and Rice, C. L. (1989). Role of neutrophils in generalized reperfusion injury associated with resuscitation from shock. *Surgery*, **106**, 509–16.

58 Mileski, W. J., Winn, R. K., Vedder, N. B., Pohlman, T. H., Harlan, J. M., and Rice, C. L. (1990). Inhibition of CD18-dependent neutrophil adherence reduces organ injury after hemorrhagic shock in primates. *Surgery*, **108**, 206–12.

59 Tuomanen, E. I., Saukkonen, K., Sande, S., Cioffe, C., and Wright, S. D. (1989). Reduction of inflammation, tissue damage, and mortality in bacterial meningitis in rabbits treated with monoclonal antibodies against adhesion-promoting receptors of leukocytes. *J. Exp. Med.*, **170**, 959–69.

60 Doerschuk, C. M., Winn, R. K., Koxson, H. O., and Harlan, J. M. (1990). CD18-dependent and independent mechanisms of neutrophil emigration in the pulmonary and systemic microcirculation of rabbits. *J. Immunol.*, **144**, 2327–33.

61 Jaeschke, H., Farhood, A., and Smith, C. W. (1990). Neutrophils contribute to ischemia/reperfusion injury in rat liver *in vivo*. *FASEB J.*, **4**, 3355–9.

62 Barton, R. W., Rothlein, R., Ksiazek, J., and Kennedy, C. (1989). The effect of anti-intercellular adhesion molecule-1 on phorbol-ester-induced rabbit lung inflammation. *J. Immunol.*, **143**, 1278–82.

63 Cosimi, A. B., Conti, D., Delmonico, F. L., Preffer, F. I., Wee, S.-L., Rothlein, R., *et al.* (1990). *In vivo* effects of monoclonal antibody to ICAM-1 (CD54) in nonhuman primates with renal allografts. *J. Immunol.*, **144**, 4604–12.

64 Flavin, T., Ivens, K., Rothlein, R., Faanes, R., Clayberger, C., Billingham, M., and Starnes, V. A. (1991). Monoclonal antibodies against intercellular adhesion molecule 1 prolong cardiac allograft survival in cynomolgus monkeys. *Transplant Proc.*, **23**, 533–4.

65 Clark, W. M., Madden, K. P., Rothlein, R., and Ziven, J. A. (1991). Reduction of central nervous system ischemic injury by monoclonal antibody to intercellular adhesion molecules. *J. Neurosurg.*, **75**, 623–7.

66 Dana, N., Fathallah, D. M., and Arnaout, M. A. (1991). Expression of a soluble and functional form of the human beta 2 integrin CD11b/CD18. *Proc. Natl. Acad. Sci. USA*, **88**, 3106–10.

67 Marlin, S. D., Staunton, D. E., Springer, T. A., Stratowa, C., Sommergruber, W., and Merluzzi, V. J. (1990). A soluble form of intercellular adhesion molecule-1 inhibits rhinovirus infection. *Nature*, **344**, 70–2.

68 Anderson, D. C., Miller, L. J., Schmalstieg, F. C., Rothlein, R., and Springer, T. A. (1986). Contributions of the Mac-1 glycoprotein family to adherence-dependent granulocyte functions: structure–function assessments employing subunit-specific monoclonal antibodies. *J. Immunol.*, **137**, 15–27.

69 Sharar, S. R., Winn, R. K., Murry, C. E., Harlan, J. M., and Rice, C. L. (1991). A CD18 monoclonal antibody increases the incidence and severity of subcutaneous abscess formation after high dose *Staphylococcus aureus* injection in rabbits. *Surgery*, **110**, 213–19.

70 Jacob, H. S., Craddock, P. R., Hammerschmidt, D. E., and Moldow, C. F. (1980). Complement-induced granulocyte aggregation: an unsuspected mechanism of disease. *N. Engl. J. Med.*, **302**, 789–94.

71 Schmid-Schonbein, G. W. (1987). Capillary plugging by granulocytes and the no-reflow phenomenon in the microcirculation. *Fed. Proc.*, **46**, 2397–401.

72 D'souza, S. E., Ginsberg, M. H., Matsueda, G. R., and Plow, E. F. (1990). A discrete sequence in a platelet integrin is involved in ligand recognition. *Nature*, **350**, 66–8.

73 Fantone, J. C., Kunkel, S. L., and Zurier, R. B. (1985). Effects of prostaglandins on *in vivo* immune and inflammatory reactions. In *Prostaglandins and immunity* (ed. J. S. Goodwin), pp. 123–46. Martinez and Nijhoff, Boston.

74 Simpson, P. J., Mickelson, J. K., and Lucchesi, B. R. (1987). Free radical scavengers in myocardial ischemia. *Fed. Proc.*, **46**, 2413–21.

75 Riva, C. M., Morganroth, M. L., Ljungman, A. G., Schoeneich, S. O., Marks, R. M., Todd III, *et al.* (1990). Iloprost inhibits neutrophil-induced lung injury in neutrophil adherence to endothelial monolayers. *Am. J. Respir. Cell Mol. Biol.*, **3**, 301–9.

76 Flynn, P. F., Becker, W. K., Vercellotti, G. M., Weisdorf, D. J., Craddock, P. R., Hammerschmidt, D. E., *et al.*, (1984). Ibuprofen inhibits granulocyte responses to inflammatory mediators: a proposed mechanism for reduction of experimental myocardial infarct size. *Inflammation*, **8**, 33–44.

77 Romson, J. L., Hook, B. G., Rigot, V. H., Schork, M. A., Swanson, D. P., and Lucchesi, B. R. (1982). The effect of ibuprofen on accumulation of indium-111-labeled platelets and leukocytes in experimental myocardial infarction. *Circulation*, **66**, 1002–11.

78 Romson, J., Bush, L., Jolly, S., and Lucchesi, B. (1982). Cardioprotective effects of ibuprofen in experimental regional and global myocardial ischemia. *J. Cardiovasc. Pharmacol.*, **4**, 187–96.

79 Cronstein, B. N., Kramer, S. B., Weissmann, G., and Hirschhorn, R. (1983). Adenosine: a physiological modulator of superoxide anion generation by human neutrophils. *J. Exp. Med.*, **158**, 1160–77.

80 Engler, R. (1987). Consequences of activation and adenosine-mediated inhibition of granulocytes during myocardial ischemia. *Fed. Proc.*, **46**, 2407–12.

81 Ward, P. A. and Varani, J. (1990). Mechanisms of neutrophil-mediated killing of endothelial cells. *J. Leukocyte Biol.*, **48**, 97–102.

82 Weiss, S. J. (1989). Tissue destruction by neutrophils. *N. Engl. J. Med.*, **320**, 365–76.

83 Crystal, R. G. and Bast, A. (1991). Proceedings of a symposium: oxidants and anti-oxidants: pathophysiologic determinants and therapeutic agents. *Am. J. Med.*, **91**, 1–145S.

84 Shlafer, M., Kane, P. F., and Kirsch, M. M. (1982). Superoxide dismutase plus catalase enhances the efficacy of hypothermic cardioplegia to protect the globally ischemic, reperfused heart. *J. Thorac. Cardiovasc. Surg.*, **83**, 830–9.

85 Stolks, S. H. and McCord, J. M. (1979). Prevention of immune complex induced glomerulonephritis by superoxide dismutase. *Alabama J. Med. Sci.*, **16**, 33.

86 Schalkwijk, J., van den Berg, W. B., van de Pute, L. B. A., Josten, L. A. B., and van den Bersselaar, L. (1985). Cationization of catalase, peroxidase, and superoxide dismutase: effect of improved intra-articular retention on experimental arthritis in mice. *J. Clin. Invest.*, **76**, 198–205.

87 Rehan, A., Wiggins, R. C., Kunkel, R. G., Till, G. O., and Johnson, K. J. (1986). Glomerular injury and proteinuria in rats after intrarenal injection of cobra ventom factor: Evidence for the role of neutrophil-derived oxygen free radicals. *Am. J. Pathol.*, **123**, 57–66.

88 Hatherill, J. R., Till, G. O., Bruner, L. H., and Ward, P. A. (1986). Thermal injury, intravascular hemolysis, and toxic oxygen products. *J. Clin. Invest.*, **78**, 629–36.

89 Jolly, S. R., Kane, W. J., Bailie, M. B., Abrams, G. D., and Lucchesi, B. R. (1984). Canine myocardial reperfusion injury: its reduction by the combined administration of superoxide dismutase and catalase. *Circ. Res.*, **54**, 277–85.

90 Werns, S. W., Shea, M. J., Driscoll, E. M., Cohen, C., Abrams, G. D., Pitt, B., and Lucchesi, B. R. (1985). The independent effects of oxygen radical scavengers on canine infarct size: reduction by superoxide dismutase but not catalase. *Circ. Res.*, **56**, 895–8.

91 Myers, M. L., Bolli, R., Lekich, R. F., Hartley, C. J., and Roberts, R. (1985). Enhancement of recovery of myocardial function by oxygen free-radical scavengers after reversible regional ischemia. *Circulation*, **72**, 915–21.

92 Ytrehus, K., Gunnes, S., Myklebust, R., and Mjos, O. D. (1987). Protection by superoxide dismutase and catalase in the isolated rat heart reperfused after prolonged cardioplegia: a combined study of metabolic, functional, and morphometric ultrastructural variables. *Cardiovasc. Res.*, **21**, 492–9.

93 Ambrosio, G., Becker, L. C., Hutchins, G. M., Weisman, H. F., and Weisfeldt, M. L. (1986). Reduction in experimental infarct size by recombinant human superoxide dismutase: insights into the patho-physiology of reperfusion injury. *Circulation*, **74**, 1424–33.

94 McCormick, J. R., Harkin, M. M., Johnson, K. J., and Ward, P. A. (1981). Suppression by superoxide dismutase of immune complex-induced pulmonary alveolitis and dermal inflammation. *Am. J. Pathol.*, **102**, 55–61.

95 Gannon, D. E., Varani, J., Phan, S. H., Award, J. H., Kaplan, J., Till, G. O., *et al.* (1987). A source of iron in neutrophil-mediated killing of endothelial cells. *Lab. Invest.*, **57**, 37–44.

96 Warren, J. S., Yabroff, K. R., Mandel, D. M., Johnson, K. J., and Ward, P. A. (1990). Role of O_2^- in neutrophil recruitment into sites of dermal and pulmonary vasculitis. *Free Radical Biol. Med.*, **8**, 163–72.

97 Ambrosio, G., Zweier, J. L., Jacobus, W. E., Weisfeldt, M. L., and Flaherty, J. T. (1987). Improvement of post-ischemic myocardial function and metabolism indexed by administration of deferoxamine at the time of reflow: the role of iron in the pathogenesis of reperfusion injury. *Circulation*, **76**, 906–15.

98 Balla, G., Balla, J., Rosenberg, K., Nath, K., Jacob, H. S., and Vercellotti, G. M. (1991). Sequestration of intracellular iron by ferritin: A crucial antioxidant stratagem of endothelium. *Clin. Res.*, **39**, 724a (abstr.).

99 Bernard, G. R. (1991). N-Acetyl cysteine in experimental and clinical acute lung injury. *Am. J. Med.*, **91**, 54S–9S.

100 Qui, Y., Bernier, M., and Hearse, D. J. (1990). The influence of N-acetyl cysteine on cardiac function and rhythm disorders during ischemia and reperfusion. *Cardioscience*, **1**, 65–74.

101 Ferrari, R., Ceconi, C., Curello, S., Cargnoni, A., Alfierio, O., Pardini, A., *et al.* (1991). Oxygen free radicals and myocardial damage: protective role of thiol-containing agents. *Am. J. Med.*, **91**, 95S–105S.

102 Mulligan, M. S., Hevel, J. M., Marletta, M. A., and Ward, P. A. (1991). Tissue injury caused by deposition of immune complexes is L-arginine dependent. *Proc. Natl Acad. Sci. USA*, **88**, 6338–42.

103 Rosenberg, S., Barr, P. J., Najarin, R. C., and Hallewell, R. A. (1984). Synthesis in yeast of a functional oxidation-resistant mutant of human alpha$_1$-antitrypsin. *Nature*, **312**, 77–80.

104 Courtney, M., Jallat, S., Tessier, L.-H., Benavente, A., Crystal, R. G., and Lecocq, J.-P. (1985). Synthesis in *E. coli* of alpha-1-antitrypsin variants of therapeutic potential for emphysema and thrombosis. *Nature*, **313**, 149–51.

105 Rice, W. G. and Weiss, S. J. (1990). Regulation of proteolysis at the neutrophil-substrate interface by secretory leukoprotease inhibitor. *Science*, **249**, 178–81.

106 Buda, A. J., Lim, M. J., Huber, A. R., and Weiss, S. J. (1991). Reduction of myocardial ischemia-reperfusion injury by recombinant neutrophil secretory leukoproteinase inhibitor. *Circulation*, **84 (suppl. 2)**, 335A.

107 Weiss, S. J., Peppin, G. J., Ortiz, X., Ragsdale, C., and Test, S. T. (1985). Oxidative autoactivation of latent collagenase by human neutrophils. *Science*, **227**, 747–9.

108 Peppin, G. J. and Weiss, S. J. (1986). Activation of the endogenous metalloproteinase, gelatinase, by triggered human neutrophils. *Proc. Natl Acad. Sci. USA*, **83**, 4322–6.

109 Ossanna, P. J., Test, S. T., Matheson, N. R., Regiani, S., and Weiss, S. J. (1986). Oxidative regulation of neutrophil elastase-alpha-1 proteinase inhibitor interactions. *J. Clin. Invest.*, **77**, 1939–51.

110 Weiss, S. J., Young, J., Lobuglio, A. F., Slivka, A., and Nimeh, N. F. (1981). Role of hydrogen peroxide in neutrophil-mediated destruction of cultured endothelial cells. *J. Clin. Invest.*, **68**, 714–20.

111 Gallagher, K. P., Buda, A. J., Pace, D., Gerren, R. A., and Shlafer, M. (1986). Failure of superoxide dismutase and catalase to alter size of infarction in conscious dogs after 3 hours of occlusion followed by reperfusion. *Circulation*, **73**, 1065–76.

112 Uraizee, A., Reimer, K. A., Murry, C. E., and Jennings, R. B. (1987). Failure of superoxide dismutase to limit size of myocardial infarction after 40 minutes of ischemia and 4 days of reperfusion in dogs. *Circulation*, **75**, 1237–48.

113 Werns, S., Brinker, J., Gruber, J., Rothbaum, D., Heuser, R., George, B., *et al.* (1989). A randomized, double-blind trial of recombinant human superoxide dismutase (SOD) in patients undergoing PTCA for acute MI. *Circulation*, **80 (suppl. 2)**, II–113 (abstr.).

114 Engler, R. and Gilpin, E. (1989). Can superoxide dismutase alter myocardial infarct size? *Circulation*, **79**, 1137–42.

115 Hearse, D. J. (1991). Prospects for anti-oxidant therapy and cardiovascular medicine. *Am. J. Med.*, **93**, 118S–21S.

116 Golde, D. W. (1990). Overview of myeloid growth factors. *Semin. Hematol.*, **27**, 1–7.

117 Boxer, L. A., Hutchinson, R., and Emerson, S. (1992). Recombinant human granulocyte colony-stimulating factor in the treatment of patients with neutropenia. *Clin. Immunol Immunopath.*, **62**, 539–46.

118 Cannistra, S. A., Groshek, P., Garlick, R., Miller, J., and Griffin, J. D. (1990). Regulation of surface expression of the granulocyte/macrophage colony-stimulating factor receptor in normal human myeloid cells. *Proc. Natl Acad. Sci. USA*, **87**, 93–7.

119 Chiba, S., Shibuya, K., Piao, Y.-F., Tojo, A., Sasaki, N., Matsuki, S., *et al.* (1990). Identification and cellular distribution of distinct proteins forming the human GM-CSF receptor. *Cell Regul.* **1**, 327–35.

120 Lopez, A. F., Eglinton, J. M., Gillis, D., Park, L. S., Clark, S., and Vadas, M. A. (1988). Reciprocal inhibition of binding between interleukin 3 and granulocyte-macrophage colony-stimulating factor to human eosinophils. *Proc. Natl Acad. Sci. USA*, **86**, 7022–6.

121 Valent, P., Besemer, J., Muhm, M., Majdic, O., Lechner, K., and Bettelheim, P. (1989). Interleukin 3 activates human blood basophils via high-affinity binding sites. *Proc. Natl Acad. Sci. USA*, **86**, 5542–6.

122 Uzumaki, H., Okabe, T., Sasaki, N., Hagiwara, K., Takaku, F., and Itoh, S. (1988). Characterization of receptor for granulocyte colony-stimulating factor of human circulating neutrophils. *Biochem. Biophys. Res. Commun.*, **156**, 1026–32.

123 Larsen, A., David T., Curtis, B. M., Gimpel, S., Sims, J. E., Cosman, D., *et al.* (1990). Expression cloning of a human granulocyte colony-stimulating factor receptor: a structural mosaic of hematopoietin receptor, immunoglobulin, and fibronectin. *J. Exp. Med.*, **173**, 1559–70.

124 Sherr, C. J. (1988). The *fms* oncogene. *Biochim. Biophys. Acta*, **948**, 225–43.

125 Sieff, C. C. (1990). Biology and clinical aspects of the hematopoietic growth factors. *Annu. Rev. Med.*, **41**, 483–96.

126 Bussolino, F., Wang, J. M., Defilippi, P., Turrini, F., Sanavio, F., Edgell, C.-J. S., *et al.* (1989). Granulocyte and granulocyte-macrophage colony-stimulating factors induce human endothelial cells to migrate and proliferate. *Nature*, **337**, 471–3.

127 Groopman, J. E., Mitsuyasu, R. T., DeLeo, M. J., Oette, D., and Golde, D. W. (1987). Effect of recombinant human granulocyte-macrophage colony-stimulating factor on myelopoiesis in the acquired immunodeficiency syndrome. *N. Engl. J. Med.*, **317**, 593–8.

128 Crawford, J., Ozer, H., Stoller, R., Johnson, D., Lyman, G., Tabbara, I., *et al.* (1991). Reduction by granulocyte-colony-stimulating factor of fever and neutropenia induced by chemotherapy in patients with small-cell lung cancer. *N. Engl. J. Med.*, **325**, 164–70.

129 Nemunaitis, J., Rabinowe, S. N., Singer, J. W., Bierman, P. J., Vose, J. M., Freedman, A. S., *et al.* (1991). Recombinant granulocyte-macrophage colony-stimulating factor after autologous bone marrow transplantation for lymphoid cancer. *N. Engl. J. Med.*, **324**, 1773–8.

130 Negrin, R. S., Haeuber, D. H., Hagler, A., Olds, L., Donlon, T.,

Souza, L. M., and Greenberg, P. L. (1989). Treatment of myelodysplastic syndromes with recombinant human granulocyte colony-stimulating factor. A phase I–II trial. *Ann. Intern. Med.*, **110**, 976–84.

131 Vadhan-Raj, S., Keating, M., LeMaistre, A., Hittelman, W. N., McCredie, K., Trujillo, J. M., *et al.* (1987). Effects of recombinant human granulocyte-macrophage colony-stimulating factor in patients with myelodysplastic syndromes. *N. Engl. J. Med.*, **317**, 1545–52.

132 Giunan, E. C., Sieff, C. A., Oette, D. H., and Nathan, D. G. (1990). A phase I/II trial of recombinant granulocyte-macrophage colony-stimulating factor for children with aplastic anemia. *Blood*, **76**, 1077–82.

133 Bonilla, M. A., Gillio, A. P., Ruggerio, M., Kernan, N. A., Brochstein, J. A., Abboud, M., *et al.* (1989). Effects of recombinant human granulocyte colony-stimulating factor or neutropenia in patients with congenital agranulocytosis. *N. Engl. J. Med.*, **320**, 1574–80.

134 Weston, B., Todd, R. F., III., Axtell, R., Balazovich, K., Stewart, J., Locey, B. J., *et al.* (1991). Severe congenital neutropenia clinical and biological effects of granulocyte-colony-stimulating factor. *J. Lab. Clin. Med.*, **117**, 282–90.

135 Jakubowski, A. A., Souza, L., Kelly, F., Fain, K., Budman, D., Clarkson, B., *et al.* (1989). Effects of human granulocyte colony-stimulating factor in a patient with idiopathic neutropenia. *N. Engl. J. Med.*, **320**, 38–42.

136 Hammond, W. P. IV, Price, T. H., Souza, L. M., and Dale, D. C. (1989). Treatment of cyclic neutropenia with granulocyte-colony stimulating factor. *N. Engl. J. Med.*, **320**, 1306–11.

137 Bonilla, M. A. and The Severe Chronic Neutropenic Study Group in Conjunction with Amgen, Inc. (1990). Clinical efficacy of recombinant human granulocyte colony stimulating factor (r-metHUG-CSF) in patients with severe chronic neutropenia. *Blood*, **76 (suppl. 1)**, 523a.

138 Dale, D. C. and Hammond, W. P. IV (1988). Cyclic neutropenia: A clinical review. *Blood Rev.*, **2**, 178–85.

139 Wright, D. G., Fauci, A. S., Dale, D. C., and Wolff, S. M. (1978). Correction of human cyclic neutropenia with prednisolone. *N. Engl. J. Med.*, **298**, 295–300.

140 Wright, D. G., Oette, D. H., and Malech, H. L. (1989). Treatment of cyclic neutropenia with recombinant human granulocyte-macrophage colony-stimulating factor (rh-GM-CSF) *Blood*, **74 (suppl. 1)**, 863a.

141 Kostmann, R. (1975). Infantile genetic agranulocytosis. A review with presentation of ten new cases. *Acta Paediatr. Scand.*, **64**, 362–8.

142 Zsebo, K. M., Cohen, A. M., Murdock, D. C., Boone, T. C., Inoue, H., Chazin, V. R., *et al.* (1986). Recombinant granulocyte colony stimulating factor: Molecular and biological characterization. *Immunobiology*, **172**, 175–84.

143 Souza, L. M., Boone, T. C., Gabrilove, J., Lai, P. H., Zsebo, K. M., Murdock, D. M., *et al.* (1986). Recombinant human granulocyte colony-stimulating factor: effects on normal and leukemic myeloid cells. *Science*, **232**, 61–5.

144 Parmley, R. T. and Crist, W. M. (1982). Childhood neutropenia. *Ala. J. Med. Sci.*, **19**, 249–60.

145 Bussel, J. B. and Abboud, M. R. (1987). Autoimmune neutropenia of childhood. *Crit. Rev. Oncol. Hematol.*, **7**, 37–51.

146 de Alacron, P. A., Goldberg, J., Nelson, D. A., and Stockman, J. A. III (1983). Chronic neutropenia. Diagnostic approach and prognosis. *Am. J. Pediatr. Hematol. Oncol.*, **5**, 3–10.

147 Danish, R., Boxer, L. A., and Emerson, S. (1990). Successful treatment of T gamma lymphoproliferative disease with G-CSF. *Clin. Res.*, **38**, 406A.

148 Weston, B. W., Axtell, R. A., Todd, R. F. III, Vincent, M., Balazovich, K. J., Suchard, S. J., and Boxer, L. A. (1991). Clinical and biologic effects of granulocyte-colony stimulating factor in the treatment of myelokathexis. *J. Pediatr.*, **118**, 229–34.

149 Balazovich, K. J., Almeida, H. I., and Boxer, L. A. (1991). Recombinant human C-CSF and GM-CSF prime human neutrophils for superoxide production through different signal transduction mechanisms. *J. Lab. Clin. Med.*, in press.

150 Brandt, S., Peters, W. P., Atwater, S. K., Kurtzberg, J., Borowitz, M. J., Jones, R. B., *et al.* (1988). Effects of recombinant human granulocyte-macrophage colony-stimulating factor on hematopoietic reconstitution after high-dose chemotherapy and autologous bone marrow transplantation. *N. Engl. J. Med.*, **318**, 869–76.

151 Welte, K., Zeidler, C., Reiter, A., Müller, W., Odenwald, E., Souza, L., and Riehm, H. (1990). Differential effects of granulocyte macrophage colony-stimulating factor and granulocyte macrophage colony-stimulating factor in children with severe congenital neutropenia. *Blood*, **75**, 1056–63.

152 Freund, M. R. F., Luft, S., Schöder, C., Heussner, P. Schrezenmaier, H., Porzsolt, F., and Welte, K. (1990). Differential effect of GM-CSF and G-CSF in cyclic neutropenia. *Lancet*, **336**, 313.

153 Alter, B. P. (1987). The bone marrow failure syndromes. In *Hematology of infancy and childhood*, third edition (ed. D. G. Nathan and F. A. Oski), pp. 195–241. W. B. Saunders Co., Philadelphia.

154 Curnutte, J. T. (1988). Classification of chronic granulomatous disease. *Hematol./Oncol. Clinics No. Amer.*, **2**, 241–52.

155 The International Chronic Granulomatous Disease Cooperative Study Group. (1991). A phase III study establishing efficacy of recombinant human interferon gamma for infection prophylaxis in chronic granulomatous disease. *N. Engl. J. Med.*, **324**, 509–16.

156 Parkinson, D. R. (1991). Biological response modifiers. In *Hematology basic principles and practice* (ed. R. Hoffman, E. J. Benz Jr, S. J. Shattil, B. Furie, and H. J. Cohen), pp. 697–707. Churchill Livingstone, New York.

157 Murray, H. W., Rubin, B. Y., Carriero, S. M., Harris, A. M., and Jaffe, E. A. (1985). Human mononuclear phagocyte antiprotozal mechanisms: oxygen-dependent versus oxygen-independent activity against intracellular *Toxoplasma gondii*. *J. Immunol.*, **134**, 1983–8.

158 Newburger, P. E., Ezekowitz, R. A. B., Whitney, C., Wright, J., and Orkin, S. H. (1988). Induction of phagocyte cytochrome b heavy chain expression by interferon γ. *Proc. Natl Acad. Sci. USA*, **85**, 5215–19.

159 Ockenhouse, C. F., Schulman, S., and Shear, H. L. (1984). Induction of crisis forms in the human malaria parasite *Plasmodium falciparum* by γ-interferon activated, monocyte-derived macrophages. *J. Immunol.*, **133**, 1601–8.

160 Rothermal, C. D., Rubin, B. Y., Jaffe, E. A., and Murray, H. W. (1986). Oxygen-independent inhibition of intracellular *Chlamydia psittaci* growth by human monocytes and interferon-γ-activated macrophages. *J. Immunol.*, **137**, 689–92.

161 Murray, J. W. (1988). Inteferon-gamma, the activated macrophage, and host defense against microbial challenge. *Ann. Intern. Med.*, **108**, 595–608.

162 Nathan, C. F., Horowitz, C. R., de la Harpe, J., Vadhan-Raj. S., Sherwin, S. A., Oettgen, H. F., and Krown, S. E. (1985). Administration of recombinant interferon γ to cancer patients enhances monocyte secretion of hydrogen peroxide. *Proc. Natl Acad. Sci. USA*, **82**, 8686–90.

163 Nathan, C. F., Kaplan, G., Levis, W. R., Nusrat, A., Witmer, M. D., Sherwin, S. A. *et al.* (1986). Local and systemic effects of intradermal recombinant interferon-γ in patients with lepromatous leprosy. *N. Engl. J. Med.*, **315**, 6–15.

164 Billiau, A. and Dijkmans, R. (1990). Inteferon-γ: mechanism of action and therapeutic potential. *Biochem. Pharmacol*, **40**, 1433–9.

165 Bonnem, E. M. and Oldham, R. K. (1987). Gamma-interferon: physiology and speculation on its role in medicine. *J. Biol. Response Modifiers*, **6**, 275–301.

166 Dijkmans, R. and Billiau, A. (1988). Interferon-γ a master key in the immune system. *Curr. Opin. Immunol.*, **13**, 269–74.

167 Izermans, J. N. M. and Marquet, R. L. (1989). Interferon-gamma: A review. *Immunobiology*, **179**, 456–73.

168 Ezekowitz, R. A. B. and Newburger, P. E. (1988). New perspectives in chronic granulomatous disease. *J. Clin. Immunol.*, **8**, 419–25.

169 Ezekowitz, R. A. B., Orkin, S. H., and Newburger, P. E. (1987).

Recombinant interferon gamma augments phagocyte superoxide production and X-linked chronic granulomatous disease gene expression X-linked variant chronic granulomatous disease. *J. Clin. Invest.*, **80,** 1009–16.

170 Ezekowitz, R. A. B., Dinauer, M. C., Jaffe, H. S., Orkin, S. H., and Newburger, P. E. (1988). Partial correction of the phagocyte defect in patients with X-linked chronic granulomatous disease by subcutaneous interferon gamma. *N. Engl. J. Med.,* **319,** 146–51.

171 Rex. J. H., Bennett, J. E., Gallin, J. I., Malech, H. L., DeCarlo, E. S., and Melnick, D. A. (1991). In vivo interferon-γ therapy augments the *in vitro* ability of chronic granulomatous disease neutrophils to damage *Aspergillus* hyphae. *J. Infect. Dis.*, **163,** 849–52.

172 Sechler, J. M. G., Malech, H. L., White, C. J., and Gallin, J. I. (1988). Recombinant human interferon-gamma reconstitutes defective phagocyte function in patients with chronic granulomatous disease of childhood. *Proc. Natl Acad. Sci.* USA, **85,** 4874–5.

173 Ezekowitz, R. A. B., Sieff, C. A., Dinauer, M. C., Nathan, D. G., Orkin, S. H., and Newburger, P. E. (1990). Restoration of phagocyte function by interferon-γ in X-linked chronic granulomatous disease occurs at the level of a progenitor cell. *Blood*, **76,** 2443–8.

174 Berton, G., Zeni, L. Cassatella, M. A., and Rossi, F. (1986). Gamma interferon is able to enhance the oxidative metabolism of human neutrophils. *Biochem. Biophys. Res. Commun.*, **183,** 1276–82.

175 Guthrie, L. A., McPhail, L. C., Henson, P. H., and Johnston, R. B., Jr (1988). Priming of neutrophils for enhanced release of oxygen metabolites by bacterial lipopolysaccharide: evidence for increased activity of the superoxide-producing enzyme. *J. Exp. Med.*, **160,** 1656–71.

176 Weening, R. S., Verhoeven, A. J., de Boer, M., and Roos, D. (1988). Development in the treatment of patients with chronic granulomatous disease. *Acta Paediatr. Hungaria*, **29,** 222–7.

Index